RECOMMENDATIONS

In a sea of conflicting information, *Food for Thought – A Healthy Temple for a Holy God* brings to light and demystifies the often intimidating subject of health and nutrition. Sylvia Ferrin's book is filled with information for Christians who are interested in being the best they can be for their Lord and Master, Jesus Christ.

Although primarily a book about nutrition, Sylvia covers a vast amount of practical information that will help anyone achieve a more balanced walk with Jesus. She dares to talk about things that not many are talking about, things that cause Christians to lack the joy that is rightfully theirs. She explains how a person's body, mind, and spirit are all connected and how that the relationship between them directly affects an individual's well-being. In an age where Christians sometimes minimize or dismiss their love of the world through humor, she is quick to point it out as a reason why we are sick and depressed.

This book presents the truth spoken in love. When you read this ͏th will set you free. If you like ͏s probably not one you want to

I am a pastoɪ ͏ɪny women who want to get he ͏better care of their families, but tney uoɪɪ ɪ aɪwɑyo ɪɪɪ.ɪw where to begin. In addition to making poor nutritional choices, many women struggle with overeating and don't know how to stop. This book will be a resource I will point them towards. It could also be used as an effective tool to guide a discussion on care of the temple for ladies groups.

I am also a home schooling mom of five children, and I would highly recommend this book for any home school library. We are living in an age of convenience our forefathers knew nothing about. For this reason, good health – achieved through a close walk with Jesus, good nutrition, and moderate exercise – is something that the next generation needs to be taught and see exemplified in the lives of their elders.

With a little bit of creativity, this book could be used for a home-schooled high school student to earn a credit in Health. So many books on this subject are written by people who also espouse non-biblical beliefs. I cannot tell you how excited I am that an apostolic has written such an exhaustive and complete work about taking care of the temple of the Living God! Finally, no more "eating the meat and throwing out the bones." It is pure filet mignon! This is a book we can hand to our children and walk away completely confident that they will not absorb anything that will cause spiritual confusion.

I know Sylvia Ferrin personally, and she is a woman who walks her talk. She is a meek, quiet, and beautiful woman of God who radiates vitality and the love of Jesus. She has a sincere desire for the holiness of God. She also has a great burden for the people of God to be free from false nutritional and medical mindsets, and the resulting burdens they create. This shines through in her book.

You will be blessed and motivated to live better by reading her book. I was!

CARMEL CAPOTOSTO
Pastor's Wife, Homemaker, Home Schooling Parent,
Student of Health and Nutrition

I love this book. When I think of the study, just plain hard work that has gone into it, I appreciate it even more. The balance between the natural and the godly examples is wonderful.

My hat is off to you Sylvia. God bless you.

LYNN HILL, N.D.
Medical Professional and Retired Pastor's Wife

Sylvia Ferrin's work on nutrition and health, and how it affects God's temple (our bodies) is a cool and refreshing drink…"in a dry and thirsty land, where no water is." How thrilling to know there is finally a book, on this subject, that covers it all for Christians. What a warm and wonderful mix of sound nutrition, health, dieting and theology, in addition to the gentle, tongue-in-cheek humor she has woven into this endeavor.

I have found Sylvia to be a warm, genuine and extremely sincere person. Her thirst for learning in this area and desire to please God with her temple, are what have fueled this book. This, coupled with her sensible and balanced approach, has made this extremely well researched book to be practical advice for the Christian who is endeavoring to make his temple a clean and pure residence for our Lord and Savior. After all, since our Lord has given us these temporal bodies to care for, is it not common sense to include nutrition in our endeavor to provide a clean house for our Lord? She has thoroughly researched every aspect of health, nutrition and dieting (even debunking some of the dieting and nutrition myths, as well as the marketing ploys claiming their products to be "healthy" foods) and has applied them all soundly with Scripture.

The challenge she issues forth should be one that we, as Christians, all accept. And by contrast, the consequences she documents in not following sound nutrition are a warning we all should heed. I am certain that all will benefit from her years of research. I am pleased and honored to highly recommend this book to all Christians seeking to honor a Holy, and Righteous, and Living God with their (or should I say His) temples.

Sylvia, thank you for the time and effort spent on this project, "your labor has not been in vain!" God bless your work for Him!

MELANIE CHANDLER, Maine
Homemaker, Home Educator and Life Long Learner

FOOD FOR THOUGHT

A Healthy Temple for a Holy God

SYLVIA FERRIN

Peace Publications

Cover design by Paul Povolni/Voppa.com

Author photograph by Michael Kinsaul Photography
www.visitmypictures.com

Peace Publications (Isaiah 52:7) – A Branch of Compassion Ministries, St. Charles, MO

To order additional copies:
Call – (314) 440-3975
E-mail – sylviaferrin@hotmail.com
Write – 1316 Pine Bluff Drive, St. Charles, MO 63304

DEDICATION

To Jesus Christ – the Lord of my life. I give you honor for every success and achievement I attain, since you are the One who makes it possible for me to accomplish anything productive. Every good thing in my life comes from you. Thank you for loving me. Without you, my life would be meaningless. It is my privilege to serve you.

I dedicate this book to you. May it bring you glory and draw many people into a deeper relationship with you.

ACKNOWLEDGEMENTS

I never could have written *Food for Thought* without the support of a team of people from near and far. I am especially grateful to the authors, ministers, and professionals who granted me permission to quote their spoken and written words.

I am indebted to all of the individuals who expressed interest in *Food for Thought* during its various gestational stages. You motivated me to continue, during times when research became tedious and tiring. Some of you helped me by providing information and directing me to resources.

Unfortunately, space will not allow me to mention each of you by name. Please be assured that I am sincerely thankful for your assistance.

BILL FERRIN
~ My Wonderful Husband ~

What a journey this project has been and you have been with me from start to finish. You have been consistently supportive of this endeavor and affirmed its validity over and over again. It would be impossible to count the hours that we spent reading, analyzing, and correcting the manuscript in its developing stages. You have had great ideas and suggestions, one of which is the subtitle that perfectly portrays the message I want to convey.

Thank you for encouraging me during the last three years and for being just as excited and enthusiastic as I was. I love you and am so glad Jesus gave you to me. Thank you for being my spiritual leader. Day-by-day I see your desire to be pleasing to God lived out through your prayer life, sincerity, honesty, compassion, and commitment. I am looking forward to what the Lord has in store for us, as we live our lives for Him.

AMOS AND CATHERINE GIBSON

Dad and Mom, your financial assistance helped my dream become reality. Thank you for supporting this endeavor.

More than anything else, thank you for introducing me to The Truth even before I was old enough to understand how wonderful Jesus is. You encouraged me to read and study the Word of God and cultivated in me a love for Bible teaching and preaching. That is the greatest gift parents can give a child.

Thank you for believing in me. The confidence that you instilled in me contributed to my belief that – with the help and guidance of the Lord – I could complete this challenging project.

It is my prayer that God will continue to bless both of you with excellent health so that you may have many more years to serve the Lord.

BEA FERRIN

Your contributions to *Food for Thought* were important ones: First, you graciously allowed us to semi-hibernate in your house during the final writing phase. Second, you willingly and promptly forwarded manuscripts and other important documents to us; you are the perfect mail liaison! And I would be remiss if I failed to mention the delicious and nutritious meals we always enjoy at your table.

I am so glad that the Lord blessed me with such a wonderful mom-in-law. You are one of the most thoughtful people I know. Thank you for being so kind to me through the years.

Long before I discovered them, you were implementing some of the principles outlined in this book. I hope that others will follow your example of good temple stewardship and I pray that the Lord will continue to bless you with superb health.

THE REVIEW CREW

Striving for accuracy, I solicited the aid of several qualified, Spirit-filled individuals to read and critique my manuscript. They brought to the table a wealth of knowledge and experience. Their thoughts and suggestions greatly enhanced this book's content and presentation. I am grateful for the time they invested. I would like to briefly commend each of them for their contributions to this work.

CARMEL CAPOTOSTO

Your commitment to feeding your seven-member family wholesome meals, regardless of additional costs and the extra effort and time required to prepare them, defies the typical American emphasis on "cheap, quick, and easy-to-prepare food."

Your table is usually filled with nutritious culinary delights that are far from mundane and commonplace. Bill and I always enjoy visiting you and your family in your home because – through your servant mentality and thoughtfulness – you have mastered the art of true hospitality. Our many discussions about various foods and aspects of healthy living have proved insightful and stimulating and your commitment to moderation and self discipline are inspiring.

Your hands-on experience and knowledge were an asset to *Food for Thought*. Thank you for understanding my vision and mission and helping me achieve my goals.

Carmel, you are one of the most Christ-like ladies I have ever met. In a world where most women are in constant turmoil because they resist God's purpose for their lives, your simplicity and sincerity are refreshing. Your gentle attitude and quiet spirit have blessed my life more than you know.

MELANIE CHANDLER

From the time I solicited your assistance with this project, you have emanated excitement and enthusiasm. You instantly understood the potential positive effects of mass-producing this information and you have unreservedly joined with me to help me fulfill my vision of sharing with others truths that can change their lives.

The reason you could so unhesitatingly grasp my vision is because for many years you have been conscious of the importance of good temple stewardship. Your husband and three children have benefited from your desire to fuel their bodies with healthy food.

You went far above and beyond the call of duty with your ideas and suggestions. Thank you for being so thorough and helpful. You are my comrade-in-arms in the fight to return wholesome, truly nutritious foods to America's kitchens.

NONA FREEMAN

My life is one among thousands that have been blessed by your life that was dedicated to serving God many years ago. You were not just a forerunner in foreign missions but you understood the food-health connection at a time when most people were unaware and uninformed.

I am honored to have your support of this book. You are living proof that good stewardship of our temples pays great dividends. The many divine healings you have received, coupled with healthy eating habits, have enabled you to minister to needy people from many walks of life. May the Lord continue to bless you with outstanding health!

LYNN HILL, N.D.

What a wonderful blessing you have been to my life. I am so grateful that the Lord allowed me to meet you. Your life has been an inspiration to me. I see in you a godly lady who has discovered the constant joy that comes from walking daily in the presence of your Savior.

You always ensure that our conversations about natural healing bring glory to God. You have not allowed your education and professional expertise to interfere with your faith in God. Your speech is constantly punctuated with praise, thanksgiving, and faith. Thank you for sharing your experiences with me and for believing in the message of *Food for Thought.*

DAVID HUSTON

For your editorial advice and patience with my countless questions regarding the technicalities of writing a book, I thank you. Your interest in the subject matter of *Food for Thought* and your affirmation of its significance were sideline applause that encouraged me during my research and writing journey.

The information you shared with me was not an asset to this book only, but will be useful in the preparation of future publications as well. Thank you for the time you have invested into our ministry. We count you and Barbara as loyal friends and fellow workers in the Kingdom of God.

JONATHAN URSHAN

Brother Urshan, you are one of the wisest men of God that have ever walked in shoe leather. I see your wisdom portrayed in your communication with people, your teaching and preaching, and the balanced way you live your life. It is my privilege for you to be my pastor.

Bill and I have been immeasurably blessed by our exposure to your ministry and Sister Urshan's consistently sweet, gentle, and kind spirit. I thank both of you for encouraging us to be all we can be for God and for enthusiastically supporting our ministry. The good that God does through us is an extension of your ministries. Through the years, your stable examples of true Christian living have been reference points for us to receive guidance. It is impossible to adequately describe how profoundly you have influenced our lives for good.

Thank you for reviewing my manuscript. Your familiarity of Bible languages and firsthand experience of the customs of Bible lands made you the most qualified person I know to examine *Food for Thought* for linguistic and cultural accuracy. Additionally, you are an excellent example of an individual who has made a lifelong commitment to moderation and self-control.

STEVE WALDRON, Th.M., Th.D.

I am grateful to you for taking time from your demanding schedule to review my manuscript. You informed me of several theological points that required modification. Thank you for utilizing your expansive store of biblical knowledge to ensure that I did not misrepresent the precious Word of God.

CONTENTS

PART II
CHANGING MINDSETS
Building a Sturdy Structure

PART III
WHOLE FOODS
Following the Blueprints

PART IV
PRACTICAL PRINCIPLES
Finishing Touches

FOREWARD

When Sylvia Ferrin asked me to write the foreward for *Food for Thought* (approximately two years ago) I readily agreed. "Eating right" is one of my favorite subjects. When the manuscript finally arrived, I decided this lady KNOWS what she is talking about! With diligence and care and great honesty, she has researched all foods, those mentioned in the Bible as well as the many variations of our modern fare --- all I can say is --- "THIS BOOK IS LONG OVERDUE." Our world desperately needs it.

I sincerely hope that all ailing people can get a copy of this book to understand how poor dietary choices can lead to a plethora of diseases. This is by far the best book I have ever read on this subject. Well done, Sylvia, dear!!

Sincerely,
Nona Freeman

FOREWARD

Sylvia Ferrin is a loyal member of Bethel Pentecostal Church in good standing. She is a woman of integrity and excellent character, devoted to her husband, who is a minister of the gospel and a member of the United Pentecostal Church International.

The contents of her book are very inspiring and will serve as excellent reading material for anyone. I have read this book and do not hesitate to recommend it to anyone.

These are thoughts that are anointed by the Lord and I commend her for writing this book.

Jonathan Urshan
Pastor, Bethel Pentecostal Church
St. Peters, MO

INTRODUCTION

There will be no more sickness and disease in Heaven, and Jesus is preparing an eternal home that will be pain-free (John 14:2; Revelation 21:4). But He desires that we have a superior quality of spiritual, physical, and emotional life right now as well. John 10:10 tells us that Jesus came to give us abundant life.

There is an undeniable link between nutrition and health. The mission of this book is to help people enjoy vibrant health through nutritional and lifestyle changes.

A LOOK INTO THE AUTHOR'S MIND AND HEART

During the formation of this book, it has been my prayer that the Lord will help me present accurate and unbiased information that is balanced by the Word of God. I do not want to lead people astray.

I pray that this book will be received in the spirit in which it was written. I do not write with an attitude of superiority but an attitude of love and compassion grounded in a sincere desire to help others. Though my sense of humor is sometimes manifested through my tongue-in-cheek writing style, it is never my intention to demean or offend others.

During my study, the Lord "gave" me a Scripture to help me maintain a proper perspective of this book and myself. It is from Romans 2:21, and I refer to it frequently to keep myself focused and to keep a right attitude: "Thou therefore which teachest another, teachest thou not thyself?"

I recognize that my diet is not perfect. I do not live in a perfect world, as do none of the readers of *Food for Thought*. The ministry the Lord has called my husband and me to frequently finds us eating at others' tables; for this reason alone it is impossible to adhere to a purist's diet. (I personally believe that very few people are true "purists," a term used to describe people that eat faultlessly all the time. Our less than ideal world and human nature do not encourage it.)

Also, though my diet at home is generally good, I am a fallible human being who sometimes indulges in foods that are contrary to the ideal. So I do not set myself up as perfect but, like my readers, am striving for perfection. To borrow Paul's statement about the spiritual life of believers, I admit that I have not yet attained, neither am I perfect (Philippians 3:12).

I do not make these transparent statements to discourage others or to lower the bar of nutritional lifestyle expectations; I state these things to 1) keep my attitude in check and 2) help readers understand that the author of this book is working to achieve and maintain the same goals they are.

I desire to have a spirit of humility that is pleasing to God, and I do not want to exalt myself to a place where I can fall.

SPECIAL NOTE

This principles-based book is the result of extensive study and research. My interest in nutrition has progressed from casual interest to a hobby to teaching others about nutrition. This book is the product of a seminar my husband asked me to teach to the church he pastored. Afterwards, he encouraged me to use my teaching notes as the basis for a book.

My life was enhanced when I began to apply nutritional principles found in the Bible. I would like to share that information with you so that you may be helped as well. It is my desire that this book will educate and equip you to make better nutrition choices that will benefit you for the rest of your life.

AN EXCITING JOURNEY

The information presented here is neither conclusive nor exhaustive. This book is intended to whet your appetite for further study of health and wellness. Use it as a launching pad for deeper exploration into achieving superior health through whole foods, natural healing, and the implementation of positive lifestyle patterns.

This book does not attempt to address all of the many diseases, syndromes, and disorders that weaken America's health. The concepts presented here are simply guidelines that will improve anyone's health, regardless of the specific malady.

For more specific information on a particular health issue or food, ask your health food store to recommend a book to you. If they don't have one on their shelves that meets your particular needs, they can usually order one for you.

Food for Thought was written to encourage the sick and to help the well stay well. Learning to nutritionally care for our bodies benefits us with the quality of life that God intended for us.

I am still in the process of learning about nutrition. It is a subject I find fascinating. The Lord has blessed me with tremendous health, and I am very grateful to Him for keeping me free of major sickness and protecting me from accidents and disease. In my 35 years of life, I have never once stayed in a hospital overnight. Compared to many people, I have taken very little medication. I give Him the credit for such providential care.

It is my very sincere desire to show my appreciation to Him by taking the best possible care of this temple, my body, that He lives in. Not only do I want it to be pure and clean spiritually, free of sin, negativity, and doubt, but I also desire to eat foods that will help me stay healthy physically. Spiritual and physical health overlap!

The Bible has much to say about food. It teaches us to eat the right foods temperately. I am still intrigued by the amount of Scriptures that address food issues. It is without doubt an important topic to God or He would not have included so many references and admonitions.

Join me as we journey into the Bible, using it as the foundation of our study of health and nutrition. Without doubt, you too will discover that God is not only interested in our spiritual well being, but our physical well being also. He has provided wholesome foods, accompanied by principles to guide our selection, preparation, and use of them, giving us an abundance of *Food for Thought.*

PART I

INTRODUCTORY CONCEPTS

Laying a Firm Foundation

ONE

JESUS FIRST

I am Alpha and Omega, the beginning and the end,
the <u>first</u> and the last.
Revelation 22:13

The Bible has a lot to say about food, health, and healing. As I was compiling information for this book, nothing really seemed to gel. I knew what subject matter I wanted to cover, but I was having difficulty determining the proper approach to use. At one point I suddenly had this thought, "I've based everything else in my life on the Bible. Why would I do any different in regards to the discussion of health, food, and nutrition?" Though I was certainly going to include biblical references throughout the book, I realized that I needed to put Jesus *first*. If I would put God and His Word *first*, then all else would fall into place. And it did.

This is an elementary principle that we must never forget. When our lives, relationships, work, decisions, *everything*, is centered around God – not ourselves, our own agendas, the people and forces that influence us – we will have true, lasting peace and contentment. We will understand our purpose, because our perspectives will have been defined by God Himself.

A marriage that is not Jesus-centered will never be happy and fulfilling, because it will be self-centered – and self-centeredness always produces unpleasant results. A church that is not truly Jesus-centered will never fulfill God's purpose and design. People who do not put Jesus first in their finances will wonder why holes seem to be in all of their pockets or why money and "stuff" never seem to bring them peace.

But when we put Jesus first, what awesome blessings result! Jesus knows that without Him, we will never be happy. We were created to live in communion with Him, listening to His voice and fulfilling His will for our lives. What a privilege and a joy it is to know God. So many people struggle with this one concept of putting Jesus first. But I have found that I'm the happiest when He is truly Number One in my life. There is no replacement for a right relationship with the One True God, our Creator. This is what people vainly search for in all sorts of things. Psalm 127:1 says "Except the LORD build the house, they labour in vain that build it."

Some people actually spiritualize food because they do not put God first. GOD is the one who created good food in the first place. Our faith should, first and foremost, rest in the fact that GOD, not the food we eat, the supplements we buy, or the doctors or health practitioners we visit, is our Healer and Provider. With this principle guiding our discussion of vitamins, whole foods, and health, all will be kept in proper perspective.

I want to always thank GOD for giving me such good health. "It is he that hath made us, and not we ourselves" (Psalm 100:3). He made my body and He can heal it. He also invented healing foods to nourish us. I give all glory to HIM and want to always remember that HE is the Source of all good things!

It is the Bible – the Word of God – that gives us great insight and instruction regarding this subject. Thousands upon thousands of books, essays, pamphlets, manuals, and research reports have been written about the subject of health and nutrition. They were written by the hands and minds of mere men and women, guided by individual personal experiences and exposure, not necessarily inspired by God. In fact, many books on the subject of nutrition actually denounce God. Since we do not share with them the basic absolute truth of God and who He is, their writings cannot be completely trusted. If the foundation is flawed, the whole structure will be crooked. Thus, our fundamental principles for study will be based upon only the Word of God. Remember, when we put Jesus first, everything else will fall into place.

TWO

OLD TESTAMENT INSIGHTS

L et's begin our journey into the Bible to see what insight God has to give us about nutrition and health.

Genesis 1:29 - And God said, Behold, I have given you every herb bearing seed, which is upon the face of all the earth, and every tree, in the which is the fruit of a tree yielding seed; to you it shall be for meat.

This is where and how it all began. In the beginning, God designed man to live in harmony with the animals (not kill them for food). Mankind lived in a perfect environment with a perfect climate. Both man and animals thrived on the herbs and fruits abundant in the Garden of Eden. When Adam and Eve sinned by eating fruit from the tree of the knowledge of good and evil, which God said they should not eat, they were expelled from the Garden, separated from both a close relationship with God and the beauty of the Garden.

Genesis 9:3 - Every moving thing that liveth shall be meat for you; even as the green herb have I given you all things.

What happened? Just a few chapters previous, Adam and Eve feasted on greens and fruit. Now God is saying that He's giving "every moving thing" to mankind to eat?

With sin came more sin and in time humanity was judged. There was a worldwide flood that destroyed everyone except Noah and his family. After Noah emerged from the ark, God made available for food "every moving thing that liveth." Since mankind was no longer in that perfect environment and his lifestyle changed, it seems reasonable that his body needed the protein and nutrition provided by animal meat and other foods.

Leviticus 11:46-47 – This is the law of the beasts, and of the fowl, and of every living creature that moveth in the waters, and of every creature that creepeth upon the earth:
To make a difference between the unclean and the clean, and between the beast that may be eaten and the beast that may not be eaten.

Whoa, wait a minute. First man ate only fruits and vegetables. Then they could eat every moving thing. Now it sounds like they're receiving stipulations on what they can and cannot eat.

That's exactly right. We've moved ahead to the time of Moses. We've passed Abraham, Isaac, and Jacob. The Israelites, God's chosen people, have been delivered from many years of slavery to the Egyptians. God gives Moses dietary laws. He defines acceptable and unacceptable foods.

These laws that the children of Israel receive from the Lord protect them from sickness and disease. They are blessed with health as a result of their adherence to these dietary standards set by God.

THREE

NEW LAWS IN THE NEW TESTAMENT

Let's progress to the New Testament. Though the moral law still applies, the ceremonial and Levitical laws are fulfilled by the death of the Passover Lamb, Jesus Christ. The death, burial, and resurrection of Jesus Christ liberated the Jews and all of humanity from the bondage of the law, providing them with a new and better law written in their hearts.

1 Timothy 4:1-5 tells us that "in the latter times some shall depart from the faith...commanding to abstain from meats, which God hath created to be received with thanksgiving of them which believe and know the truth. For every creature of God is good, and nothing to be refused, if it be received with thanksgiving: For it is sanctified [cleansed] by the word of God and prayer."

Following the dietary laws given to Moses is no longer a mandate; however, there are great blessings in following them. I Timothy 4:1-5 does not negate, or cancel out, the tremendous health benefits we will experience if we choose to follow those dietary laws. So, though we are permitted to eat all things, it would be wise to stick as closely as possible to the guidelines of Leviticus 11. I believe God's wisdom is unsurpassed. It is no longer a sin to eat pork, for instance, yet God had very good reasons for deeming it "unclean" and forbidding the Israelites to eat it.

This is an excellent place to address an issue that I feel is very, very important. I Timothy 4:4 tells us that "every creature of God is good, and nothing to be refused, if it be received with thanksgiving." Jesus gave instructions to His disciples when He commissioned them to go and minister: "And into whatsoever city ye enter, and they receive you, eat such things as are set before you" (Luke 10:8).

In my own kitchen I can control the type of food I prepare and eat. Though I am free according to the Word to eat anything as long as I receive it with thanksgiving, because I understand that some foods are better than others, I mostly choose more nutritive foods for domestic use.

When I enter another's home, however, the tables are turned. When I am invited to someone else's home, *they* are the ones that have spent their time, effort, and resources to share a meal with me. It would be an insult to their hospitality and potentially offensive to refuse to eat what they place before me just because I know that it is unhealthy. It is more important to not offend than it is to make a scene for the benefit of the food on my plate.

In *The Front Row*, Gwyn Oakes wrote a somewhat humorous story about an evangelist that came to minister to the church that her husband pastored. It is a hilarious example of the temptation to impose on our hostess our personal beliefs about healthy living at the expense of being a gracious and grateful guest. Fortunately, Gwyn Oakes must have been an easygoing pastor's wife, for it seems that she was not insulted or offended by the evangelist, merely amused.

"There was this evangelist who planted himself at the kitchen table three times a day at about an hour before the meal. First of all, he wanted to make sure that I didn't use anything but stainless steel – no aluminum and no iron skillets!

"Secondly, he needed to watch how I prepared the food to see how much of the vitamins would be lost by paring or overcooking. Thirdly, after determining exactly what the fare for the meal was to be, he began to spread out his stash of vitamins to see which he would need to supplement his meal.

"One midmorning, I went into the church for something and there he was – no, not having a peanut butter and jelly sandwich on the sly – he was standing on his head on the platform of the church! I was afraid to ask what he was doing, so I said nothing. He said, 'Do you know what I am doing?' It was obvious what he was doing, but I bit and said, 'No.' He said, 'Well, if you stand on your head for a certain amount of time each day, you are able to think more clearly.'

"He then explained all the reasons it was good to stand on your head. By the time the revival was over, I was ready to try almost anything. After he left, I gave it a try, but could never manage to get my feet to stay in the air. Who knows, maybe it works. He really was a very good evangelist. I cannot recommend standing on your head, even though you might be able to think more clearly, because it would be very unladylike!

"Oh, I forgot to mention he was also a very good stainless cookware salesman. Mine are still in good shape after thirty years! I use my iron skillet though because another minister said cooking in iron was very healthy! Who knows, someone may come along who wants food cooked only in ironware!"[1]

When conversation turns toward nutrition is the ideal time to contribute your thoughts non-judgmentally. Don't go overboard unless others show sincere interest; some people can only take nutrition information in small doses. Being right never justifies a wrong attitude. You may need to inform your hostess of specific dietary restrictions for such things as diabetes or food allergies. Otherwise, unless she sincerely offers to tailor-prepare your food, don't demand that your hostess alter her plans for you. Put yourself in her shoes and don't jeopardize your relationships with those you love.

Self righteousness is never an acceptable attitude for an individual who is striving to be like Jesus. It reeks of a better-than-thou mentality. In our desire to see people take better care of their temples, it is possible to be overly zealous and pushy. Instead of arousing people's curiosity, this method will repel them. We will get more "converts" when we are kind and considerate.

Self righteousness stems from an unwillingness to be honest with self. When it comes to eating healthily, education and understanding of proper nutrition is never an excuse to look down on others. For most of us, eating healthy has not been a lifelong endeavor; we realized its importance as adults. As such, we should stop and remember that all good things, even the understanding of how to properly care for our temples, comes from God and not ourselves. This will prevent bad attitudes and keep us off our "don't you know that stuff is bad for you" soapbox when others are not ready to learn about a better way of eating and living.

When you are eating at your own table, which is probably most of the time, you can cook as healthy as you want. Chances are, if you have a mostly healthy lifestyle and diet, a meal out now and then will have little negative impact on your overall good health. I've sat in restaurants where someone else was graciously paying the bill and thought, "Yikes! This food is filled with nothing but chemicals and additives." Do you know what I did? I enjoyed it! I received it with thanksgiving. Show your appreciation to those who provide food for you, no matter what or where it is. Remember, it is sanctified by the Word of God and by prayer.

At this juncture, some people will invariably think or say, "If I pray over the food I eat, then what is the point of monitoring what I eat?" I know a missionary who gained fifty pounds during his deputation travels. Without doubt, he was thankful and prayed before he ate. I have met very godly people who voluntarily admitted that their sicknesses were a direct result of their eating and lifestyle habits.

The point is that we must balance I Timothy 4:5 with the many Scriptural references that teach us about our responsibility to take care of our bodies. Faith coupled with works is a biblical concept that is the key to superior stewardship of our bodies – God's temples.

FOUR

OUR BODIES – GOD'S TEMPLES

Beloved, I wish above all things that thou mayest prosper and be in health, even as thy soul prospereth.
III John 1:2

King Solomon was the general contractor for the building of the temple in Jerusalem, the first fully permanent temple dedicated to the worship of Jehovah. It was such a magnificent structure that its glory and beauty gave it great acclaim throughout the then-known world.

Solomon followed the instructions of David his father regarding the temple's design and architecture. David had already accumulated many of the supplies and materials needed for the building of the temple. Everything used to build the temple was the best available. Solomon went to elaborate means to ensure a superior grade of materials and craftsmanship. He contracted skilled workers from afar and also used the manpower of his own kingdom to construct this magnificent edifice.

Inside the temple, the walls were made of cedar and the floors were made of cypress. Both the walls and the doors were very ornate and overlaid with gold. Every piece of furniture that was placed in the temple of the Lord was the product of the finest raw materials combined with excellence in detailed labor.

Careful, time-consuming thought and planning was put into constructing this temple for the presence of the Lord to dwell in. Great sums of money were raised and designated for this massive project. Men worked intricately and carefully to create this house for God. It was a house of glory and beauty – a reflection of the very best that man could give to the One True God of glory and beauty.

When we are filled with the Holy Ghost, our bodies become the temples of God (I Corinthians 3:16; 6:19-20). God no longer dwells in temples made with man's hands but in people who allow Him to dwell within them (Acts 7:47-49). Our bodies house the Spirit of the Almighty God. Pause a moment and consider the wonder of God taking up residence in mere mortals like us. Think about the implications of the created housing the Creator. *God* created *us* and then filled us with His Spirit!

If you made something for someone – a beautiful quilt, a handcrafted piece of furniture, or a lovely flower arrangement – would you appreciate them uncaringly tossing it in the basement or shed amongst grime and dust? Probably not! If you give someone a gift that you have carefully and lovingly made, it is theirs to do with as they please. But it might bother you if, after all of the work and love you put into creating it especially for them, they misuse it and fail to properly appreciate it.

Psalm 139:14 says that we are "fearfully and wonderfully made." God is thorough and meticulous. He puts a lot of thought and detail into His original creations. It is not unreasonable for Him to expect us to take care of our bodies; they are His gift to us.

We go to great lengths to safeguard and protect something that is valuable to us, such as a special gift from a special person, a car, a house, a family heirloom. We will carefully protect and preserve it and maybe even sacrifice our time or money in order to keep it in pristine condition.

How much do you value your body as the gift and temple of God? You see, not only did God bless us with bodies that are absolutely fascinating in their operation, but when He fills us with His Spirit, we become recipients of royalty. The King comes to live in our houses.

"When you think of a temple, you probably visualize a work of beauty – something that has been skillfully and carefully handcrafted to give honor to the One who is to be worshiped within. In the same way, it brings honor to God when you take care of *your* temple, making sure you look and feel your best as you live your life for Him.

"Consider the position you are in as a Christian. So many people around you do not understand spiritual things and therefore make judgments according to your natural, outward appearance. That is why the "natural you" that everyone sees should radiate outwardly with health and vitality even as the beauty of Jesus shines forth from within."[1]

It is God's design that He receives glory from our lives. If we are sick, constantly fatigued, irritable, and fearful, just how much glory does He get from our lives? God has called each of us to work for Him. The quality and quantity of work that we do for Him can be severely limited by poor health and failure to apply His Word to our lives. While there are many important factors that create healthy, vibrant temples, spiritually and biblically speaking, our focus here is on the care of our bodies.

In spite of America's advances in technology, science, and medicine, overall it is one of the unhealthiest nations on the planet. It is a basic anthropological and historical fact that modern health challenges such as cancer, heart disease, obesity, and diabetes are relatively new and their mass development coincides with the extensive production and use of refined foods. While some sicknesses and diseases are not avoidable and may be produced by our environment or heredity, most are preventable. If we are healthy, we are more effective in Kingdom work and of more benefit to God.

The American Cancer Society informs us that 50% of men and 33% of women will develop some type of cancer during their lifetime. While this statistic is alarming, most medical experts agree that about 65% of all cancers are preventable. That means that by making wise day-to-day choices and a few lifestyle changes, we can, with God's help, greatly decrease our odds of getting cancer. The biggest causes of cancer are within our power to control: Poor diet and obesity (account for 30% of cancer cases), smoking (30%), lack of exercise (5%), and alcohol consumption (3%). The remaining causes that we have no or little control over are genetics (10%), viruses (5%), carcinogens in the workplace (5%), family history (5%), as well as reproductive factors, socioeconomic status, and environmental pollution.

Some people, especially young people, think, "I hear the statistics but it won't happen to me. That only happens to other people." This thinking is reminiscent of the attitude of a 16-year-old boy who thinks he is invincible and exempt from the repercussions other people experience when they engage in behavior similar to his. He drives fast and lives loose, all the time thinking, "It won't happen to me." Yet all too often we hear reports of teenagers dying in tragic speed-related car wrecks and it is all too common for boys to become fathers at age 16. Many people live in this same state of live-for-today denial in regards to their health.

The fact is that, for the most part, God did not pre-select some people to enjoy good health and pre-select others to suffer with poor health. To a great extent, our present health is the result of yesterday's decisions, and today's decisions determine our future health. While good health is a wonderful blessing from the Lord, it is possible for us to thwart His blessings by our behavior. God wants to bless us, but sometimes He needs our cooperation. "There is a humorous and very relevant story told of Reverend Jones, who was working in his garden one bright summer day, when along came a parishioner and commented: 'My, my Reverend, doesn't God make a nice garden?' And the Reverend replied: 'Yes, but you should have seen it before I got here.' The point is, God does His work, and we are expected to do our work."[2]

If you knew you could avoid a terrible disease, would you change? No matter how much you love XYZ food, if you knew that it was detrimental to your health, would you be willing to replace it with a more nutritious food? If you knew that your eating habits and/or lack of exercise would interfere with your future work for God, would you be willing to do things differently?

We have three choices:

1) We can resign ourselves to sickness and disease, thinking that we might be predestined to endure unavoidable physical problems, regardless of our lifestyle and dietary changes.

2) We can act as though we will escape health issues regardless of our reckless behavior because those things only happen to others but not us.

3) We can show our appreciation to God by being good stewards of our temples as we trust in Him as the Source of health and wellness.

I propose that the third choice is the best.

We have been entrusted to be caretakers of the residence of divine royalty. Royalty deserves the best. We should strive to glorify God in our bodies and in our spirits, which are God's (I Corinthians 6:20). A building that is not properly maintained will decay (Ecclesiastes 10:18). But a building that is lovingly and carefully maintained is a tribute to the owner of the house.

The builder of the house is worthy of greater honor than the caretaker of the house or the house itself (Hebrews 3:3). Everything we do should bring glory to God. Our pleasant attitudes, smiles, selflessness, and well-maintained temples should inspire people to desire to meet the One who lives inside us. Everything about our lives should bring glory to God, to the very best of our ability.

In addition to being the temple of the Holy Ghost, we are called to be God's ambassadors (II Corinthians 5:20). This world is only the place of our natural birth. When we were born again, it was a spiritual birth and we were born into a heavenly kingdom. We are only on this earth temporarily. One day soon our King will call us home. While we are here we are His ambassadors, His representatives.

An American ambassador represents America, its government, and its president in a foreign land. While there, he must conduct himself in a manner that accurately represents our nation to people that may never visit America and may never meet our president. As spiritual ambassadors, we are required to represent Jesus Christ and His kingdom. Vibrant spiritual, emotional, and physical health should emanate from us to others. We should shine with excitement and vitality.

We are comprised of body, soul, and spirit. As such, what we do in the physical realm affects the spiritual realm and vice versa. The overlapping connectivity of our being demands that we not disregard our responsibility to care for our bodies, the temples of God.

I Thessalonians 5:23 says "And the very God of peace sanctify you wholly; and I pray God your whole spirit and soul and body be preserved blameless unto the coming of our Lord Jesus Christ." Paul had a comprehensive outlook toward pleasing God. I don't think it is a stretch to conclude that Paul was including care of our physical bodies in this passage. Sometimes we are guilty of diminishing the importance of physical fitness and health because of our busyness with spiritual activities. Paul prayed that our spirits, souls, *and* bodies would be preserved blameless. He advocated a synergistic balance.

WHOSE HOUSE?[3]
Nona Freeman

We're given temporary residence
In a vulnerable house of clay,
Without a lease or promise of time
Eviction could come any day.

Since the longest residency is brief,
How careful and wise we should be
To occupy each short golden moment
In the light of eternity.

And nurture the clay house diligently
Even though it comes from a clod,
For the King graces it with His presence
To become the Temple of God!

FIVE

WHAT'S THE DIFFERENCE?

Milk, butter, cheese, bread, grains, meat, fish, herbs, fruit, dried fruit, honey, oil, vegetables, vinegar, and salt are all foods repeatedly mentioned in the Bible.

Disparity occurs when we think, "Oh great, I can eat dairy products, bread, fruit, and honey!" without considering that the forms of these foods differ greatly from how they were eaten in Bible times.

For instance, did you know that the cheese that David's father had him carry to his soldier-brothers was not a cooler full of neatly packaged 8-ounce plastic bags of dyed-yellow shredded cheese that he picked up at the supermarket on his way out of town? It was actually slightly pressed milk, more like what we would think of as curds, carried in rush baskets (I Samuel 17:18).

When the Lord appeared to Abraham in the form of a theophany, Abraham and Sarah served Him water, bread, butter, milk, and calf meat. Sarah did not run to her breadbox for a loaf of fluffy white bread and defrost some calf meat in her microwave oven as she pulled a rectangular-shaped pound of butter and a gallon of 1% milk out of her refrigerator.

Abraham told Sarah to take "three measures of fine meal, knead it, and make cakes upon the hearth" (Genesis 18:6-8). Sounds labor intensive if you ask me, but bread was baked daily, and those ladies had the process down to a fine science. They mixed the flour with water, made it into dough, and rolled it out into small cakes. Then they placed the cakes on the dirt floor, which was hot from a previous fire, and covered them with hot embers. The bread was eaten as soon as it was done baking.

You probably would not have identified Sarah's butter as butter and the milk they served was curdled or sour milk, fermented for preservation. (Yum! Would you like one glass of milk or two?!) The calf Abraham killed for this special occasion was probably beef. (Hopefully you don't mind meat with a gamy taste.) They roasted the fresh meat over a fire, either whole or on skewers. (Fresh rotisserized kabobs – now *that* might actually be edible!)

And one last illustration to drive home the point that we don't eat the way they did in Bible days:

Remember the story of Jesus multiplying the loaves and fishes to feed thousands of hungry people? Yes, truly a miracle. Yet I just have to shatter the dreamy illusion some of you sweet Southerners may have about this account.

You're in the very back of the multitude yet the aroma of a down home fish fry is wafting through the air. Your mouth salivates as you hurry through the crowd toward Jesus, picturing huge kettles filled with hot oil. Grandmas hover around, swatting flies and children away from the picnic tables. Chattering and laughing kinfolk are bringing all sorts of covered dishes and setting them on the tables. You can hardly wait to uncover them. Mounds of batter-fried catfish fill huge platters. And the hushpuppies! What is a fish fry without hushpuppies, cornbread, and rolls – the more the better! Then there's all the fixins' – malt vinegar, ketchup, tartar sauce. You're almost to Jesus now and the sound of ice cubes tinkling in tall glasses of sweet iced tea fill your ears as your eyes light up in anticipation of the coming feast.

Suddenly you stop dead in your tracks. You have just caught sight of Jesus and disappointment floods your taste buds. What's this? From your vantage point, what Jesus is serving looks like little more than sardines and crackers! What happened to the hot fried fish and crunchy hushpuppies?!

I guess you get the point, right? The Standard American Diet (SAD) is just not the same as the diet practiced by Jesus and the Bible figures of old.

(By the way, all you good Southerners will just have to forgive my being a little tongue-in-cheek. I have a right to pick at you – my mother is a Southerner to the core!)

You may now be asking: "So what is a dyed-in-the-wool, soda drinking, candy bar eating, fast-food addicted body to do? I'm getting the idea that our food consumption quality is far inferior to God's ideal. Should I buy goats, camels, and cows and move to Nowhereville, North Dakota and start a health guru commune? I can grow all of our own food. I'll get plenty of exercise working on the farm. Man, just shivering in the winter will help me burn calories! I won't have all that stress of fighting traffic and if I get hot during a summer day while I'm weeding the garden, making cheese, and baking bread, all I have to do is walk down to my mountain spring for a drink of pure, refreshing, cold water."

Very few people are capable of actually doing such a thing and even that would not guarantee good health. Our society is totally different from that of Bible days. We don't use camels and donkeys to get from place to place. We use cars and airplanes. Extended families don't usually live and work among one another every day. Many of us live states and even countries away from one another and communicate infrequently. And neither do we have the means to perfectly duplicate the dietary culture of days of old.

Everything that was eaten then was eaten fresh or in its naturally preserved state, usually by the process of fermentation. This is what most of us cannot relate to. Even a tomato you buy in the produce section of the supermarket was chemically grown, plucked green, and transported from who-knows-where, irradiated along the way.

But don't let that be cause for despair! There are many things we can do to improve our health by implementing biblical principles into our lives. Hopefully, you are starting to change the way you think about your health and nutrition. This book will empower you to change the way you view food and equip you to alter your eating habits for the better.

But next, let's take a look at the epidemic that is overtaking the health and vibrancy of America and see if we, one person at a time, can do something to stop and reverse the trend – at least in our lives!

SIX

OVERFED AND UNDERNOURISHED

64.5% of American adults are overweight or obese.

At the root of many major sicknesses and diseases in America is obesity, a problem of nearly pandemic proportions. Most Americans are aware that the state of being overweight or obese is a common challenge for many people. It is frequently discussed via the public media system. Still, for all of the attention it receives, most people are miserably unsuccessful at losing weight and keeping it off.

Fad diets, get-thin-quick plans, and weight loss pills promise a perfect body in a short amount of time with little effort. These slick advertisements appeal to people desperate to be healthier and thinner. In a society that greatly values outward appearance, it is paradoxical that the majority of Americans fall far short of achieving "perfection" as defined by societal standards.

Young teenage girls especially use the figures of models and movie stars to gauge their self worth. But in spite of Hollywood's emphasis on extreme thinness, these girls find it nearly impossible to emulate the world of the unreal. Instead they settle for looking like those around them. For many of them, that entails finding themselves in an overweight or obese condition.

Because in reality, we get our concepts of what is acceptable by our own personal worlds. If Mom and Dad are overweight, then it is perceived as somewhat acceptable and maybe even normal to children. If Uncle Dave eats five candy bars a day and overdoses on coffee and soft drinks, then Nephew Joey will perceive such excessive consumption as just fine. After all, he adores his uncle who can "do no wrong."

As well as children, most adults are followers and unthinkingly reflect the lifestyles and habits of those closest to them. So as contradictory as it may seem, Americans really find extra weight quite acceptable.

America is one of the few countries where this mindset it prevalent. But America's prosperity and power have made us quite egocentric, and we erroneously think that a little pot belly is the norm all over the world. But few countries are as overweight as America.

Unfortunately, in every country where a "modern" western diet replaces the native diets of primitive societies, the health of the people diminishes. Asians are typically thin and fit people. But move them to America and their physical form and health change drastically. It is unfortunate that America, which has the potential to be the healthiest nation in the world, is instead leading the world astray into a fast-food, processed food, nutrient deficient food lifestyle.

An overweight condition is defined as an unhealthy excess of body fat. Obesity is the state of being 20 percent above ideal weight. Between 6 and 7 million Americans are "morbidly obese." This means that they are 100 or more pounds beyond their ideal weight.

You might ask, "Why is it such a big deal if I have a few extra pounds hanging around?" One reason it is a big deal is because "obesity is viewed as the cause of 400,000 premature deaths a year."[1]

Why die before you have to? Obesity can be the visible sign of inwardly developing health problems such as high blood pressure, heart disease, strokes, colon cancer, breast cancer, even asthma. Obesity greatly diminishes quality of life. Excess weight places pressure on the heart, legs, and knees, hinders mobility, makes breathing laborious, and strains all systems of the body, greatly hampering the ability to thrive and excel in all areas of life. I know from experience that when I gain just a few pounds, I have shortness of breath, reduced energy level, backaches, fatigue, and less agility. If I gained a substantial amount of weight, the problems would only increase.

In his book entitled *Chew on This*, Eric Schlosser gives a simple explanation of why being overweight is detrimental: "A typical person has 25 to 35 billion fat cells. The body needs those fat cells to stay healthy. They communicate with the brain, signaling how much energy has been stored and when it's time to eat. They also play an important role in the immune system, helping the body protect itself from cancer and diseases. Fat cells are good for you. But in this case, you don't want too much of a good thing. An obese person can develop as many as 275 billion fat cells. That's almost eight times the normal amount. All those fat cells don't just sit there. They require new blood vessels and place new demands on vital organs. They create chemical imbalances. Instead of helping the immune system, these billions of new fat cells make the body much more vulnerable to illnesses. Once you've got so many fat cells, it's hard to get rid of them. Going on a diet only shrinks them. That may be one of the reasons why many people go on a diet, lose weight – and then gain back all the weight a few months later. Their fat cells rarely vanish. They just shrivel for a while, like empty little balloons, and then fill up with fat again. Becoming obese early in life may fundamentally change a person's body chemistry, making it difficult to become thin. If you are obese by the age of thirteen, there's a 90 percent chance you will be overweight in your midthirties."[2]

"If you need another reason to maintain a healthy weight, consider this: The number of inconclusive diagnostic imaging exams doubled in the U.S. between 1989 and 2003, despite advances in technology. The cause is obesity, which makes interpreting results difficult, especially when fatty tissue is very dense. This can result in serious health consequences including misdiagnosis or lack of a diagnosis altogether. While power can be increased in standard machines for higher-quality images in x-rays and CT scans, doing so could expose obese patients to increases in radiation."[3]

In third world countries a little bit of fat on the bones is a sign of wealth. It means that you can afford to eat on a regular basis. In America, however, overweight and obesity are not signs of prosperous health; they are the results of overfed but undernourished bodies, because the food we eat makes us fat but does not actually nourish us.

TRUTH – THE KEY TO FREEDOM

My husband, Bill, worked in a hospital as a chaplain's assistant. While there, he met a man who was very large. In fact, this man was so large that when he needed to go to the hospital, he could not fit through the door of his trailer. A crew cut through the wall to make an opening big enough for him to fit through. This man told my husband, "People think that I am this large because I just eat all the time. That's not my problem. I have a very large non-cancerous tumor that keeps me from being able to move around at all. The doctors remove it and it just grows back again." This is a very sad example of an obese individual whose weight was determined by something out of his control.

Because of uncontrollable obstacles, a small amount of people find losing weight more challenging than others. Successful weight loss and maintenance may be determined by factors such as body shape tendencies, metabolism, age, certain health issues, and familial support.

Too often, however, people fall back on one of these factors without honestly examining if their crutch is really valid. If you think you are powerless to change, then you won't change. If you think you are destined to be overweight, then you will be overweight. The truth is that very few people have such extreme complications as this man with the tumor. We simply find it easier to use a crutch than to change.

The object of this book is not to embarrass, shame, or isolate the reader, but to empower you. Empowerment comes through embracing truth and being honest. If losing weight is a challenge for you, take some time in prayer with the Lord. Ask Him to help you identify and confront the things that keep you from achieving a healthy weight. Ask Him to give you the courage and consistency necessary to lean on His strength, instead of using easy excuses that require no accountability. If you will seek God's assistance, this whole process will be a lot less difficult and you will grow closer to Him as a result.

I am not unsympathetic towards the challenge that people face in order to lose weight and keep it off. Some people think that thin people are thin naturally. In America, where there are restaurants on every corner and food is an obsession, that is not the case. In most cases, thin people are thin because they consciously make the effort to be and stay thin. Very few Americans can eat the Standard American Diet, have unhealthy lifestyles and still enjoy good health. There is no doubt in my mind that if I had not consciously taken control of my eating habits (and I'm still working to better them) I would be twice the size I am now. But before I could change, I had to examine when and why I adopted erroneous ideas about my body size, food, and exercise.

Think about it this way. You leave New Orleans, Louisiana, with Los Angeles, California as your destination. You drive steadily until you suddenly realize that you are on the outskirts of Birmingham, Alabama. You are driving in the opposite direction of where you want to go. In order to reach Los Angeles, you will have to consult a roadmap or activate your GPS and determine what you did wrong. What wrong turn did you make? What was so distracting that you did not notice a long time ago that you were on the wrong road? Do you have a poor sense of direction and need a knowledgeable person to help you navigate your way to Los Angeles? Did someone unintentionally give you the wrong directions, leading you astray? Once you figure out what went wrong, you can properly plan and change directions.

For most of us, this defines our weight issues. We drive in the wrong direction for years until we are unkindly confronted with a health or social issue because of our condition. At this point many people choose to ignore the signs and continue driving in the wrong direction, because they think they are powerless to change their lives. Think logically and ask yourself, "Just how much sense does that make?"

All of us want to be fit and healthy. No one really wants to be overweight and suffer from the toll it usually exacts from not just our health, but our relationships, careers, and emotions. Desire is not enough, though. There were signs along the way telling us that we were headed down the wrong road, but we didn't see them because we were distracted or else we purposely chose to ignore them. We must add a plan of action, commitment to change, and honesty to our desire.

In the presence of the Lord, identify the root problem of your overweight condition. Remember, obesity is only the symptom of deeper problems that need to be addressed. Were you taught poor eating habits by your parents, grandparents, or siblings? Were you more sedentary than active as a child and carried that behavior into adulthood? Do you lack self control in not just the area of physical stewardship but other areas as well? Did food become an emotional escape for you because of a tragic or painful incident sometime during your life? Were you verbally abused or sexually molested and you use extra weight as a shield so that you won't have to be emotionally and sexually vulnerable? Do you have a defiant attitude and don't want anybody telling you what you can and can't eat and how you should look? If so, when and why did that defiant attitude originate?

Is looking at these things easy? No. In fact, it may be very painful. When you start asking yourself why you are overweight, you may unearth things you haven't consciously thought about in years. They've been affecting you, though, in more ways than just weight management. If you are going to change your direction, you will have to determine in your mind that where you want to go is worth confronting what went wrong in your past and worth the changes that you must make.

Truth (which is called honesty when it is applied to our own lives) and understanding are crucial in order to make lasting changes. Jeff Arnold once said, "Ignorance is not bliss; ignorance is bondage." Some people would rather not closely examine why they are the way they are, resting instead on easy crutches. That is choosing to remain in bondage. Jesus said that liberation is the result of truth (John 8:32).

If you really want to be free of the control you allow food to have over you, you must evaluate how and why you surrendered yourself to its power in the first place. Is doing this hard work? Yes. Is it worth it? Yes. Things that are valuable to us are worth working hard for. It's easier to make excuses, but it's 1,000 times more satisfying to change direction and arrive at our intended destination. Seek truth – it is the key to freedom.

DEBUNKING MYTHS ABOUT OBESITY
Myth #1
"Obesity is a byproduct of physical disorders."

In most cases, obesity is the *cause* of physical malfunctions. Acid reflux, chronic fatigue, joint pain, sleep apnea – the list is endless – are all caused or exacerbated by excess weight.

Think about it this way. If you owned a horse and you added 200 pounds to that horse for it to carry around all day and all night, never giving it a break, don't you think it would develop some health problems? Sure it would. Horses are natural burden-bearers, yet they would have problems under these circumstances.

We were not designed to carry heavy loads 24 hours a day. When we add excess amounts, even small amounts, of weight to our bodies, we are only hurting ourselves.

Myth #2
"There are these great surgeries that will help me lose

weight. If I get too fat, I can always resort to that."

Radical bariatric surgery is performed over 45,000 times a year. 80% of these surgeries are administered to women. For a few morbidly obese patients, this surgery may be the only thing that stands between them and death.

Though there are undoubtedly times when surgery is in order, many times it is nothing more than an escape from personal accountability. This thinking is a reflection of the mindset of our culture. We are too careless, self-indulgent, and irresponsible. We simply put too much in our temples. Then we rely on an expensive quick fix to remedy our poor behavior. At some point we ought to take inventory of our behavior and change instead of relying on a surgeon to fix our mistakes.

People think that they can't change their behavior. We can change our behavior; the human mind and will are very powerful. The fact is that we are *unwilling* to change because we are too accustomed to pampering ourselves.

There are many problematic issues with weight loss surgery.

First, most patients are doomed to live on synthetic vitamins for the rest of their lives, because they can no longer absorb adequate nutrition from food. Because of the vitamin deficiencies and protein malnutrition that results from surgery, the nutrition they should be getting from food will come from a pill. This is not how God intended things. God did not design us to get our nutrition from pills, but from the food He created. During Creation, He did not step back, fold His arms and say, "It is good" as He gazed at the vitamin assembly line He created. Rather, He was pleased by His creation of fruit trees, herbs, and vegetation (Genesis 1:11-12).

Second, people turn to weight loss surgery because they think nothing else will work. Self-discipline, wise eating choices, and exercise would work for the vast majority of people. I know a lady who was told by a doctor that she would never be able to lose weight on her own. Yet he wanted her to lose a certain amount of weight before the surgery – and she did. What's up with that? It has the ring of a money making scheme. If she could lose weight *before* the surgery, why couldn't she lose weight *without* the surgery? To add insult to injury, after the surgery, she began religiously exercising an hour every night. There would have been no need for surgery if she would have reduced her portion sizes and exercised while her stomach was yet untouched by the surgeon's knife.

Third, surgery patients can eat only small amounts of certain foods. A rounded diet is out of the picture. God designed for us to enjoy (but not overly enjoy) the taste of food and the entire eating process. This surgery thwarts God's thoughtfulness when he prepared such a wide variety of delicious foods for us to enjoy and gain nourishment from. These stringent limitations adversely affect many patients mentally and socially.

And last, the patient puts himself at risk for surgery side effects such as malnutrition, infection, bowel and gallbladder problems. Some patients even die as a result of complications of the surgery. The patient is forced to adopt new habits, because eating too much too fast will make him sick and could even result in death. These forced behavior changes leave the patient without a choice and can create psychological and emotional crises. Additionally, some patients that do not strictly follow the post-surgery regimen can stretch their stomachs by overeating and again become overweight. This is very dangerous for the gastric bypass surgery patient.

Myth #3

"I can't do anything about my weight. It's all genetic."

Genetics receive overrated attention for their link to obesity. For the most part, our own choices and temperance, or lack thereof, determine our body size. It's time to quit passing the buck in an attempt to eliminate personal responsibility. The satisfaction you will receive by properly caring for your temple in a responsible way is incredible.

The following quotes are from Dr. Will Clower, author of *The Fat Fallacy*. "The wide belief that your genes determine your weight leaves us believing that there's nothing we can do about it, that there is no training your body or your brain. If you're fat, you're fat. It's out of your hands and onto your hips because it's your genes' fault. ...it has only been over the past 30 years or so – an eye blink for your genes – since American weight problems have really exploded onto the national health radar. We got fatter. Our genes stayed exactly the same.

"Americans are almost all of immigrant stock, so nothing in our genetic makeup would predispose U.S. citizens to be any more gigantic than anybody else on the planet. Clearly the concept that a single gene or chemical controls our weight is far too naïve. Your weight results from a raucous combination of personal, social, familial routines, mixed here and there with unknown quantities of hormonal signals, neural impulses, and emotional baggage.

"More than 250 genes and at least 40 neurochemicals regulate metabolism and appetite in still strange and unpredictable ways."[4] Scientists have isolated *one* gene from our complex genetic makeup and simplistically conclude that *one* gene is the reason 65% of Americans are overweight or obese. People would rather believe in the questionable power of a single "fat gene" and suffer poor health all of their lives than change. The "fat gene" idea feeds into America's shift toward the escapism mentality: escape from responsibility and play the blame game. It's easier to blame our ancestry than it is to admit our weaknesses and change our ways.

This of course leads to the classic "nature versus nurture" debate. If we embrace the "fat gene" theory, then maybe scientists should start looking for an "alcoholic gene," a "murderer gene," and a "manipulator gene." Maybe they will even find a "lazy gene." Occasionally the "nature" train of thought is applicable to certain scenarios, but America's out-of-control obesity is not one of those cases. Most of our problems result from learned behaviors which can be changed. Surely Philippians 4:13, which tells me that "I can do all things through Christ which strengtheneth me" wasn't written just so the apostle Paul could practice his penmanship.

According to the fat gene theory, if you have this special gene then you are doomed to be fat, regardless of what you do. If the "fat gene" theory is true, then why do people lose weight when they change the poor eating habits they adopted as children? If the "fat gene" theory is true, then why do people lose weight when they implement exercise into their daily routine? If the "fat gene" theory is true, then why do people lose weight when they fast for an extended period? If the "fat gene" theory is true, then why do people lose weight after gastric bypass surgery?

There's a skunk in the woodpile; the "fat gene" idea just doesn't make sense. If our weight problems really are a result of genetics, then nothing should be able to make us lose weight; after all, we can't change our genes.

There may be some things about us that we have no control over, but for the vast majority of people, weight is not one of those problems. It's easier to believe in genetic predisposition than to change behavior patterns that we are comfortable with. But you are not powerless to change.

THE FAT BELONGS TO THE LORD

Maybe you have heard someone laughingly use Leviticus 3:16, which says that "all the fat is the LORD's," to make light of their excess weight. By this glib statement, which takes the Scripture out of context, obesity is equated with godliness. As he pats his tummy, a man might say, "The Bible says that the fat belongs to the Lord. All of this belongs to Him."

I met a sweet young lady who had recently been baptized in Jesus' name and filled with the Holy Ghost.

She was brimming with excitement and wonder at all God was doing in her life. Being newly exposed to apostolic truth, she was noticing all kinds of things about the Church. One thing she noticed was the percentage of people who were overweight. In her naiveté she said, "I suppose so many of them are overweight because they fast so much that they mess up their metabolism." Very gently I broke the news to her that, unfortunately, fasting is not the cause of our plump condition.

Clay Jackson, MD, wrote a timely article about obesity for the *Pentecostal Herald*. His statements provide us with clear understanding and wise advice. "Our convictions regarding a godly lifestyle tend to help us live a healthy lifestyle. That includes prohibitions against promiscuous behavior and the abuse of addictive substances, including nicotine and alcohol. But some elements of a healthy lifestyle encouraged by Scripture may have been overlooked and de-emphasized. I am thinking about the epidemic of overweight and obesity that is occurring in the United States. Pentecostals are not immune; we might be worse off than the general population. We have not emphasized proper nutrition and exercise nearly so much as we have other aspects of healthy living. We often quote I Corinthians 6:19-20 in defense of our position against smoking tobacco and drinking alcohol because they tear down the well-being of our bodies, the temples of the Spirit. I agree with that, but if smoking and drinking are not good ideas because they harm our bodies, how can we overlook eating to excess or not exercising properly? Paul wrote in Galatians that temperance, or personal self-control, is part of the fruit of the Spirit of God. If our pursuit of health is rooted in the concept of stewardship, then everything we do (and are) is to bring glory to God."[5]

Is it so wrong to think that those of us who are filled with the Holy Ghost, the very Spirit of Almighty God, should need to take care of our temples? It seems that if anybody should be mindful and respectful of the physical state of their bodies, it should be those who house the Spirit of God.

FIGURATIVE FAT IS WHERE IT'S AT

Today, we think of excess body fat as something dangerous to our health, which it generally is. Our biblical predecessors did not think of fat in the same way. Generally, having so much excess fat that their health was compromised was not an issue with them. Being well acquainted with famines and unpredictable harvests, they used the word fat to refer to healthfulness and prosperity.

In the Bible, whenever the word fat is used in a negative context it appears to be referring to obesity or the dark spiritual condition of the Israelites (Deuteronomy 31:20; 32:15; Judges 3:17-22; Job 15:27).

For the most part, though, the passages that use the word "fat" in positive contexts teaches that it is proper actions that make us "fat." In other words, a productive, fulfilling, successful, prosperous life are direct results of our choices.

Psalm 92:12-14 says that the people that plant themselves in the house of the Lord (i.e. they have committed their entire lives to God and serving Him) shall be "fat and flourishing." Proverbs 13:4 tells us that those that are diligent in their work "shall be made fat." Proverbs 15:30 encourages us to speak uplifting words and talk about things that are enriching: "A good report maketh the bones fat." Proverbs 28:25 emphasizes the importance of trusting God: "He that putteth his trust in the LORD shall be made fat."

A LIGHT APPROACH TO A HEAVY SUBJECT

Overweight and obese people often use humor to deal with their condition, because they are emotionally sensitive about it. They figure they will make fun of themselves before someone else does. I've heard it said, "People can tell that I'm on the level because my bubble is in the middle." Humor is a defense mechanism for them, a way of dealing with a very painful issue that they are unwilling to confront or have been unsuccessful at overcoming.

I was watching people file through a buffet line. One rather large lady was conscientiously filling her plate with generous helpings of an assortment of food. Someone in the line behind her said, "Hurry up. You're holding up the line." She jokingly responded, "I'm taking my time. This is important business I'm taking care of here." As she patted her bloated stomach, she laughed and said, "I have invested a lot into my figure and I need to take care of it."

This kind of humor is only a diversion to keep us from dealing with something we know is harming us. It distracts us from examining how we came to be in this state in the first place and prevents us from doing something about it. Being overweight is not a laughing matter. It is a dangerous matter, one that should not be dismissed with a joke.

The latest medical trend is to label obesity a "disease." Obesity is no more a disease than alcoholism is a disease. Labeling such things as "diseases" gives the mistaken impression that an individual contracted obesity or alcoholism similar to the way one would contract malaria. This conveniently removes personal responsibility from the equation. "If I did nothing to create the problem, then of course there's nothing I can do to remedy the problem."

Obesity is not a disease and you are not doomed to endure it for the rest of your life. You have the power to do something about your condition. Don't just give in to how you feel, thinking that you will always be sick and overweight, masking your fears and discomfort with a joke. If you think that you will always be overweight and that there is nothing you can do about it, then chances are you will remain miserable. But if you will grasp onto God's principles of wise stewardship, you will be laughing because you enjoy life, you feel good, and you are free from the bondage of food, not because you are attempting to cope with a painful issue.

OBESITY AND CHILDREN

One-sixth of American children are overweight or obese. Children should not be held responsible for an overweight or obese condition; the parent(s) should be held responsible. Children mimic their parents' eating habits. Children do not have the ability to buy healthy groceries. They are at the mercy of their parents' preferences. It is the parents that develop in their children a taste for sweets and junk food. Parents lead children in their food addictions – by their example and enablement. Habits and lifestyle are far more responsible for obesity than genetics. Children take on the shape of their parents, not primarily because of inherited genes, but because they eat and live the same way as their parents.

Consider for a minute. Most families look alike. If the parents are overweight, the children usually are too. Again, genetics play only a very minute role in this; lifestyle is much more the reason. If the parents are relatively physically fit, the children usually are too. What is important to parents will be important to children.

Parents err when they think that they are the only ones affected by their poor choices. Children take with them into adulthood, which comes in seemingly the blink of an eye, more than obesity and poor health. They take mindsets that they consider normal because the two most influential people in their lives – Mom and Dad – have taught them how to think.

Read the following story and ponder it in relation to the example you are setting for your children.

The King's Highway
Author Unknown

Once a king had a great highway built for the members of his kingdom. After it was completed, but before it was opened to the public, the king decided to have a contest. He invited as many as desired to participate. Their challenge was to see who could travel the highway best.

On the day of the contest the people came. Some of them had fine chariots, some had fine clothing, fine hairdos, or great goods. Some young men came in their track clothes and ran along the highway. People traveled the highway all day, but each one, when he arrived at the end, complained to the king that there was a large pile of rocks and debris left on the road at one spot, and this got in their way and hindered their travel.

At the end of the day, a lone traveler crossed the finish line and wearily walked over to the king. He was tired and dirty but he addressed the king with great respect and handed him a bag of gold. He explained, "I stopped along the way to clear away a pile of rocks and debris that was blocking the road. This bag of gold was under it all, and I want you to return it to its rightful owner."

The king replied, "You are the rightful owner."

The traveler replied, "Oh no, that is not mine. I've never known such money."

"Oh yes," said the king, "you've earned this gold, for you won my contest. He who travels the road best is he who makes the road smoother for those who will follow."

It is not easy for parents to move obstacles out of their children's way. Doing so requires introspective, confrontational, personal change that can be difficult. Parents must weigh their desires. Do they desire to continue doing the same things they have always done just because change is hard, no matter how it may damage their children? Or do they see the greater good of setting an example for their children that will positively influence them for life and make their journeys easier?

Children follow. Clear their paths of the poor habits you model before them that will cause their walk through life to be challenged by unnecessary physical maladies that can be avoided by exercising self-discipline and common sense. No, we don't have control over everything that may physically influence our children (toxic environmental exposure or accidents, for example), and we can't make their adult choices for them, but we need to do what we are capable of doing.

If parents exercise, play outdoor games, take walks after dinner, and stay fit, the children will usually follow in their footsteps. If parents are sedentary, overweight, inactive, and gluttonous, the children will usually follow. If parents reach for candy bars and junk food, so will their children. If parents reach for apples, salads, and yogurt, the children will be much more likely to do the same. Children eat what parents eat. Children emulate the habits of their parents and make them their own.

In the Bible, the fleeting days of youth were synonymous with strength, vitality, energy, and heroism. Unfortunately, many of today's youth are tired, listless, and unmotivated. The formative years of a child's life determines his future. Parents set the pattern. If a child wishes to deviate from poor examples set before him, he must work hard to change the habits that have been inbred in him. On the other hand, positive role models who eat temperately and healthily will encourage children to make eating right a lifestyle. Children will see the benefits of it because the parents modeled it. We are only as good as our environment – usually – because most of us are followers, not leaders. Don't expect your kids to be healthy if you're not. Don't demand that they eat right if you don't. Remember, in America good health has to be worked at; it will not come naturally if we eat the Standard American Diet.

Take inventory of the subtle patterns in your home that contribute to unhealthy lifestyles. Do you cave in every time your child begs you for candy at the checkout line? Do you find it easier to pacify your child with food than to deal with behavior issues? Have you forgotten that you are the parent, not your child? Because you are the parent, it is your responsibility to do what is best for your child, in spite of what he might want. Children don't usually know what is good for them; they just want to be in control. Do you use media as a babysitter? If so, you are doing more than destroying them morally. You are setting them up for food failure. Erik Steele, D.O. wrote that the average child sees an astonishing 10,000 ads for food each year.[6] And it is highly unlikely that even a minute percentage of those ads are for anything remotely healthy.

A sedentary lifestyle diet of TV, video games, and Internet usage is anathema to the health of children. Help your children really live. Take them camping, hiking, bicycling – anything that is active. To substitute unnecessary eating, try some new activities, such as a new board game or outdoor sport. Involve them in physically active chores such as gardening, mowing the lawn, and washing the car. Turn necessary tasks into fun, quality family time. Check with your local tourist information bureau for things to do in your area. You may find that there is a really neat museum or park that you never even knew about that can provide you with fun things to do other than overeating.

STOP THE CYCLE

It's a cycle. We become overweight because we are gluttonous, lack self control, and do not eat responsibly. Then we develop serious health problems due to our obesity. Those health problems create more health problems. These conditions linger and make it difficult for us to exercise, thus we accumulate more pounds, worsening our situation.

It's time to stop the cycle.

Because it's not just about us. It's about our children. It's about generations following. It's about longevity. It's about the health of our marital relationship. It's about our productivity on the job and our fulfillment of the Great Commission. It's about our Kingdom work.

There are a lot of things to motivate us to change. No matter how hard it may seem, in the long run one small change at a time will pay off big dividends.

SEVEN

THE "ACCEPTABLE" SIN

Hast thou found honey?
eat so much as is sufficient for thee,
lest thou be filled therewith, and vomit it.
Proverbs 25:16

Gluttony is the acceptable sin. Well, *we* think it is acceptable. Unfortunately, God doesn't find it acceptable at all. But think about it: When was the last time you heard a sermon devoted to the sin of gluttony? I cannot recall *one.*

Gluttony, however, is mentioned numerous times, and temperance is a prevailing theme throughout the Word of God. It is necessary to eat to live, but many of us fail to differentiate between eating for survival and overeating for pleasure. We sanction the sin of gluttony, because it is something most of us participate in.

Gluttony is eating more than our bodies actually need. One of the biblical definitions of the word "glutton" describes one who wastes his own body.[1] Gluttony is an unharnessed appetite, an unrestrained desire to eat to excess. Gluttony is a lack of self-control and temperance. In the Bible it is always mentioned as a shameful activity.

I used to work at a restaurant that had an all-you-can-eat buffet. One regular customer was a very large man with a peculiar sense of humor. One day he told me that he used to be a lot bigger, which was hard to imagine. He told me that when he was a kid he would eat two dozen eggs for breakfast. He said, "My mom always told me that I ate too much, so I cut back to one dozen eggs. That's how I lost weight." This man never knew what it was like to enjoy a reasonable, healthy weight, because he was a glutton from childhood.

I have a friend who is as thin as a stick. A donut shop opened just a couple of blocks from her house. She loved these donuts and would frequently eat a dozen at a time. She was very energetic to begin with, and she worked out several hours a day. These donuts did not add a miniscule bump to her figure. One day she asked me, "Sylvia, do you think it's a sin to overeat if you don't gain weight from it?" I had to laughingly answer in the affirmative.

Although overweight and obese conditions are usually accurate indicators of inner health problems, occasionally a person may be moderately overweight and yet be relatively healthy. Conversely, not all skinny people are necessarily healthy.

If you are one of those rare individuals who can eat large quantities of whatever you want and never gain an ounce, please keep in mind that you are not exempt from the admonitions of Scripture. You may say, "I'm healthy and I'm at an ideal weight. I don't need to watch what I eat." Two adages come to mind: "An ounce of prevention is worth a pound of cure" and "You reap what you sow." Sooner or later, our habits, whether they are good or bad, will produce a crop of some sort. If we want to reap health and vitality, then we must sow seeds of health and vitality.

Don't just live for today. Have a far-reaching vision of your future, the future of your children and grandchildren. Grandparents should never underestimate the influence they have on their grandchildren. Not only do grandchildren need role models who will teach them by example to temperately eat healthy foods, they need grandparents who will maintain their health so that the grandchildren can enjoy their grandparents for many, many years.

We must remember that just because our gluttonous behavior doesn't show up on the scale right away doesn't mean that it might not come back to haunt us in the future.

Our bodies were not created for us to see how much food we can stuff inside them. Yet often we feel as though we have not really done a meal justice unless we leave the table with actual physical pain in our stomachs because we have overloaded them. What happens to a computer that is overloaded with information? It shuts down and quits working. Hopefully, the computer doctor can revive it, but some valuable information may have been lost in the process.

If you have poor eating habits and tend to overeat on a regular basis, examine your close acquaintances. Chances are good that they also overeat. Don't abandon those friends but make some new ones who are temperate and will help you to be temperate. Daniel Segraves has an enlightening commentary on Proverbs 23:20-21: "Since we tend to become like those with whom we associate, it is important to associate with those who exemplify the highest character qualities. It is a mistake to associate with the self-indulgent. Self-indulgence often manifests itself in drinking alcoholic beverages and an unhealthy fascination with food. But both drunkenness and gluttony will lead to poverty. They produce drowsiness, and drowsiness is one of the chief traits contributing to poverty. Conversely, one of the most important steps toward prosperity is alertness."[2]

If we want to prosper, not just financially but in all areas of life, we must exercise self-control. Eating is a good place to start, since gluttony seem to be the acceptable sin that most of us red-blooded Americans yield to on a regular basis. Why not begin stopping before you're stuffed? It is a wonderful feeling to know that you are in control of your food instead of allowing it to control you. My pastor, Jonathan Urshan, routinely leaves a small amount of food on his plate. He does this because he doesn't want food to control him. By leaving a small portion of food on his plate, he is continually exercising discipline and restraint. Food does not control him.

"When thou sittest to eat with a ruler, consider

diligently what is before thee: And put a knife to thy throat, if thou be a man given to appetite. Be not desirous of his dainties: for they are deceitful meat" (Proverbs 23:1-3). The phrase "consider diligently" means to mentally separate or distinguish. In other words, "think before you eat."

A lifestyle of gluttony is an imbedded mindset. Only when we decide that we will stop participating in the sin of gluttony will we be successful at portion control.

EIGHT

PORTION CONTROL

Remove far from me vanity and lies: give me neither poverty
nor riches; <u>feed me with food convenient for me</u>: Lest I be full,
and deny thee, and say, Who is the LORD? or lest I be poor,
and steal, and take the name of my God in vain.
Proverbs 30:8-9

"Do you want fries with your cheeseburger today?"
"Would you like to super-size your meal?"
"We have a special today. The all-you-can-eat buffet is
only $8.99."

Every day we are bombarded with the "more-is-better" sales pitch. When it comes to food portions, America has been lied to and has believed the lie. We are all too willing to believe that "bigger is better" when it comes to the amount of food that can be piled on our plates. All-you-can-eat buffets attract us like a mouse to cheese. But when that little metal bar on the mousetrap snaps across a mouse's body, it discovers too late that the cheese on the mousetrap is not what it thought it was. And sooner or later, we too realize that our consistent overindulgence has a darker side.

I once knew two sisters who, though not remarkably thin, were fairly fit and healthy during their growing-up years. When they went to fast-food restaurants, they each ordered a cheeseburger and a small order of fries. One of the sisters continued eating relatively small portions of food into her adulthood. The other sister started ordering a double cheeseburger and a large fry instead of the single cheeseburger and small fry. Soon she lost control over her eating habits. Her health began to decline as her weight increased. She became unhappy and her relationships suffered as a result.

It is a proven fact that we Americans routinely consume more calories than we think we do. We eat more than we realize. We start in the morning with a breakfast pastry and a mug of coffee as we head out the door. A quick snack from the vending machine during mid-morning break keeps us going until lunch, when we head to a fast food joint. We get a jumbo soda refill on the way out of the restaurant and sip on that through the afternoon. Dinner fare varies depending on our schedule. It could be a big, heavy meal concluded with a large slice of pie, or it could be an extra-large pizza delivered to our door, followed by ice cream and late night snacks. You put all that food (most of it non-nutritious) together and you have a whopping calorie count big enough to give the federal deficit a run for its money.

People put away more calories than they think, especially when they are eating a food that they perceive to be healthy because it is labeled "low-fat." "'People indulge a lot more in low-fat versions of processed foods than in their regular counterparts, and overweight people seem especially vulnerable. Such products are seemingly designed to improve health, but they may actually contribute to weight problems,' says Brian Wansink of Cornell University's Food and Brand Lab in Ithaca, N.Y. 'We're a nation of low-fat foods and high-fat people.'"[1]

There are many people in the world that feel blessed if they get one meal a day. God has blessed the United States with an abundance of food and plenty of jobs. Most of us have no idea what it would be like to have an empty refrigerator or no money to buy food. So we have the opposite problem of nations that are poverty-stricken and impoverished. Instead of wishing that our hunger pangs would go away, we wish that our overindulged, swollen stomachs would magically disappear. We have to consciously exercise discipline in order to stay fit. Solomon asked to be fed with food "convenient" for him. "Convenient" refers to a specific portion or measure of food. The Wise Man, speaking to us from millennia past, understood the need for portion control!

The Lord provided manna for the children of Israel to eat during their wilderness sojourn (Exodus 16:14-18). The Israelites called this small, round food "manna" because they had never seen it before. "Manna" simply means "What is this?" Whatever it was, manna must have contained a terrific balance of nutrients because it kept men, women, and children healthy and strong for 40 years.

The Lord gave the Israelites specific instructions about the manna: "Gather of it every man according to his eating." Each morning, every person was to gather only as much as he or she could eat during that one day. The next morning, there would be fresh manna. There was always extra manna but God wanted them to gather just enough for each person, no more. This was divine portion control.

Exercise your ability to reduce intake by consciously and deliberately choosing your food portions. Too often an individual finishes a meal, leans back in his chair, pats his bloated tummy and says, "I am stuffed! I think my eyes were bigger than my stomach!" Sometimes we order or prepare much more food than we actually need. Keep this in mind when ordering food at a restaurant. Order a half-portion, if possible. If you are still hungry, you can always order a little something more. But chances are, you will probably be quite satisfied with a smaller portion and your tummy will thank you for not stuffing it with more than it was designed to receive and digest.

If you're at a restaurant and the waitress brings you a plate with an enormous amount of pasta on it, ask for a takeout box before you ever start eating. Put half of the pasta in the box. You can eat your leftovers the next day. If you don't do this and you are an individual who was raised to finish all of the food on your plate, you will feel obligated to try to eat every last noodle, regardless of how stuffed you are.

Try ordering one meal and sharing it with a friend or family member. This not only helps you control your portions, it also saves you money. Don't order or serve yourself more than you really need and stop eating before you are stuffed to the gills. Don't load up your desk at work with candy, chocolate, and chips. Use smaller plates and don't refill them. *Think* about what and why you are eating before you eat. Many times we eat just to be eating; we aren't really hungry at all. Instead of super-sizing, down size and your temple will thank you.

It is important to keep in mind that, as we become disciplined in controlling our portions of food, there may be some foods we have to abstain from altogether. Most Americans do everything to excess and learning to live with "all things in moderation" takes time. Confession is good for the soul so I'll admit that if I buy a half gallon of my favorite ice cream, it is highly likely that I will eat all of that ice cream within a 48 hour period. It is wisdom to recognize our areas of weakness. Since I know that I will want to quickly devour that much ice cream, common sense tells me to not bring it into my house very often. If I could be moderate and enjoy a small scoop now and then, great. But until I can achieve self control with that particular food, the best thing to do is abstain, refrain, refuse it altogether. If I don't start, I won't get into trouble. You may have a weakness – coffee, candy bars, potato chips. While working towards moderation, do without until you are strong enough to control that food, instead of it controlling you.

Avoid all-you-can-eat buffets. Buffets encourage even the most disciplined to overindulge. Don't fall for the "I must get my money's worth" mentality. Some restaurants are legendary for their giant-sized food portions. Bigger is not necessarily better, either taste or health wise.

Eating well and moderation tend to go hand in hand. Hence, the adage "The better you eat, the less you eat; the worse you eat, the more you eat."

I have observed that more upscale restaurants usually serve smaller portions. That is because the food is typically very flavorful and designed to be savored. Quality, rather than quantity, is emphasized. I have been to restaurants where the flavors of the food were so stupendous that I would take a bite and wait several moments before taking another bite, letting the flavor linger on my tongue. Good chefs are trained to create culinary masterpieces that you won't get at chain restaurants or from precooked frozen dinners.

Granted, good food eaten out usually comes with a price, but it is a wonderful way to create memories with a loved one. A meal with several courses means that there's not so much food on the table at one time that you feel compelled to eat it all in a hurry before it gets cold. Several, smaller courses also allow you to enjoy the company of your family and/or friends.

As you begin to control your portion amounts, you will enjoy the benefits of discipline. Instead of your taste buds and your love for food dictating to you how much you eat, you will turn the tables on your "flesh" and be fulfilled and happy because you exercised restraint.

NINE

ON THE LIGHTER SIDE

HAPPY BIRTHDAY!
Question: What do angels serve at their
birthday parties?
Answer: Angel food cake!

FOUR-STEP ITALIAN PASTA DIET
Inventor Unknown
Step 1 – You walka pasta da bakery.
Step 2 – You walka pasta da candy store.
Step 3 – You walka pasta da ice cream shop.
Step 4 – You walka pasta da refrigerator.

THE UNTOLD STORY OF THE WORLD'S FIRST
DIETERS: ADAM AND EVE
Author Unknown
In the beginning, God created the heaven and the earth and populated the earth with colorful fruits and vegetables of all kinds so that Man and Woman could live long and healthy lives. Then Satan created doughnuts and ice cream. And Man and Woman ate of them. And Satan smiled.

And God created healthy yogurt that Woman might keep the figure that Man found so fair. And Satan brought forth white flour from the wheat and sugar from the cane and combined them. And Woman gained in size.

So God said, "Try my fresh green salad." And Satan presented thick creamy dressing, buttery croutons, and garlic toast on the side. And Man and Woman loosened their coverings.

God then said, "Behold, I have sent you heart-healthy vegetables and olive oil in which to cook them." And Satan brought forth deep-fried fish and chicken-fried steak. And Man's cholesterol reached toward the heavens.

God then created a light, fluffy white cake and named it "Manna." And Satan created chocolate cake and named it "Devil's Food."

God then brought forth running shoes for His children. And Satan gave them cable TV with a remote control. And Man and Woman became lazy and gained pounds.

Then God brought forth the potato, naturally brimming with nutrition. And Satan peeled off the healthful skin, sliced the starchy center into chips and deep-fried them. And Man continued to grow in size.

God created lean beef so that Man might consume fewer calories and fat. And Satan created the 99-cent double bacon cheeseburger and asked, "Do you want to super-size those fries?" And Man went into cardiac arrest.

God sighed and created quadruple bypass surgery. And Satan created HMOs.

ELBOW BENDS

Elbow Bends are one of the easiest exercises to do. Anyone, even young children, can do them. Simply set a heaping plate of food on the table in front of you. Place a fork in your hand. Bend your elbow down to the plate, pick up a forkful of food, and bend your elbow again to carry the fork to your mouth. Empty the food into your mouth and chew. Do this repeatedly until the plate is empty, then fill the plate and repeat the entire exercise. Do this as many times as desired.

Note: Your goal will determine the number of Elbow Bends you do each day and your consistency. If your goal is to become more fit, it is advised that you carefully monitor the frequency of your elbow bends and not place too much weight on the fork. If your goal is to stockpile great stores of excess fat, then more elbow bends will help you achieve this.

THE FIRST BOTTLED WATER

You probably think that bottled water is a new invention, the brainchild of modern entrepreneurs with a great marketing plan. It seems, however, that Abraham was thousands of years ahead of the current bottled water trend. Genesis 21:14 tells us that "Abraham rose up early in the morning, and took bread, and *a bottle of water*, and gave it unto Hagar, putting it on her shoulder, and the child, and sent her away: and she departed, and wandered in the wilderness of Beersheba" (emphasis added). Abraham equipped Hagar and her son with provisions for her directionless journey: whole grain bread and bottled water!

(Of course we know that this water was not in a convenient plastic bottle with a quick-pop sports top. The "bottle" was a container made from the skin of an animal.)

PART II

CHANGING MINDSETS

Building a Sturdy Structure

TEN

AN INTERVIEW WITH MOSHE MYEROWITZ

Following is an interview conducted with Dr. Moshe Myerowitz (D.C., C.C.Ac, C.C.N.) of Myerowitz Chiropractic Natural Care.[1] For almost 50 years he has been helping people achieve better health through non-invasive, natural methods. I appreciated his willingness to share his time and expertise with us. His openness and sense of humor made our interview insightful and pleasant.

SF: From your experience, is there a definite link between nutrition and health?

MM: The short answer is "yes." You cannot be healthy unless you have good nutrition. But nutrition is only one component of the health pie. You need exercise, a properly functioning nervous system, good rest, and low stress levels. Hormones, which are affected by nutrition and the aging process, are pieces of the pie. All ingredients are important for optimum health.

SF: What are some of the top killers of Americans today?

MM: Heart disease, stroke, cancer and iatrogenic conditions. Iatrogenic conditions are caused by medical drugs and medical treatments.

SF: What forms of treatment do you utilize to help people achieve better health?

MM: In no particular order, I use homeopathy, chiropractic, herbs, nutrition, chiropractic acupuncture and auriculotherapy. I am a board certified clinical nutritionist.

Auriculotherapy is a healing method used by the military at selected sites, although many people are unaware of that. The ear has many points that can influence health. The premise of auriculotherapy is that treatment of appropriate active ear points can favorably affect distant organs and tissues within the body.

SF: In degree of effectiveness, how do these treatments differ from conventional treatments, with which most people are familiar, such as prescription medication and invasive surgeries?

MM: Once we experience symptoms, we are no longer healthy. Medical doctors are wonderfully trained in medicine and surgery. They are poorly trained in anything else. Most will admit they know little about the many modalities used in alternative care including supplements and homeopathy.

The drug and surgery methods used by conventional medicine and the alternative measures used by alternative doctors are worlds apart. Drugs do little to restore health; the sickness is ongoing. When as much as 8, 10, 12 drugs together are prescribed for the same patient, as is done frequently with senior citizens, no one knows what the effects will be. All drugs have downsides. Generally, they do not restore the patient back to health; they make the patient more comfortable. When it comes to surgery, the good Lord did not supply the body with spare parts. When parts are removed, a burden is placed on the rest of the body.

Drugs create nutritional deficiencies. Some third world countries are healthier than us. They don't live longer, civil wars and such take a heavy toll, but they are healthier overall.

SF: What motivated you to pursue a career in alternative medicine?

MM: I had my own miracle. Actually, I had three miracles. One started when I was young. According to the ophthalmologist, I was going to be legally blind by the time I was twenty. When I was 12-years-old, I went to a chiropractor four times a week for four months. After that period of treatment, I returned to the ophthalmologist. He examined me and said that I did not even need glasses. It was then that I knew I wanted to be a chiropractor.

SF: What results have you seen as a consequence of your work?

MM: There are as many different conditions as there are people. We analyze people individually and base treatment upon the findings. Most everyone who has followed their prescribed plan has improved. I see people with incurable diseases: IBS, Crohn's disease, Hodgkin's lymphoma. I do not treat these conditions. Essentially my approach is to return the body to normal biochemistry. As this occurs, most of these conditions improve.

People are looking for treatments that are target specific for their condition. They need to forget the condition. They need to consider correcting the biochemistry of the body. The body tissue is the soil from which new tissues and cells are grown. If you want to grow good vegetables, you must nurture the soil. Abnormal soil conditions enable abnormal cells to grow. Food is the fertilizer for the human body.

There are hundreds if not thousands of conditions and they confound people if they only look at conditions and symptoms. The difference between an allopathic and an alternative practitioner is that the alternative practitioner moves to correct the soil and put it back into balance. All I try to do is bring the human body back into biological equilibrium, the equilibrium that most of us are born with.

During conception and the period of pregnancy, if the mother is healthy, the child will be born into this world without deficiencies and abnormalities. Whatever the child is fed that is bad will change the quality of the soil. Conditions will develop which will produce symptoms.

Pesticides, artificial flavors, etc. are not indigenous to nature and the body has to deal with them. We are putting things into the soil that do not belong there. There are an overwhelmingly abundant number of chemicals that we are exposed to daily, such as the heavy metals mercury, arsenic, lead, and aluminum.

We are inundated with chemicals. No wonder we grow tumors; our bodies are out of balance. At this point in time, it is nearly impossible to go from the cradle to the grave without getting sick. We must be vigilant and pay attention to the early warning signs that our body is communicating to us in the form of early symptoms. If we do not pay attention these symptoms will worsen until a serious condition develops.

SF: Do you advocate one diet in particular or a whole foods lifestyle?

MM: I advocate diets that are based upon the individual need. No two people are exactly the same. Even identical twins are not the same; they have their own biological individuality.

SF: What key advice would you give to people who desire to improve their health by lifestyle and dietary changes?

MM: Eat organic foods. Anything that is not organic has chemicals in it. Eat less often and chew your food more. Intake of foods needs to be more alkaline than acidic. Eat omega 3 and omega 6 fatty acids foods in a 3 to 1 ratio or less. Doing these things will have a positive effect on the body; for some dramatically.

SF: What is the best method of determining individual vitamin and mineral deficiencies?

MM: There is no best method. There are many methods. Blood tests are a resource. They can be expensive. I use galvanic skin response testing, electrodermal screening.

SF: What is your opinion of a biblically based whole foods diet, a diet based on whole grains, fresh, raw dairy products, healthy meats, fruits and vegetables, olive oil, etc.?

MM: I don't have any disagreement with what the Bible says. There is tremendous wisdom in the Bible. If you follow what the Bible says, you'll do well.

ELEVEN

WHY DO WE EAT?

*Whether therefore ye eat, or drink, or whatsoever ye do,
do all to the glory of God.*
I Corinthians 10:31

You might say, "Well, that's easy. We eat because we need food to live." And you would be right. But most of us eat much more food than our bodies can utilize. And the excess does not just disappear into thin air; instead, our bodies store up the unused food as fat and we become overweight, then obese. Along with these extra pounds comes sluggishness, fatigue, limited mobility, joint pain, and a host of physical ailments. The organs and muscles in our bodies are simply not designed to accommodate large amounts of fat. Our bodies suffer when we overload them.

I once made a list of the reasons I eat or overeat. It was startling how long the list became. And most of the things on my list were not legitimate reasons to eat. Below is my list, presented in a slightly lighthearted manner to cushion the blow of some of the statements that you might identify with. (Change is sometimes hard. A little humor goes a long way.)

It might be beneficial for you to create your own list. Some of your reasons may be the same as mine but no doubt you will have different ones as well. The next time you open your refrigerator, look at your list and ask yourself, "Am I really hungry? Does my body really need food right now? Or am I eating for some other reason?" It is good to pinpoint the reason and identify the *root* of the problem in order to overcome it.

1. I eat out of habit.
Obviously, eating is a habit because we do it every day. But sometimes we eat just to be eating, not because we're hungry or our bodies need the food.

2. I have a little idle time and eating just seems like the thing to do.
We are part of such a busy society that when we have some free time with nothing to do, we think we need to fill it with eating food.

3. I enjoy baking and cooking, and of course, I must partake of the fruits of my labor.
You can tell who the cook in the family is by the loosened apron strings and the sample spoon in the hand. Too many samples make for a rotund tummy.

4. I'm tired and want something to perk me up.
This "something" is usually sweet and sugary, which will only send our blood sugar on a roller coaster ride. If we're tired, maybe our body is telling us it needs some sleep. What a novel idea!

5. I'm with others who are eating so I eat too, though I'm not really hungry.
Monkey see, monkey do. We must learn to enjoy the company and conversation of others and pass on the food if we don't really need it. Or try eating just a *little*.

6. I lack energy.
Again, when I lack energy, I usually reach for caffeine or sugar – quick pick-me-ups. Unfortunately, they are also quick let-me-downs. I should eat complex carbohydrates and protein for lasting energy. Drinking a glass of water might be all I need to boost my energy. And ironically, nothing chases away the energy blues like exercise.

7. I get slightly lightheaded or dizzy.
I need to rest or eat something with iron or protein – *not*

sugar or caffeine. My lightheadedness may be due to going too long without stable food and filling up on sugar and junk food instead.

8. I don't want to waste food.

This is a commendable view, but when I have to choose between the refrigerator, trashcan, or my body to be the storage facility for excess food, I need to choose the refrigerator or the trashcan. When Jesus miraculously fed 5,000 hungry men, he told His disciples, "Gather up the fragments that remain, that nothing be lost." They gathered enough leftovers to fill twelve baskets. This is what "remained over and above unto them that had eaten" (John 6:12-13). Notice that Jesus did *not* say, "Even though you guys are stuffed, make sure you eat every last fragment of every last barley loaf." No, He did not endorse gluttony; He encouraged the conservation of leftovers for a later time. If it is not feasible to store excess food as leftovers, throw it away. Choose the waste can over your waistline.

9. I'm used to feeling full or overfull.

Push away from the table before you actually feel full. If we let a short amount of time pass, the food will reach our stomachs and signal our brains that they have enough food in them. We need to learn to stop eating before we're satiated and our stomachs are in pain.

10. I'm upset about something and eating is an emotional outlet for me.

Food can mask pain and distract us from dealing with painful emotions. We must learn that food will not fix our problems. Emotion-based eating only creates more problems.

11. I overeat at one meal and it escalates into overeating at the next meal.

Again, gluttony can become a habit; habits can be broken. If we can train ourselves to overeat, then we can also train ourselves to eat temperately.

12. People tell me that I'm thin, so I think it won't hurt to eat more than I need.

Other people should not set the gauge for us. Sometimes people might tell us that we are okay being overweight because they are overweight too and they don't want to change. Or maybe in comparison to them I'm thin, but I know that I have unnecessary pounds hanging around that are stealing my energy.

13. Food just tastes good and I like to eat it!

The lure of this universal human passion no doubt besets us all. We just like the taste of food and enjoy the eating process. We must learn to enjoy eating but tell ourselves that we will get to eat again at a later time, so we don't overindulge, thinking that we will never get another good meal like this one. Sometimes we must reason with ourselves!

14. Sweets are enjoyable to eat.

It is possible to alter the foods our bodies crave. I used to drink soda all the time and now I can hardly tolerate two swallows of the awful stuff. It's far too sweet to me now, since I have been without it for such a long time. I love water instead.

15. Food shopping is a pastime.

When I married, I found out that my husband finds grocery shopping enjoyable and relaxing. At first I went to the store with my detailed list and was frustrated when he wanted to dilly-dally around sampling cheeses or inspecting exotic fruits. When I figured out that he was grocery shopping for recreation, I slowed down. It's okay to enjoy food shopping (after all, it has to be done so we might as well try to enjoy it!), but we must keep in the back of our minds that food is not our god.

16. When I'm getting ready to fast, I overeat to "store up."

This is bad, very bad. I've found that the hardest part of

a fast is not the fast itself but the time before and after the fast. Greater discipline is required.

17. I know that a certain food is good for me, so I think I can overindulge because it is healthy.
Once I sat at someone's table and ate fresh blueberries (albeit with fruit dip) until I was nearly sick. I love beans, especially lentils, and they are a great source of folic acid, but enough is enough. Even if we eat very healthy foods, we can still gain weight if we overindulge.

18. I'm thirsty.
Sometimes we eat when our bodies are crying out for nothing but water.

19. I get bored and have idle time when traveling long distances, so I snack.
When I want a snack, it helps to be prepared with a small cooler containing some fresh veggies, dried or fresh fruit, or raw nuts. If candy bars or cookies are available, that is what I'll eat, so I must plan our snacks.

20. I feel obligated to eat what people give me or prepare for me.
Here I must exercise discretion. Under nearly all circumstances, it is better to not offend than it is to throw away a triple layer chocolate cake. An alternative would be to have a slice of cake and then share the rest with a friend or neighbor. There is a fine balance between offending someone and maintaining a healthy lifestyle.

21. I'm playing a board game with family and friends and snacking seems in order.
The key to surviving recreational evenings is to choose healthy snacks. Make a fruit salad instead of brownies. Buy raw pecans or almonds (delicious!) instead of M&Ms.

22. I'm at a social event and there is an enormous amount and variety of food to eat. I want to eat it all and try everything.
What church social event is not centered around food? The key to surviving church suppers is to eat only one plate and not fill that one plate a foot high. Enjoy but don't over-do it. Skimp on the desserts and drink water, not soda.

23. I'm truly hungry.
Ah, finally! The best reason to eat! My body says, "I'm hungry. I need some fuel. Please feed me some good food and I will treat you right." Some people say that we should not wait until we are extremely hungry to eat and I agree with this. At that point, your body wants to eat mountains of food. But if we eat temperately, we will be more in tune with what our bodies really need and when it needs to eat.

CHANGE – IT'S WORTH IT

Many people resist change even when it is for their own good, for the betterment of their lives and the lives of their family. Many people would rather be habitually sick and feel lousy than make the necessary changes that would make them feel better. They prefer poor health to doing something different from what they have always done. They would rather feel bad than feel good, if feeling good requires them to change.

I read an article about a Floridian police chief who was fired from his position because he was trying to stop the cycle of obesity among the Winter Haven police force, the men that citizens rely on to protect them. "Police Chief Paul Goward was only looking out for the welfare of his officers and the community they served. He was concerned about the health and fitness of the police force of Winter Haven, Florida and how it was affecting their jobs. He sent them a straightforward but tactful memo, encouraging them to lose weight, stop smoking, and limit alcohol consumption. He provided a list of 10 reasons police officers should be in shape. He said overweight police poorly represent the profession. He said out-of-shape cops are a liability to the city and their families. Because of the physical activity involved when pursuing criminals or handling tough situations, policemen should be as fit as possible. Unfortunately, the policemen didn't think so. Instead of seeing their chief's advice as a motivation to better themselves, they took offense and took measures to oust him from his job."[1]

This is an example of the intense way people resist change, even if changing promises to improve their quality of life. Some people, such as these policemen, go to ridiculous extremes to defend and justify their unhealthy and/or obese conditions.

It takes effort, sometimes great effort, to change eating patterns. If we do not analyze why we are putting in our mouths what we are putting in them, we will continue to overload our bodies.

We must truly *want* to change our ways. I once heard someone say that most people give up what they *really* want for what they want right now. Our desire must catapult us into making changes that will affect our futures.

I read about a man who was very overweight. He got to a point in his life where he was truly ready to change. He was tired of being obese. He started asking himself a question when he was getting ready to eat something unhealthy. He would say, "I have a candy bar here. I can eat it if I want to. What do I want *more*? Do I want this candy bar or do I want to lose weight?" He repeatedly chose to pass by the momentary emotional pleasure and quick sugar rush the candy bar provided. Losing weight and regaining his health was more important to him. He eventually lost over 100 pounds and reclaimed his health.

Our health is a result of a lot of little choices that form habits in our lives. These habits can be good or bad; the process is the same. If we are consistent in our positive choices we will form positive habits and be rewarded with positive results. Consistency is the key that unlocks the door to a lifetime of health.

We must come to a place where we desire physical well-being, a healthy weight, and increased energy levels more than we want to resist change. We must want freedom from chronic sickness, allergies, and colds more than we want to maintain our destructive habits and emotional attachment to food. What do *you* want more?

Everyone *desires* to be fit, trim, in shape, and healthy. Nevertheless, desire in itself is not enough. What makes the difference between the achievers and non-achievers is determination, a vision of good health, and consistency. Little by little, they make the necessary changes to do things differently than they've always done them. They set goals, become accountable to someone who can help them, identify the root cause of their overeating, change their direction, and don't look back.

Desire alone for better health is not enough. Knowledge without application is useless knowledge. Knowing that we need to make changes, exercise more, think biblically and positively, is not enough. Desire must catapult us to action. Some people will only succeed with an accountability partner or group. Recognize your weaknesses and deficiencies in reaching your goal. If you know you need help, seek it out. James 2:26 tells us that "faith without works is dead."

American culture and food enthusiasts tell us that we need to enjoy our food. I believe that God wants us to enjoy eating or he would not have made food so delicious. After all, He's the one who gave us our taste buds. We shouldn't feel guilty for enjoying the taste of our food. But problems arise when our pleasure in eating escalates to the point of misusing our bodies, these temples that God lives in. We must learn to eat to live and not live to eat.

TWELVE

EXCUSES, EXCUSES, EXCUSES!

I saw few die of hunger – of eating, a hundred thousand.
Benjamin Franklin

Through the years I have repeatedly heard the same excuses given for not taking responsibility for the condition of our bodies, these temples of God. They are listed here. Each is followed by a logical refutation.

"Everyone has to die of something. I might as well eat what I want and enjoy myself. Eat, drink, and be merry for tomorrow we die."

This concept has been around for millennia. People who live out this notion are usually obese, tired, stressed, and unhealthy. They refuse to confront their gluttony, lack of discipline, and disregard for their bodies.

"This tastes good. It must be bad for me. Nothing that tastes good is good for me."

This is frequently heard while an individual is wolfing down a triple scoop hot fudge sundae or diving into a mega-meal at a fast food restaurant. When most Americans make food choices they don't consider what foods are good for them; rather, their taste buds control their choices.

Aside from being false (What tastes better than a crisp, juicy apple or a bowlful of fresh, ripe raspberries?), this concept reveals that an individual's taste buds have become so inundated by artificial flavors that it is difficult for him to appreciate the natural flavors that God put into the foods He created.

"My physical problem is hereditary. I can't do anything about it."

While our genes predispose us to a certain height and determine our eye and skin color, obesity and the vast majority of diseases are unrelated to heredity. Believing this concept only enables us to justify and continue poor habits. I have noticed that when many people discover they have a disease or terrible sickness, they rarely stop to think of *why* they are sick; it's easier to dismiss it as hereditary. They simply accept the sickness, never honestly analyzing how the sickness came to be. As a result, they do not change their habits and behavior that may have produced the sickness in the first place. Therefore, many times the sickness visits them again.

I do not eliminate altogether the role genetics plays in our health. However, the truth is that most families look alike because they eat alike. They have similar health problems because they practice the same lifestyles. Our parents' health problems are not our destiny. If you have family members that battle cancer or heart disease, don't limply accept that as your lot. Genetics plays a role, but it is usually a small role. Examine your habits and diet and change to a more health-friendly lifestyle and you will greatly reduce your chances of having the same problems they have.

"I don't have *time* to exercise and prepare healthy meals."

We take time for the things that are important to us. If you don't schedule time for your health, it simply means you consider other things to be more important. It is productive to honestly examine our priorities often to see if they are in order, so that we can adjust them as needed.

"I can't *afford* to eat healthy and buy workout equipment."

Actually, eating healthy *saves* money in the long run. You'll save on doctors' bills, prescription drugs, and missed days from work. You don't need a $5,000.00 home gym set to be healthy. Use your two legs to go for a walk, do stretches, or buy a small indoor trampoline.

Most people understand the value of paying a little more for a quality car versus a cheaper, less reliable, poorly crafted vehicle that will require more repairs and not last as long as the more expensive car. In the long run, the extra up-front expense is a much wiser investment. So it is with purchasing healthy food.

Some of the same people, who dismiss eating healthy food because they think it is too expensive, think nothing of spending a substantial amount of money eating out each week. For the amount needed to take a family out to dinner just once a week, a week's worth of organic produce could be purchased.

"My sickness is to the glory of God."

For those who espouse this line of thought, I have a question: *"How* does God get glory out of your sickness?"

In the New Testament, when Jesus healed people, He did not receive glory until the healing occurred. It is when He does what no one else can do that He receives glory.

Besides, if your sickness is to the glory of God, then why do you go to the doctor, take prescription drugs, and receive medical treatment? If you truly believe that God is getting glory out of your illness, then why try to get better using medical means? If God is getting glory from your sickness, then why are you trying to get better?

I know a few people who have become very sick. Instead of getting bitter and depressed, their deepened consecration and faith became a blessing and inspiration to others. God certainly gets glory when we praise Him in the midst of trials.

There may be occasions when God has a bigger plan than we can perceive in allowing a sickness to linger in an individual's life but such cases are exceptions, not the rule. In John 9, Jesus healed a man that had been blind since birth. When Jesus' disciples asked why the man had been born blind, Jesus said that his blindness was so "that the works of God should be made manifest in him." Even in this extreme case, it was a supernatural healing that manifested the glory of God, not years of blindness.

We need to be sure that saying, "My sickness is to the glory of God" is not just an easy crutch to excuse our unbelief in divine healing or our unwillingness to take responsibility for properly caring for our temples.

"I've tried to lose weight and get healthy before and it just didn't work."

Chances are, you've tried fad diet after fad diet without lifestyle changes and have been repeatedly disappointed. Or, you lacked consistency. Or, you lacked an accountability partner and proper understanding.

"Nobody else in my family wants to eat healthy. It's hard to eat carrot sticks while they're eating ice cream and cookies."

Most people are followers by nature and don't like to go against the flow. You will, however, take a stand for your health and physical well-being when it becomes important enough to you.

"I don't *feel* like preparing healthy meals and exercising."

Productivity is not realized by feelings. It would get pretty interesting if all of the police officers in the United States woke up one morning and didn't go to work because they just didn't *feel* like it. The mechanic responsible for safety inspections of the airplane I'm about to board may *feel* like taking an early lunch break without completing his inspection. But I sure hope he doesn't give in to his feelings.

Children allow their feelings to dictate to them. Eventually, we should grow out of this behavior. We must be motivated enough to overcome our feelings with habit changes. We must learn to base our actions and behavior on doing what is right, not on our feelings. I have found that though I may not feel like exercising or putting much effort into healthy food preparation, if I will just do it, I will start feeling better and be motivated by good results to make these things habits.

"It's just too hard to change."

Certainly, change is never easy. But you *will* change when it becomes easier to change than it is to reap the painful, uncomfortable, and expensive consequences of mismanaging your temple. It has been said that everyone will have pain in life – either pain of regret or pain of change and self-discipline.

"I don't see what difference it makes. Even "health nuts" get diabetes, cancer, and die of heart attacks."

While it is very true that health-conscious people do occasionally have severe health problems, statistically, they are at much less risk than others. And although thinness is not a guarantee of perfect health, it certainly eliminates the dangerous side effects of obesity. I'm not going to help the process of degeneration to my health if I can help it. And I can.

Furthermore, while no one is exempt from death and people who are health-conscious will be just as dead as junk food junkies, chances are very good that the health-conscious people will live more active, mobile lives for longer periods of time.

"I'm too old to worry about changing my bad habits."

If you are in the twilight years of your life, that is all the more reason to eat a little healthier and take care of yourself. Younger generations need the wisdom, stability, and example your years of experience have given you. They need you to help make happy memories for them and influence their lives for the good. Preserve your good health as long as you can.

"Eating provides an emotional escape for me."

Jesus wants us to learn to cast all of our cares upon Him. Nothing, food included, should be a god to us in place of the Lord. If you find yourself escaping to food, ask the Lord to help you deal with and overcome your insecurities, fears, and inhibitions. Seek out someone who can use biblical truths to help you become whole, both spiritually and emotionally.

NO MORE EXCUSES

My wise pastor, Jonathan Urshan, says, "An excuse is nothing more than a white-washed lie." While blunt, this statement is very true. If any of these excuses have hit home with you, please take a moment to ask the Lord to help you change your mind-set. The first step to better health is a change of mind-set. Change the way you think about nutrition and exercise, and you will enjoy your journey to vibrant health.

Picture yourself 10, 20, 30 years ahead. If you continue in the direction you are going now, where do you think you will be then? For instance, if you gain just 10 pounds a year, which is easy to do on the Standard American Diet, 10 years from now you will be 100 pounds overweight. Does that sound like fun to you? The byproducts of obesity are alarming, to say the least.

Stop the trend now. You don't have to accept ill health, sickness, and disease as inevitable. You have the power to control your health through the principles of the Word of God.

THIRTEEN

THE MIND-BODY CONNECTION

A merry heart doeth good like a medicine:
but a broken spirit drieth the bones.
Proverbs 17:22

Our minds directly influence our health. The first step down the road to better health and greater energy is to change the way we think.

FEAR OR FAITH?

Do you often worry about your future health? Do you fear getting a certain disease because your mom, aunt, or brother had that same disease? Do you resignedly accept the doctor's prognosis, never giving God an opportunity to heal you because of your lack of faith?

Faith and fear are polar opposites. If you are afraid that you will get cancer or have a heart attack, you live in a state of worry and faithlessness. It is not God's will that our thoughts be filled with fear. This type of thinking produces irrational behavior, stress, and headaches. Again, it is not the will of God that we live one second of our lives being fearful. "For God hath not given us the spirit of fear; but of power, and of love, and of a sound mind" (II Timothy 1:7).

If unbelief accompanies our sicknesses, our minds will be tormented with depression and fear. Sick people must allow the Word to encourage them. They must not exalt the problem; they must exalt the Problem Solver. They must speak words of faith, not fear. They must allow Spirit-filled believers to speak words of assurance to them and accept the prayer of faith that is prayed. It is difficult for Jesus to work amidst negativity, doubt, and self-centeredness.

Job said, "For the thing which I greatly feared is come upon me, and that which I was afraid of is come unto me" (Job 3:25). The Hebrew translation of this verse is, "I feared a fear, and it came upon me." Fear is very powerful. We must banish our fears and replace them with thoughts and words of faith in God, His Word, His abilities, and the work that He is doing in our lives – even if we can't see what He is doing at the time.

As was the case with Job, sickness can actually serve to bring us closer to God. It is not the *absence* of problems in life that makes a person successful and joyful. Rather, it is perseverance *through* problems that makes a person successful. Having the proper perspective when dealing with physical challenges determines whether or not we learn valuable lessons from our trials.

THE SIN FACTOR

In Psalm 38:3 David wrote, "There is no soundness in my flesh because of thine anger; neither is there any rest in my bones because of my sin." The word "rest" in this passage refers to peace and health. It is possible for sin and its accompanying feelings of guilt and shame to affect us mentally and physically. People who live with unresolved sin will have an absence of peace in their minds.

David recognized the futility of covering and justifying his sin. He realized that he had to admit his sin to God. He said, "I will declare mine iniquity; I will be sorry for my sin" (Psalm 38:18). I John 1:9 tells born again believers how to take care of sin: "If we confess our sins, he is faithful and just to forgive us our sins, and to cleanse us from all unrighteousness."

We can avoid sin and its mental, spiritual, and physical repercussions by simply obeying the Word of God and consulting the Word when faced with temptation. But when we do sin, if we confess our sin to Him in humility and sincerity, He cleanses us and purifies us.

Oftentimes our sin is related to our poor relationships with others. If we harbor bitterness, hold grudges, and are critical of others, we are involved in sin and we will never be happy until we acknowledge our sin and humble ourselves before God. Only then will we know true peace and be free from the bondage of self-will.

STRESS NOT

Cortisol is a stress hormone. When people are overly stressed, their bodies release greater amounts of cortisol, which can create various health problems and cause weight gain.

There are some circumstances that life brings us that will never make sense. Answers will evade us just as they did Job. Some people go through their entire lives allowing circumstances to dictate their joy or lack thereof. They don't realize that worrying and fretting about circumstances is just a method of control. When we simply trust God to take care of us, whether we see our circumstances change or not, we are relinquishing control to Him.

Our busy-ness is not an indication of our success or importance. Some people can't imagine what life would be like without always being in a hurry and stressed to the max. They are comfortable with it.

Jesus desires that we live stress-free lives. I love what He said in Matthew 11:28-30: "Come unto me, all ye that labour and are heavy laden, and I will give you rest. Take my yoke upon you, and learn of me; for I am meek and lowly in heart: and ye shall find rest unto your souls. For my yoke is easy, and my burden is light." We will have burdens to bear but when we are yoked together with the All Mighty One, how much easier can the journey get?

It is God's design that we live calm, peaceful lives. If you are overwhelmed with stress, relinquish it to the Lord. He can handle it and He doesn't want you to bear it. He cares for you (I Peter 5:7).

THE POWER OF WORDS

From time to time, I hear people make very unusual statements about food such as "This chocolate cake is divine" or "The entrees at that new restaurant are to die for."

I know that these are just phrases of exaggeration. I tend to say things like, "I must have rewritten that sentence ten million times!" In reality I only rewrote it four times but in my excitement and/or exasperation, I exaggerate for emphasis. I want the listener to understand the depth of my thoughts and emotions. Exaggeration is unnecessary and can actually be detrimental to our credibility.

The words that come out of our mouth are very powerful. "I'll always be overweight." "My mom had diabetes so I guess I'll get it too." "My aching back is killing me."

Ecclesiastes 5:2 says, "Be not rash with thy mouth, and let not thine heart be hasty to utter any thing before God: for God is in heaven, and thou upon earth: therefore let thy words be few." It is better to be silent than to speak untrue words. Like David, we should desire that the words we speak and the thoughts we think will be acceptable to God (Psalm 19:14).

THE POWER OF THOUGHTS

Someone said, "You are what you think about all day long." Abraham Lincoln said, "I am about as happy as I make up in my mind to be." Someone else summed up the power of our perspective: "Two men looked through the same prison bars; one saw the mud, the other saw the stars."

Your thoughts, whether negative or positive, will determine victory or defeat, joy or depression, sickness or health. Our lives are in many ways a result of where our thoughts have taken us.

If you think you can't lose weight, then you won't. If you think you will always have a certain disease or problem, then most likely you will. This is called the mind-body connection. Instead of thinking, "I've tried and failed so I don't think I will try again," think, "If at first I don't succeed, I'll try, try again. Eventually, I *will* succeed."

Paul Harvey said, "I have never seen a monument erected to a pessimist." Envision yourself energetic, happier, lighter, and healthier – your thoughts will motivate you to do the things that will make your vision reality. Change your thoughts and you will change your world.

A sense of humor that is never far from the surface of life's circumstances is an indispensable asset. I like what LaJoyce Martin says: "Bad times manufacture themselves. If we're going to have good times, we will have to manufacture them ourselves in our own good times factory." Jesus never promised us exemption from tragedies and rough times but He gave us a wonderful promise to carry us through whatever life may bring our way. "In the world ye shall have tribulation: but be of good cheer; I have overcome the world" (John 16:33). Shift your focus from the shifting sands of life's circumstances and place your life in God's unchanging hand.

Instead of Thinking: It's not fun to eat healthy and exercise.

Think: It's not fun to be sick, constipated, listless, fatigued, and irritable due to excess sugar consumption, obesity, and unnecessary health problems.

Principle: It's more fun to exercise some responsibility and enjoy good health than it is to participate in "sin for a season" and be miserable. Not everything in life is fun, but good health is a great reward for eating wisely. In time, as our taste buds change, we actually will enjoy eating healthy foods. We will love the results of exercising.

Instead of Thinking: I can't help myself. I have food cravings that I can't control.

Think: "A craving is a feeling – not a command. Feelings pass. There'll be no pain, no blood loss. I will not have to

call 911 for the rescue squad. Studies show that cravings pass in minutes. If I don't negotiate or equivocate, isn't thin worth a few minutes?"[1]
Principle: Resisting food cravings is the product of self control. Our bodies don't need everything that we think they need.

Instead of Thinking: How quickly can I prepare this meal?
Think: How healthy can I prepare this meal?
Principle: Speed in meal preparation does not necessarily equal quality.

Instead of Thinking: I can't afford to eat healthy foods.
Think: I can't afford to eat unhealthy foods.
Principle: Bargain-priced food does not always equal quality food.

Instead of Thinking: I'll eat however I want and go to the doctor when I get sick.
Think: I'll eat healthy and take care of my temple, so I don't have to waste my time and money at the hospital, doctor's office, and pharmacy.
Principle: The availability of doctors and medicine does not guarantee good health.

Instead of Thinking: I will always be sick. It is my lot in life.
Think: God wants me to live a life of optimal health. He wants to use my life for His glory, and I need to be as healthy and energetic as possible for His purpose to be fulfilled in my life.
Principle: God is our Healer and He *wants* to heal us. He will also honor our biblically based disease-prevention methods to keep our bodies healthy and free from sickness and disease.

What thought patterns keep you debilitated by unhealthy living? Identify them and change them.

Keep your mind free of the clutter of negativity and fear. Meditate instead on the good things of God, His faithfulness, His power. Solomon instructed, "My son, attend to my words; incline thine ear unto my sayings. Let them not depart from thine eyes; keep them in the midst of thine heart. For they are life unto those that find them, and health to all their flesh" (Proverbs 4:20-22).

Pray – it's the ultimate stress reliever. Choose friends who will lift you up, not pull you down. Keep your mind and vision stayed on Jesus. Focusing on God is the key to abundant spiritual, emotional, and physical life.

FOURTEEN

THE MEDICAL WORLD AND YOUR HEALTH

And Asa in the thirty and ninth year of his reign was diseased in his feet, until his disease was exceeding great: yet in his disease he sought not to the LORD, but to the physicians.
II Chronicles 16:12

The facts are alarming.

Conventional healthcare – meaning prescription drugs, surgeries, and medical treatment – is not a guarantee of good health. Spending a lot of money on care does not mean that we will live long, healthy, disease-free lives. Per capita, the United States spends more money on healthcare than any other country in the world, yet the state of our health does not yield a good return when compared with such elevated expenditures. Some experts believe that the reason for this disparity is that, instead of disease prevention, we espouse a "we can buy our cures" attitude.

"Americans pay more when they get sick than people in other Western nations and receive more confused, error-prone treatment, according to the largest survey to compare U.S. health care with other nations. While patients in every nation sometimes run into obstacles in getting care and deficiencies in treatment, the United States stood out for having the highest error rates, most disorganized care and highest costs, the survey found. Americans also reported the greatest number of medical errors. Thirty-four percent reported getting the wrong medication or dose, incorrect test results, a mistake in their treatment or care, or being notified late about abnormal test results."[1]

PRESCRIPTION DRUGS

While there are without doubt many well-meaning people in the pharmaceutical industry, the driving force behind the health agenda of drug companies is money. "There's a cure for whatever ails you, even if it's not a disease. The *British Medical Journal* reports that a poll of its physician-readers identified almost 200 conditions that aren't real diseases – ranging from baldness to jet lag – but which have commercially available 'cures.' The report suggests that some drug companies are 'disease-mongering' by widening the boundaries of treatable diseases in order to boost their markets. BMJ editor Richard Smith says it's easy to create new diseases out of many ordinary life processes such as aging. 'Global pharmaceutical companies have a clear interest in medicalizing life's problems, and there's now an ill for every pill,' he writes."[2]

How about that? Drug companies are using every means imaginable to make another buck, all at the expense of your bank account and your health. Not only are prescriptions expensive, but there is not a single drug without potential side effects, many of them serious.

Prescription drugs are not all they're cracked up to be. "An estimated 4.5 million Americans have Alzheimer's disease, and the pharmaceutical industry has responded with a variety of prescription drugs. Four commonly used drugs that increase acetylcholine (a neurotransmitter that's low in AD patients) carry significant side effects and may lead to 'sudden worsening' of symptoms. One of these drugs, galantamine (Reminyl), was recently found to increase mortality due to heart attack and stroke in a placebo-controlled study of AD patients in 16 countries. Even the U.S. FDA medical officer who reviewed this drug claims that 'the beneficial effects of Reminyl are small [and] only a small minority of patients [taking it] actually improve.'"[3]

This story line is repeated over and over with different drugs prescribed for different ailments. A Greek named Hippocrates, the "Father of Medicine," is famous for the phrase "Let food be your medicine and medicine be your food." He lived several centuries before Christ and his prescriptions were simple and natural. "In the Egyptian pharmacopoeia are the names of many plants which cannot be identified, but most of the remedies used by them were dietetic, such as honey, milk, meal, oil, vinegar."[4] Food and the natural remedies directly derived from them have been mainstay medicines for thousands of years.

Yet the FDA resists natural remedies, saying that they are dangerous, though few of them have side effects and they really do work. The FDA prefers to approve pharmaceuticals and then remove them from the market when patients experience terrible problems because of them. Personally, I'm not interested in volunteering my temple for their experiments.

Some pharmaceutical drugs are highly addictive. The problem of medical drug addiction is all too common. One of the saddest things I have ever heard is the hopelessness and remorse that is voiced by people who would never do street drugs, yet their addiction to legal medical drugs is with them all day, every day.

Natural healing is viewed with skepticism. But that is nothing new. Dr. Steinke, a dentist, wrote of the historical and current effectiveness of natural treatment versus prescription medicine. "In the 1700's one of the most common methods of eliminating toxins from the body was 'bloodletting' in which they removed blood with a theory that the poisons were in the blood. They also used toxic materials such as mercury in high concentration to drive out infection. Presently, we would think this is crazy.

"Those who vigorously promoted healthy eating and lifestyle and utilizing small doses of natural plants have been ridiculed and chastised. From the 1600's through today, naturopaths, osteopaths and homeopaths have been ridiculed for their natural philosophies which all promoted knowing that your body is being fed properly. Those physicians that were "bloodletting" and giving heavy metal toxins were the same ones that were condemning the natural health practitioners for their views.

"It is wonderful to have drugs when we need them. For so many maladies in our world our medicines have allowed us to have longer, more active lives with more quality in each day. The line we must walk though, is that prescription medicine should ONLY be used after we have this healthy lifestyle.

"The health practitioners who have been promoting nutrition and healthy lifestyles are most correct. 70% of all our modern diseases can be prevented with optimum nutrition and lifestyle, so should we treat cavities with a drill or with limiting refined sugars from snacks? Should we treat gastric reflux with a pill or with eliminating fatty foods and eating healthier overall? Should we treat blood pressure with a pill or with optimal weight, nutrition and exercise? Should we treat diabetes and osteoporosis later in life or should we prevent it early on by limiting carbonated drinks and high sugared diets and prevent obesity in our children?"[5]

Common sense tells us that a few dietary and lifestyle changes are much better remedies than prescription drugs. It is a path that few choose to follow, yet it has prevailed through the centuries, used by commoners, midwives, and laypeople as the most effective method of treatment for a great variety of conditions.

MEDIA MANIA

The latest news is that a "revolutionary new study" shows that XYZ food is very unhealthy. A couple of years later the cutting edge news is that "revolutionary new studies" have found the same XYZ food to be one of the healthiest foods you can eat. Such inconsistent, unreliable, conflicting reports create unwarranted food phobias and cause the public to be misled, skeptical, and disillusioned.

Have you ever heard the children's lullaby:

Rock-a-bye baby, in the tree top
When the wind blows, the cradle will rock
When the bough breaks, the cradle will fall
Down will come baby, cradle and all.

Sung in a soothing, quiet, calming manner, how many mothers have put their children to sleep to the words of this lullaby? Yet, think about the words. In the first place, why is a baby in the top of a tree? Why isn't the baby at home where it can be safe? Why would you sing a song about a baby falling out of a tree?

There are numerous legends about the origin of this lullaby, yet the fact remains that most modern mothers have no need to jeopardize their babies' lives by placing them in trees. Yet, untold numbers of mothers have *repeated* this lullaby, never stopping to analyze the words. If they really listened to what they were singing, they would probably be furious. After all, no loving mother would want her helpless baby to fall out of the top of a tree.

Diets. Pharmaceutical claims. Before and after pictures. Food manufacturers' gimmicks. All of these are brought to our attention through some form of media – usually television, but also the Internet, magazines, and newspapers. Like robots, we repeat what we hear. I've done it; we've probably all done it. We do not analyze what we hear to find out the truth. We are easily swayed by the gloss and professionalism that packages the words we hear. We subconsciously think, "These people know what they are talking about. They must be right so I need to believe them. Surely the media isn't swayed by money, politics, and ulterior motives that cause them to be biased."

Think about it this way. When is the last time you heard about the media coming to an apostolic church to get information for a broadcast after God has healed someone of cancer or helped someone narrowly escape a car accident? When is the last time the media visited an apostolic church to film a worship service where the Spirit of God was "moving" among us and the preaching of the Word went forth with power and anointing? Only rarely do we hear of the media portraying the glorious church in a favorable light. However, the media is always eager to spotlight a minister or church that is in trouble. They seem to have plenty of room to showcase God's people in a negative light. Reporters and cameramen always seem to find time in their busy days to go to the scene of a church problem.

Just as the media has hidden agendas religiously and spiritually speaking, they are not always unbiased regarding health and nutrition reports.

MEDICAL ADVERTISING

Advertising rules the roost of the media. The media frequently reports on new drugs, medical breakthroughs, and the latest medical technologies. Sometimes what is presented as factual medical news may in reality be nothing more than unpaid advertising. You see, pharmaceutical companies spend billions of dollars on advertising annually. Is it possible that money talks to the media networks, helping them decide what information they should present to the public?

Convincing drug ads conclude with the words, "Ask your doctor if XYZ drug is right for you." The goal of advertising is to sell products. Unwary citizens never question the motives of advertisers. They simply buy the product, convinced by the smooth voices and well-placed words of professional actors that it is effective and safe. "TV advertising is about selling you a drug, not about making you a smarter consumer."[6]

BIG BUCKS

"Approximately 130 million Americans – many of them healthy – take prescription drugs regularly. No wonder this country is the world's largest user of pharmaceuticals. Unfortunately, these medications may be the fourth leading cause of death in the U.S. this year.

While a few drugs definitely save lives, 'we are taking way too many drugs for dubious and exaggerated ailments,' claims Marcia Angell MD, former editor of the *New England Journal of Medicine.* The dollar value of drug company sales last year approximately equaled that of sales at all U.S. gas stations combined."[7] Try finding that piece of news in mainstream media. Your search will be unsuccessful, because the prescription world has an enormous amount of influence on the media.

A FEW STATS

Consider these following statistics from *Energy Times*:

80% - Percentage of ear infections that clear up in seven days on their own without antibiotics.

0 – Number of over-the counter cough medicines that recent research has found to be effective for kids or adults.

40% - Percentage of antibiotics prescribed by doctors for virus infections even though viruses are not affected by antibiotics.

65% - Percentage of times doctors write antibiotic prescriptions for kids whose parents want this medicine.[8]

KIDS ON DRUGS

Over five percent of American children are routinely administered Ritalin. "Some 29 million prescriptions for methylphenidate (sold under brand names Concerta and Ritalin, among others) were written in this country last year even though this stimulant family has long carried warnings for psychiatric side effects, including agitation, psychosis, and transient depression. A routine FDA review of children taking Concerta, a long acting form of methylphenidate, found more reports of hallucinations, suicidal thoughts, and violent behavior than anticipated, and a similar review of other methylphenidate products has turned up similar findings. Even more frightening, a small study at the University of

Texas Medical Branch and the M.D. Anderson Cancer Center discovered chromosome damage in 12 children who had taken Ritalin for three months. With Concerta linked to severe liver damage in a few patients, larger clinical studies of these controversial drugs are clearly warranted. No drug company in its literature mentions the fact that 40 years of research [finds] no long-term benefit of [ADHD] medications."[9]

"There is no test to diagnose ADHD. Instead, doctors use input from places like the child's home, school and social environments to make the diagnosis."[10] Symptoms of ADHD are similar to other disorders such as learning disabilities. If there is no biological test to prove that a child has ADHD, is it not little more than experimentation to give them dangerous drugs and label them with something they may not even have?

Many children exhibit hyperactivity just because they are active and excited kids. Others lack the boundaries of discipline and are seeking safety and approval from adults. Some may subsist on nothing other than sugar and processed food, so the highs and lows of their blood sugar fuel hyperactive and irrational behavior. Still others have such dysfunctional domestic lives that they react in the only ways they know how, not being equipped to deal constructively with the turmoil in their homes. You're not going to fix that with medication.

A drug, however, sometimes combined with group counseling or life skill training, is the best the medical world can offer. They can prescribe a pill, but that pill can't fix a brokenhearted child or bring peace to his home. That is something only Jesus can do, and a pill will never be a suitable substitute for His ability to mend, soothe, and heal deep, inner wounds.

UNHEALTHY HEALTHCARE

"I am thankful for all of the wonderful medical breakthroughs and excellent emergency medical care available in this country. Most doctors are sincere, hardworking professionals who try to do their jobs well.

However, the American healthcare system is not healthy. It is downright unhealthy at times because it has skewed its entire care system toward dispensing health out of a drug container. Dr. Barbara Starfield of the Johns Hopkins School of Hygiene and Public Health noted that a quarter of a million deaths occurred due to a physician's activity, manner, or therapy – including 12,000 unnecessary surgeries, 7,000 medication errors in hospitals, 20,000 'other errors' in hospitals, 80,000 infections acquired in hospitals, and 106,000 'non-error, negative effects of drugs' (And these are the low estimates.)."[11]

In an article entitled "Lawmakers Take Notice of Hospital Infections" "KMBC's Maria Antonia reported that an estimated 2 million patients get an infection while in health care and about 90,000 die because of the infections."[12]

If you want to get sick, take a vacation to your local hospital.

"MY" DOCTOR

Some people find a warped comfort in taking drugs (prescription and otherwise) and get reassurance from a physician's attention. They refer to the doctor they visit as "my" doctor or "my" surgeon as though he belongs to them. Doctors do not belong to you! They are not infallible. Their word is not law. They do not have all the answers. They are not right all the time. They are not immune from errors and mistakes. Many doctors won't even acknowledge the possibility of the power of prayer or natural healing. Yet we accept their word as though it is the gospel truth. They say, "Your mother has 6-8 months to live" and we accept their decree without question. What's wrong with this picture?

The next time you hear someone say, "My doctor has given me six to eight months to live," ask him which doctor made that proclamation. Was it Doctor Jones or Doctor Jesus? Doctor Jones may have accurate information about the medical case, but Doctor Jesus is the one that gives life and takes it away (I Samuel 2:6).

The human doctor's word is not divine. Though his prognosis may be accurate, it is not necessarily the end of the line for you if you have Jesus to turn to. He's the one that made you and knows you inside and out. He will never misdiagnose you or give you the wrong prescription. He can perform a surgery and not even leave a scar. Respect medical doctors but respect Jesus more. Your ultimate trust should be in Him!

While driving through a large city, I noticed a billboard advertising a health insurance company. The ad said, "The wealthy and wise part is up to you. Leave the rest to us." Their sales line was borrowed from Benjamin Franklin, who coined the adage, "Early to bed, early to rise makes a man healthy, wealthy, and wise." I thought it a bit audacious that the company would take such conclusive responsibility for an individual's health. It is slightly demeaning for someone to imply, "Just send us a check every month and we'll make sure all of your health needs are covered," as though it would be silly of us to think of living without buying their health insurance. Health insurance ads capitalize on people's fear of becoming terribly sick. Medical care is so expensive that it seems reasonable to insure yourself in the event of an emergency, medical crisis, or long-term illness.

People sometimes ask my husband and me, "Do you have health insurance?" My husband used to answer "no" until he realized that we do have health insurance, but it's not a typical plan. For nine years we have not paid a single dime to a health insurance company, yet not one time have we needed to visit a doctor for anything other than a routine physical check-up. We have not needed the services of an ambulance, emergency room, or life-flight helicopter. The Lord has kept us well. He has provided for us so that we can feed our bodies healthy food and has healed us several times. He is the best and greatest Physician, on call 24-7.

If we should ever need medical care, I am convinced that the Lord will provide a way for our bills to be paid. After all, He is the same yesterday, today, and forever. If He was Jehovah-Jireh (My Provider) yesterday then He will be Jehovah-Jireh today and tomorrow (Hebrews 13:8; Genesis 22:14). Some people might think this mentality reflects irresponsibility, but that is not the case. My husband and I pay tithe, give offerings, sometimes sacrificially, to the work of the Lord. We have put Him first and He promises to see that all of our needs are met. It's really that simple.

While I acknowledge that this may not be the choice everyone can make due to previous health problems, needs of children, etc., I can experientially say that it is a joy to be able to completely rely on the Lord as we do. He has never let us down, and I am 100% convinced He never will.

NOT GOOD-FOR-NOTHING

Am I implying that the entire medical arena is useless? No. I am not lambasting the knowledge and education of doctors, nurses, therapists, and medical emergency personnel. We should not be anti-doctors altogether. The medical world provides a tremendous service in times of emergencies, health crises, and necessary surgical procedures. I must sincerely say that I appreciate the expertise, dedication, professionalism, and desire to help that most in the medical profession demonstrate.

When I was 18 years old and 1500 miles away from home, I contracted blood poisoning. Several days passed before I realized the severity of my problem. In the middle of the night, unable to sleep because of the worst pain of my life, a blue streak started running up the back of my leg. I literally crawled, slowly and painfully, to the bedroom of the lady I was staying with. She took me to the emergency room and within a short time the blue streak was receding and the medical personnel had me on my way.

A few years ago my mother went to the emergency room thinking that she had a severe case of the stomach flu. Instead of the flu, she was informed that she had colon cancer. She received emergency surgery and thanks to quick thinking and acting doctors and the direction of the Lord, I still have my mother with me today.

We should not criticize people that utilize doctors' expertise. My goal is not to turn people against doctors and conventional medicine altogether, though they are fallible and their procedures are not foolproof. We should not expect the medical world to do for us what we can do for ourselves: Keep ourselves out of their offices.

My goal is to help us realize that our ultimate faith and trust should rest in Jesus to heal us when needed and to redirect our minds to disease prevention through God-given nutrition.

King Asa's error was not so much that he sought to the physicians but that He did not seek the Lord. That he sought help from the doctors of his day and rejected the Lord was a revelation of who he trusted in the most.

The type of relationship we build with God in good times will be manifested by our reaction to emergencies and crises. If the first thing we do is turn to the world to make use of their expertise and we never turn to God, we trust Him very little, regardless of what we may say.

If you choose to seek medical attention, don't make the mistake that Asa made. Keep all of your trust in God and His ability. Magnify His power and ability in your mind. Talk about Him and give Him glory for His healing power.

Many people have encountered terrible health crises and, because they immediately sought God's help, were the recipients of divine miracles and heavenly intervention. Years ago, when medical technology was limited and inaccessible, people sought God because they knew that He was their only hope. Today, with the accessibility of hospitals and drugs, it has become easy to turn to the doctors we can see with our human eyes. Yet, Jesus is the Perfect Physician. Though you can't see

Him, He is always on call and willing to help His children whom He loves so much.

PEACE IN A PILL

Some people are thrilled when a doctor prescribes a pill for a mental condition, such as bi-polar disorder, depression – the list is endless. The doctor, by issuing a prescription drug for a labeled mental disorder, is saying that the problem is biological and physical in nature. This removes responsibility from an individual to investigate the real cause of their mental problems, which usually result from extremely dysfunctional lives, abuse during formative years, irresponsibility, poor diet, and unresolved emotional issues. In cases such as these, the best doctors can do is prescribe pills or administer shock treatment, which often worsens the situation. For the most part, they simply cannot provide solutions to children and adults with confused minds, broken hearts, and feelings of rejection, abandonment, and shame.

Spiritual sickness cannot be cured by medical means. A clogged up line between God and us because of bitterness, grudges, and anger must be cleared before we can be cured. Drugs cannot remedy diseases of the mind.

There is, however, One who can "bind up the brokenhearted" and heal the inner wounds to our fragile and damaged spirits (Isaiah 61:1). He will address the root cause, not merely patch up the symptoms. But we must be willing to let Him begin His healing process. We must identify the source of our fears and problems and begin addressing them, no matter how painful the process may be. Medication will only divert our attention away from the real issues. You can't package peace in a pill.

THE FAITH FACTOR

We should not take the approach "I'll eat and live however I want and when I get sick, I'll ask God to heal me." God is very merciful, kind, and longsuffering, and

He responds to faith. Thus, many times He does heal us even when, because of our ignorance, inability, or unwillingness to change our ways, we create our own problems. He is a gracious, compassionate, and patient Father who loves His children more than we can comprehend.

But that is not the preferred method. Instead, we should responsibly take care of our temples to the best of our ability. Despite our best efforts, however, we do live in an imperfect world. Sometimes things happen that we have little or no control over – things like diseases (malaria, for example) contracted because of overseas travel, car accidents, and environmental toxin exposure. If life should bring sickness or disease our way, we have many wonderful promises from the Lord regarding His willingness to heal His children.

Some people believe that God no longer heals, that He only healed people in Bible days. They've come too late to try to convince me of that, though. Since I was just a child to the present time I have seen God heal people of "little things" like headaches and "big things" like heart disease. I have been divinely healed. God is still just as interested in His people and their health as He was thousands of years ago.

The Lord is not a respecter of persons (Acts 10:34). Matthew 8:16 says that everyone that was brought to Jesus was healed. Jesus bore our sicknesses so that we don't have to carry them (Matthew 8:17). Unbelief was the only factor that prevented Jesus from being able to heal people (Matthew 13:58).

Neither is one sickness more of a challenge to God than others. Psalm 103:3 tells us that the Lord heals all diseases. We categorize sicknesses and diseases as "big" and "little" but to God, healing cancer is just as easy as healing a headache.

In the Old Testament, little reference is made to doctors. The Israelites relied on God to heal them when needed and the dietary laws He gave them kept them healthy. In Exodus 15:26 God said, "If thou wilt diligently hearken to the voice of the LORD thy God, and wilt do that which is right in his sight, and wilt give ear to his commandments, and keep all his statutes, I will put none of these diseases upon thee, which I have brought upon the Egyptians: for I am the LORD that healeth thee."

God is the Great Physician. He created our bodies and knows them better than any human doctor is capable of ever knowing them. When we are sick, prayer should not be our last resort, our last-ditch effort when the doctors have done all they can. Remember, we reveal who we trust the most by who we turn to first with our problems. Prayer should be the first thought on our minds when we hear a negative diagnosis from a doctor. And our faith should reside in God and the prayer that has been prayed, despite how we feel physically or emotionally and despite what further depressing words the doctor, our family, or friends might dispense to us.

The work of a doctor is called "medical *practice*," where "theoretical knowledge is put to practical use."[13] This practice occasionally leads to malpractice because doctors are just human beings. They get tired and make mistakes just like the rest of us.

Part of the problem is that a lot of people wait until they are desperately sick before they see a doctor. Then they say, "Please fix me" and expect a doctor to repair what they have spent years messing up. Most of the time doctors do a commendable job, yet they simply don't have the resources to fix everything.

Some (wise) doctors, some of whom are not Christians, will nevertheless readily admit that the scope of their capabilities is limited. They realize the power of faith and prayer. They encourage people to trust in God to help them. Born again believers should not do any less.

When God heals, He's not practicing. He does all things perfectly and His healing methods are complete. He will never leave an instrument or a piece of gauze inside you when He's done operating. He won't get tired and make a mistake during surgery. All of His medication is side-effect-free. If you get sick, place all of your faith in Doctor Jesus. If a doctor gives you a firm diagnosis, don't despair. Just use the information to pray specifically. Take the diagnosis to God. He specializes in everything.

Believe the Word of God more than you believe the words of a doctor. "Is there any sick among you? Let him call for the elders of the church; and let them pray over him, anointing him with oil in the name of the Lord: And the prayer of faith shall save the sick, and the Lord shall raise Him up" (James 5:14-15). This Scripture and many more leaves no room for doubt. If you will do your part, God will do His part. Exercise faith and obedience by requesting the elders of the church to pray for you. It says that the prayer of faith *shall* save the sick. The word "shall" leaves no room for question or possibility of failure. Our God is a Healer! I have seen many divine healings throughout my life. If you are sick, believe the Word! When a doctor diagnoses, he does not usually factor in your faith, which rests in the power of God that can alter his diagnosis. YOU have to do that. Use God's long track record of healings to keep your faith strong.

HEALING HERBS AND FOODS

Thomas Edison hoped for a vastly different medical world than the expensive and complex health care labyrinth of our day. He said, "The doctor of the future will give no medicine, but rather will instruct his patients in the care of the human frame, in diet and in the cause and prevention of disease."

We get sick and diseased and never trace it to the root. Proverbs 26:2 tells us that "the curse causeless shall not come." Drugs treat symptoms. If we don't trace sickness to its root (instead of masking the symptoms), we will probably get sick again. The culprit is usually poor nutrition and an unhealthy lifestyle.

"America has the most expensive and technologically advanced health care system in the world. For acute critical care, no medical system in the world can match ours. Yet, oftentimes we fight the symptoms of degenerative diseases with drugs and surgery in a futile losing battle, when the real answer to the patient's health problems might have been something as simple as diet improvement, or gentle herbal healers, or a sympathetic ear. Think of a sink overflowing with a mess of water all over the floor. Our medical system spends an incredible amount of time and money trying to wipe up the mess on the floor when the easiest solution is to turn off the faucet that produces the diseases." [14]

God has provided us with natural medicine. This is a means of divine healing, since it is God who created it. Ezekiel 47:12 tells us that the leaf is medicinal. God made a wide variety of fruits, vegetables, grains, and herbs, and each of them has different enzymes, vitamins, and minerals that benefit us physically when we consume them as He created them (i.e., eat the potato, not the potato chips!). Foods as God created them are actually healing foods. Many herbs and oils have wonderful healing properties that should not be shunned in favor of synthetic man-made drugs.

Luke, the writer of the Gospel of Luke and the Book of Acts, was a physician, though we know that medical practices of his day were far different from ours. He would have relied on poultices and treatments made from botanical, not chemical and man-made sources. In our day, he would be considered an herbalist or naturopathic physician, as he resourced the world of nature around him for healing remedies.

When my husband and I visited Singapore, we stepped inside a "pharmacy." Instead of bottles of pills and little white packages, the room was filled with herbs and mushrooms. A customer was sitting at the counter with his prescription from the doctor in front of him. The pharmacist read the prescription, then took several canisters off of the shelf. He measured the herbs, placed them on a paper, wrapped them up, and handed the package to the customer. The customer then went home to make teas or tinctures out of the prescribed herbs.

Unlike mainstream medicine, natural medicine addresses the problems instead of treating the symptoms. It is a synergistic approach, viewing a sickness in a balanced way through the use of all-natural botanical (plant based), herbal, and homeopathic (mostly plant and mineral derived) remedies.

Isn't this a better way? Wouldn't divine and natural methods of healing be easier on our bodies?

A BETTER WAY

If you knew that 20, 10, or just 5 years from now you would be sitting in a doctor's office hearing the chilling words "You have cancer," and you knew that if you made certain changes you could keep that conversation from occurring, would you be willing to make those changes? If you knew that you could greatly reduce your chances of becoming a diabetic, would you be interested in knowing how to do that? If you knew that by discontinuing use of a tanning bed you would greatly lower your risk of cancer, would you do it? If several of your family members died young of heart disease, and symptoms were warning you that if you did not make some dietary and lifestyle changes you would follow in their footsteps, which path would you choose?

The fact of the matter is that you do have the ability to choose good or bad health. It is not all genetics. It is, for the most part, totally in your control to be healthy or unhealthy. You don't have to simply resign yourself to chronic sickness, disease, seasonal allergies, and obesity unless you just don't want to exchange your bad habits such as smoking, poor eating habits, and a sedentary lifestyle for lasting cures. It's your choice. You have to decide what you want. Do you want to be sick or well?

It's easy to be sick. Just continue embracing the Standard American Diet, refuse to exercise, shun taking personal responsibility for your health, and expect a doctor to "fix" you when you get sick. Don't take seriously the statement "An ounce of prevention is worth a pound of cure." Living with disease and sickness is easy. It's like going downstream; it takes little effort and work, and it's all a joy ride until you crash over the waterfall of disease. Be assured: Bad habits *will* catch up with you.

On the other hand, in American society, health and wellness require consistent, conscientious effort. You have to make changes that may be uncomfortable, because you have been doing things a certain way for so long.

You will have to take responsibility for your health and quit expecting a doctor or a pill to repair the damage you have done. You'll have to quit making excuses for why you can't eat healthy and exercise. You'll have to take an honest look at the way you eat and evaluate if it is benefiting or harming your body. You'll have to address the nebulous self-deception in your mind that has you believing that it really doesn't matter what you put in your body. You'll have to quit procrastinating, putting off until tomorrow eating right and exercising. You'll have to change the way you think – about yourself, about food, about life, about being the temple of God, if you are filled with the Holy Ghost. You'll have to force yourself to do what you know you need to do instead of doing what you want to do.

To avoid and escape the onslaught of sickness and disease that seems to be so normal and acceptable in mainstream America, you must make active, deliberate changes.

FIFTEEN

WHAT ARE WE EATING?

To eat is a necessity, but to eat intelligently is an art.
Francois de La Rochefoucauld

An apple a day keeps the doctor away, right? Well, maybe. It all depends on the apple. If the apple was grown in nutrient depleted soil, sprayed with chemicals during its growth, and irradiated while being transported, chances are good that eating too many of them might send you *to* the doctor instead of keeping him away.

No one in their right mind would walk into the laboratory of a chemist and guzzle down a vial of artificial flavoring or demand a bowlful of MSG. Anyone who did would be escorted to the nearest mental hospital. People aren't supposed to eat chemicals. Yet we eat them all the time and think nothing about it. We pay good money for them too. They're so nicely packaged and taste so good.

PURE AND SIMPLE

God puts a high premium on purity. He required that the tabernacle and temple and everything in them be pure. One of the Hebrew words used to describe the gold, furnishings, and spices used in the house of the Lord is *cagar*. This means "to surrender, to enclose." Many of the objects and furnishings were overlaid (enclosed, covered, encased) with gold, which provided protection from decay and deterioration. The gold was not to be mixed with silver. Its purity was not to be compromised in any way.

Spiritually speaking, when we participate in things that are unholy, we expose ourselves to harm. Purity is a state of containment unto God and separation from sin. When we pursue purity, we separate ourselves from behaviors, attitudes, and thoughts that are unclean and impure.

This brings us into closer communion with God, who is pure and holy, and will not ally Himself with that which is defiled. His holiness will not change. He will not compromise His purity to gratify us. His Word is pure and He expects us to align ourselves with it, rather than Him altering His Word to suit us. That is because He knows what is good for us. He knows that purity of mind and spirit provides us with safety, security, and peace. He wants us to be clothed with His righteousness and covered with His holiness so that we will be protected and safe.

TAINTED AND COMPLICATED

When God created mankind, He created him with the need to eat to survive. He specially prepared food that would nourish and sustain man. As Creator, He understood man's body and what he needed to thrive and be healthy. His plan was simple: provide pure, wholesome food for man to eat.

Today's grocery stores are not exactly the Garden of Eden. Food additives are in almost everything from hot dogs to canned goods to cereal. To make more money, fillers are added to make a product go farther. This strips food products of their optimal nutrition.

"A food additive is any substance that a food manufacturer intentionally puts into a food product in order to achieve a specific desired effect during production or processing. While many additives are helpful and have no known side effects, others can be harmful."[1]

There are currently about 3,000 additives in use in the United States, some of which have been outlawed in other countries. Entire volumes have been written on the single subject of food additives, their origin and uses, and their level of safety. Food additives are found in just about all processed foods from bottled spices and packaged seasonings to potato chips and cookies to canned soups, broths, and sauces. The foods that contain the most additives are microwaveable, packaged, and frozen foods.

No longer is food pure and its preparation simple. As the family farm gave way to big industry, food became tainted and contaminated. The processing and manufacture of food is complicated and beset by the seeming necessity of food additives such as preservatives, artificial colors, artificial flavors, and processing aids. Irradiation is used on some foods, adding insult to injury.

PRESERVATIVES

The need to preserve food is nothing new. The history of preservatives stretches back through generations and transcends cultures. But the preservation methods of yesteryear are vastly different from those of modern society. For example, unrefined salt, an organic element of the earth and sea, used to be one of the preferred methods of preserving food. Today some preservatives, such as natural and unaltered tocopherols (vitamin E) and ascorbic acid (vitamin C), are derived from plant sources and do not pose risks to human health; actually, some of these preservatives may benefit and complement the nutrient level of the food to which they are added.

Unfortunately however, many of the preservatives used today are chemical in nature and are harmful to human health. Mass production relies heavily on these artificial preservatives. They prevent spoilage, preserve the flavor and color of foods, and keep oils from going rancid. Sulfites, BHA, BHT, sodium nitrites, and sodium nitrates are preservatives that should be avoided.

Sulfites are widely used to prevent discoloration. Because they destroy the vitamin B1 (thiamine) in foods the FDA prohibits their use in foods that are naturally high in vitamin B1. Sulfur dioxide, sodium sulfite, sodium and potassium bisulfite, and sodium and potassium metabisulfite are all sulfiting agents.

Some people are more sensitive to sulfites than others. For these people, sulfites can be dangerous. Among other things, sulfites have been known to trigger asthmatic attacks in susceptible people. Even more alarming is that, "there have been seventeen deaths that the FDA has determined were 'probably or possibly' associated with sulfites."[2] Conventional fruit juice concentrates and conventional dried fruit are the hardest hit by sulfur dioxide and should be especially avoided.

BHA (butylated hydroxyanisole) and BHT (butylated hydroxytoluene) are chemical cousins. They are suspected of being toxic to the kidneys. England does not permit BHT to be used as a food additive and California recently listed BHA and BHT as carcinogens.

Propyl gallate is a preservative that is best avoided due to its questionable safety. It is often found in products that contain BHA and BHT, as it works synergistically with them.

Any food that contains sodium nitrate or sodium nitrite should be avoided. In conventional processing, nitrates and nitrites are used in meat products such as bacon, bologna, ham, dried sausage, smoked fish such as salmon and tuna, deviled ham, meat spread, potted meat, Vienna sausages, and delicatessen lunch meat.

Also, certain vegetables like beets, celery, collards, eggplant, lettuce, spinach, and turnip greens contain dangerous amounts of nitrates due to their inability to resist absorption of nitrate fertilizers. (This is one more great reason to invest in organic and biodynamically grown produce.) Unfortunately, drinking water can also contain unhealthy levels of nitrates due to runoff from farms where these chemicals are used.

In the human body, nitrates and nitrites become nitrosamines, which are cancer causing agents. The USDA now requires manufacturers to add sodium ascorbate (a form of ascorbic acid, or vitamin C) or sodium erythorbate (similar to vitamin C minus vitamin C's nutritional value) when using nitrites to help counteract the formation of nitrosamines.

When eating nitrate-laced foods, eat a piece of fruit high in vitamin C for added protection. Good choices are fresh, organic berries and citrus fruits.

ARTIFICIAL COLORS

Coloring agents lend eye appeal to a product. Americans have grown accustomed to certain processed foods being certain colors, never pausing to wonder what turned that product neon green or bright pink. Children especially are lured by the dazzling colors found in such foods as bubble gum, frozen treats, candy, breakfast cereals, and sugary juice.

Food dyes are sometimes identified as FD and C (food, drug, and cosmetic) colors. Many food colorings are derived from coal tar. Many of them cause allergic reactions, from mild to severe, in some people.

Some of the most commonly used artificial colors are Yellow 5, Yellow 6, Blue 1, Blue 2, Red 3, Red 40, and Citrus Red 1. Yellow 5 and 6 can cause anaphylactoid reactions (abdominal pain, rashes, faintness, swelling in throat), angioedema (swelling of the skin), and contact dermatitis. Yellow 5 can cross react with aspirin, acetaminophen, and sodium benzoate. Blue 1 and Blue 2 are triphenylmethane dyes that can cause bronchoconstriction. Red 3 is a neurotoxin that is found in a wide variety of common products from toothpaste to barbequed potato chips to hot dogs. Scientists have determined it to be carcinogenic and may contribute to breast cancer in particular. Red 40 is one of the most popular dyes of processed food manufacturers. Even some fruits are the victims of coloring agents to appeal to the consumer as seen by the use of Citrus Red 2, which is used to brighten the skin of some Florida oranges. Fortunately, the dye does not seep through the skin into the pulp, as studies indicate that Citrus Red 2 is carcinogenic. Just don't use conventional orange peel in your cooking and baking endeavors!

Of special note is cochineal extract. (Labels sometimes list carmine or carminic acid as colorings, both of which are derived from cochineal extract.) Cochineal extract is sourced from the cochineal beetle. These beetles are harvested in Peru, Mexico, Central America, and the Canary Islands. The pink, red, and purple colors that come from these dead insects are used in candy, yogurt, ice cream, beverages, some meats, some spices, and many other foods. Cochineal extract has been known to cause allergic reactions that range from hives to anaphylactic shock, a life-threatening condition. Even if this coloring agent was perfectly safe to the human body, which it is not, who wants to eat dead insects?

Breakfast cereals, jelly, ice cream, baked goods, spaghetti, cheddar cheese – you name it and almost any processed food for sale at the supermarket has artificial coloring added to it.

ARTIFICIAL FLAVORS

Instead of accompanying delicious foods harvested from gardens or orchards, which are carefully prepared in gourmet kitchens, the smells and flavors of most processed foods are created in laboratories. "The flavor industry is highly secretive. Its leading companies will not disclose the formulas of their flavor compounds or the names of their clients. These secrets help protect the reputations of beloved brands. The fast-food chains would like people to think that the taste of their food comes from the cooking in their restaurant kitchens, not from distant factories run by other firms. The heart of the flavor industry lies between Exit 4 and Exit 19 of the New Jersey Turnpike, a part of the state dotted with oil refineries and chemical plants. More than fifty companies manufacture flavors along that stretch of the New Jersey Turnpike."[3]

About two-thirds of all additives are flavoring agents. That equates to 2,000 artificial flavors available for use to food manufacturers. 500 of these are considered natural; the rest are artificial. Natural flavors are from natural sources, like the oil extracted from oranges and lemons. They may or may not still be altogether pure by the time the processors are finished with them, but they are generally much safer than artificial flavors. Artificial flavors are chemicals that simulate the real flavors of real foods. These laboratory created flavors replace the true flavors of foods that are lost during processing. Some artificial flavors have their origin in nature, but production convolutes and destroys any benefit that may have originally been present.

Obviously, flavorings are too numerous to discuss in much detail. Amyl acetate, benzaldehyde, ethyl acetate, ethyl butyrate, and methyl salicylate are a few to avoid. Many artificial flavorings act as central nervous system depressants. Benzaldehyde is one flavoring that is positively known to be highly toxic. It affects the central nervous system and can cause convulsions. Watch out for benzaldehyde in imitation vanilla flavoring.

Flavor enhancers are used to enhance the taste of foods, improve texture, and prolong shelf life. They enable manufacturers to reduce the amount of real food used, compensating for real food flavors with enhancers. Canned chicken soup is a prime example. Examine the ingredients list on a can of chicken soup and then think about just how much chicken is in the can. There's very little chicken and a long list of other stuff.

MSG (monosodium glutamate) is by far the most well-known flavor enhancer. It has no flavor of its own but brings out the flavor of the food to which it is added. MSG originated in Japan in the early 1900s. It is 78% processed free glutamic acid and 22% sodium (salt). Processed free glutamic acid, unlike the glutamic acid that occurs naturally in foods such as homemade meat broth, fermented soy sauce, and miso, causes adverse reactions in sensitive prone people. These people may experience headaches, dizziness, nausea, weakness, numbness, or a burning sensation in their necks and forearms when eating foods that contain MSG. Some people complain of wheezing, heart rate changes, and difficulty breathing. MSG can aggravate asthma. Even more alarming is the possibility that MSG may be a contributor to very serious diseases: "MSG has now been implicated in a number of the neurodegenerative diseases, including ALS (Lou Gehrig's disease), Parkinson's disease, Alzheimer's disease, multiple sclerosis, and Huntington's disease."[4] Some people are aware of the overuse of MSG in many Chinese restaurants and ask to have meals prepared without the addition of this special ingredient. Food manufacturers rely heavily on MSG. Be sure to read labels.

Hydrolyzed vegetable protein (HVP) consists of vegetable (usually soybean) protein that has been chemically broken down. It is used to bring out the natural flavors of foods. It contains MSG and should be avoided.

PROCESSING AIDS

Manufacturers take advantage of a wide variety of processing aids in order to generate products. These processing aids are classified as emulsifiers, stabilizers, texturizers, binders, and thickeners, and they do what their names imply. By giving and/or maintaining desired texture, body, form, color, and flavor, they ensure consistency in processed foods. Quite a few of these agents serve more than one purpose. For example, carrageenan is both a stabilizer and an emulsifier. In addition to these processing aids, sanitizing and clarifying agents are used to clean dirt and bacteria from products.

Here are a few miscellaneous tidbits of information about some commonly used processing aids:

- Alginates (ammonium, calcium, potassium, sodium) are substances derived from seaweed. They stabilize, de-foam, emulsify, clarify, and give texture to many products such as ice cream, baked goods, chocolate milk, and cheese spreads.
- Amylopectin is corn derived starch that serves as a texturizer.
- Calcium chloride, a common thickener and texturizer, is what keeps canned tomatoes from falling apart.

- Casein (sodium caseinate) is a milk protein that both texturizes and whitens.
- Gelatin is protein derived from animal bones, skin, tendons, and ligaments. It is frequently used as a thickener and stabilizer. The capsules of vitamins are made of gelatin. If you prefer to not consume animal gelatin, look for products that say they are made with "vegetable cellulose capsules" or "vegetarian gelatin capsules."
- Gums serve as emulsifiers, stabilizers, and thickeners. Some of them are the resin from plants; others are derived from seaweed or from moss harvested from various areas of the world. Carrageenan, sometimes called Irish moss, is a commonly used gum. Furcellaran (sodium, calcium, potassium, ammonium) is made from northern European seaweed. Agar-agar is seaweed that is harvested from the Sea of Japan and the Pacific and Indian Oceans. Some of these gums have histories that stretch back hundreds, even thousands of years. A couple of them, such as gum tragacanth and gum arabic, have their origins in Bible lands. (Gum arabic, or acacia gum, is made from acacia trees. The "shittim wood" used in the Bible was from these trees.) Other gums are gum karaya, gum benzoin, gum guaiac, ghatti gum, and guar gum. Also, cellulose gums (CMC) are synthetic gums made from cotton byproducts; they are often used in processed foods.
- Modified starch is a thickening agent that helps processed foods "gel." It is mostly derived from wheat, potatoes, rice, corn, and beans.
- Pectin is derived from the fruits, roots, and stems of plants. It serves as a stabilizer, thickener, and texturizer and is used in foods that lack natural pectin.
- Sorbitan monostearate is an emulsifier that, among other things, keeps white spots from forming on chocolate products. Other common emul-

sifiers are lecithin, polysorbate 60, diglycerides, monoglycerides, and propylene glycol alginate. Emulsifiers maintain consistency in volume and serve as anti-caking agents. They keep ingredients in foods, such as oil and water, from separating. They ensure the uniformity and fineness of grain. Sometimes called surfactants or surface-active agents, they are used in many products, a few of which are cake mixes, mayonnaise, salad dressing, and candy.

* Sorbitol is a multi-purpose processing aid derived from berries, seaweed, and algae. It is a thickener, sequestrant, stabilizer, sweetener, humectant, and texturizer. It is favored in foods marketed for diabetics because it is absorbed slowly into the bloodstream. However, it should be used with caution by sensitive individuals as it has been known to cause diarrhea and gastrointestinal problems.

MORE PROCESSING AIDS
Acids and Alkalis

Acids, alkalis, buffers, and neutralizing agents are added to food to control acidity and alkalinity levels. A proper acid-alkaline balance is essential for good health. A balanced and healthy whole foods diet will yield proper intake of electrolytes, which carry minerals and amino acids to all areas of the body and help regulate the pH (measure of acidity and alkalinity) of the body.

The nature of processed foods demands the addition of balancing agents. Utilized for this purpose are ammonium bicarbonate, calcium carbonate, potassium acid tartrate, tartaric acid, sodium aluminum phosphate, sodium bicarbonate, sodium hydroxide, and the enzyme hydrochloric acid.

Bleaching and Maturing Agents

Bleaching and maturing agents whiten food or

make it colorless so that artificial color will be better absorbed. They also help products mature at a faster rate than normal. Their usage runs the gamut from refined vegetable oils to maraschino cherries, but they are especially useful to the commercial dairy and flour industries.

Hydrogen peroxide is applied to eggs, butter, and cheese, particularly cheddar and Swiss cheeses. Benzoyl peroxide bleaches blue cheese, Gorgonzola cheese, and milk.

Benzoyl peroxide, calcium peroxide, chlorine dioxide, and nitrosyl chloride are all used to bleach flour and cause it to age faster than it normally would. These dough conditioners are a boon for commercial bakeries, because they make dough rise faster and improve the texture of the finished product.

Oxidizers are substances which cause oxygen to form. The flour industry relies heavily on oxidizers because they improve bread quality. These oxidizers contain potassium bromate, potassium iodate, and calcium peroxide. Potassium bromate is banned in every country except the United States, Great Britain, and Japan. The oxidizers also contain inorganic salts such as ammonium sulfate, calcium sulfate (Plaster of Paris) and ammonium phosphates.

Chelating Agents
Chelating agents, sometimes called sequestering agents, remove or disable trace minerals to prevent rancidity and discoloration and to maintain flavor, texture, and appearance. They are used in a variety of foods such as canned pears, salad dressing, shellfish, corn, and carbonated beverages.

Enzymes
Enzymes are used to tenderize meat, alter starches, remove oxygen to slow or prevent oxidation, clarify fruit juices, clean shellfish, degrease bones, and remove bleaching agents (as hydrogen peroxide from cheese). They are used in the production of cheese and

bakery products. Enzymes are vital to human health and, in the production of manufactured foods, need to be added to aid digestion.

Humectants

Humectants absorb and retain water, preventing food from drying out. Humectants are used in the production of a diversity of foods such as ham, poultry, marshmallows, candy, chocolate products, shredded coconut, baked goods, and beverages. Glycerin, mannitol, propylene glycol, and sorbitol are frequently used humectants. Polyphosphate solutions, ingredients of humectants, are added to meat.

Nutritional Supplements

Nutritional supplements fortify foods that have been robbed of their vitamins and minerals during processing or supply a semblance of nutrition to fake foods. For example, vitamin D is added to milk, vitamin A is added to margarine, and vitamin C is added to orange drinks.

"A common statement made on processed foods is that the product has been enriched by adding vitamins and minerals. Rarely are these vitamins and minerals in a form that can be easily utilized by the human body."[5]

Waxes

Waxes are used to give shine to many fruits and vegetables such as apples, cantaloupes, cucumbers, eggplants, grapefruits, oranges, peaches, persimmons, rutabagas, squash, sweet potatoes, and tomatoes. In addition to cosmetic appeal, waxes also keep produce from drying out during its long production, travel, and shelf life. Waxes made in the United States are derived from plants, insects, and petroleum. Imported fruit may have animal-based wax on them. Carnauba is one of the most common waxes. It is made from the leaves of Brazilian palm trees.

WHOLE FOODS NEED NO "IMPROVEMENT"

Many of these processing aids are naturally sourced. Some of them are actually beneficial to our health. Others are neutral, neither dangerous nor healthful. Still others are questionable at best and highly detrimental at worst. The FDA, however, awards nearly all of them GRAS (Generally Recognized as Safe) status.

Though the FDA claims that these manufacturing marvels are safe for use in the processed food made for human consumption, many of them are chemically altered in order to create desired effects. Some are combined with other agents, which may or may not be natural in origin. Allergic reactions can plague susceptible people. Additives can counteract one another and interfere with pharmaceuticals.

If you are particularly sensitive to certain processing aids and are concerned about possible problems, the best thing to do is avoid processed foods as much as possible. By so doing, you can minimize any possible unpleasant repercussions. Since space does not permit a conclusive discussion of these processing aids, you are encouraged to do further personal research to determine which additives you personally should and should not ingest.

Keep in mind that processing aids are found in some of the least nutritive foods – those which are highly processed, not whole foods. (For example, a fresh grapefruit is not in need of chemically altered flavorings and preservatives to improve its taste and increase shelf life. It is a whole food and needs no improvement.) It is difficult to go wrong by choosing additive-free whole foods that have not been altered by implanted processing aids.

THE CIDES

The suffix "cide" means "to kill." Think homicide and genocide. Also think pesticide. Those we entrust to grow our food for us routinely use pesticides – chemicals used to kill crop pests such as insects, rodents, and weeds. These chemicals are classified as insecticides, herbicides, rodenticides, fungicides, and fumigants. According to the Environmental Protection Agency (EPA) there are over 80,000 manmade chemicals in use in America today.

People who think that these toxic chemicals just disappear into thin air and don't affect our food supply are living with their heads in the clouds. Pesticide residues are routinely found in food. Over the last several decades, several pesticides were banned after they were found to be very dangerous.

Pesticides contaminate our soil and water, including drinking water. Pesticide runoff is a big problem, as rivers and streams are contaminated as well as the fish that live in them. We eat the fish and voilà we too consume the pesticides.

Many of the pesticides that are routinely applied to crops are carcinogenic. They disrupt the cellular function of humans and are particularly threatening to small children.

Some may resign themselves to eating food that is the product of modern industrial practices, considering them to be necessary evils utilized to feed millions of people. Yet, though I am not a farmer, chemist, or agriculturist, common sense seems to indicate that natural methods that have been used for centuries are a better way to go. The problem lies in the fact that small farms which choose to operate simply and pesticide-free are being overrun and bought out by massive companies with power, money, and clout. We can help keep our food supply pure by seeking out and supporting small farmers that are using natural, organic, and/or biodynamic (soil sustaining) methods of food production.

My husband and I met a farmer who refused to use any chemical sprays on his land. He used age-old methods for pest control, such as planting certain pest repelling plants beside the ones he was growing for harvest. To be sure, this method is probably more time consuming and labor intensive, but he was eating the food he grew, as well as selling it, and he wanted it to be pure. If small farmers such as this man, and many others we have met, can produce great harvests that contain nature's bounty of nutrition, then large corporate farms could do the same thing if America's health was their chief aim instead of high profits.

In the days of family run farms, crop rotation and soil fertilization (usually manure, compost, and lime) were normal farming techniques. These procedures allowed the soil to rest and be replenished. Today, corporate farms use synthetic fertilizers, which are a far cry from the old-time methods of soil replenishment, which nurtured the soil and ensured a healthy supply of trace minerals. The result is fewer nutrients in the soil and fewer nutrients in the food grown in that soil.

Also, farmers used to allow produce to ripen on the tree or vine before they picked it. Today, food grown in California is transported to New York. Farmers send their unripened crop thousands of miles and sometimes spray the produce to prevent it from ripening before it reaches its destination. This adversely affects the vitamin and mineral content of the food.

IRRADIATION

Irradiation, used to control insects, bacteria, and parasites, is something few Americans are aware of, yet it affects much of the food we eat. "Irradiation is a process by which food is exposed to beams of electrons from an X-ray machine or to gamma rays from radioactive material such as cobalt 60 or cesium 137."[6] "Foods that the FDA has approved for irradiation include wheat, flour, red meat, poultry, pork, fresh shell eggs, vegetables, and spices as well as refrigerated and frozen uncooked meat, meat by-products, and certain other meat products."[7] (Irradiation cannot be used on some foods such as lettuce, grapes, tomatoes, and cucumbers, because it makes them mushy and inedible.)

Dr. Gabriel Cousens, author of *Conscious Eating*, expounds on the potential dangers of eating irradiated food. "There is no solid evidence to show that eating irradiated food is safe, but there is some evidence to show that it has specific dangers. Food is irradiated with gamma rays. The gamma rays break up the molecular structure of the food and create free radicals. The free radicals react with the food to form new chemical substances called 'radiolytic products.' Some of these include formaldehyde, benzene, formic acid, and quinines, which are known to be harmful to human health. In one experiment, for example, benzene, a known carcinogen, was seven times higher in the irradiated beef than in the non-irradiated beef. Some of these radiolytic products are unique to the irradiation process and have not been adequately identified or tested for toxicity. Irradiating the food destroys somewhere between 20% and 80% of the vitamins including A, B2, B3, B6, B12, folic acid, C, E, and K. Amino acids and essential fatty acids are also destroyed. Enzymes, of course, are destroyed as are the bio-photons."[8]

Dr. Cousens explains why irradiation is not the panacea for producing quality, pathogen-free food. "The once publicly defeated issue of food irradiation has re-emerged after Hudson Foods' recall of 25 million pounds of beef due to E. coli contamination. For reasons that are typical of American corporate thinking, the press came out with some pro-food-irradiation articles. The thinking basically goes like this: Since the food supply is contaminated, food irradiation is a quick and easy way to fix the problem. They have failed to address the deeper issues. How did the food supply become so contaminated? What are the ramifications of building hundreds of nuclear irradiation plants? What are the damaging effects of nuclear irradiation on the food and the people who end up eating it?"[9] "Food irradiation does not solve the problem, it only gives the illusion of helping. It actually makes the situation worse because it makes possible the conditions for lowering the hygiene standards even further."[10] The solution to producing clean, quality food is not found in irradiation. Irradiation cannot prevent the problem; it can only help curtail it once it has begun. The source of the problem is poor sanitation, inadequate inspection, and the fast pace required at beef and poultry slaughterhouses. All of these promote the spread of disease.

Dr. Cousens explains the danger of future high-use irradiation: "To irradiate all the flesh food alone, hundreds of facilities would be needed. The only radioactive isotope available for this level of usage is cesium-137, which is not only deadly today, but remains dangerous for approximately six hundred years."[11] This raises an important safety issue for those who live in the vicinity of irradiation plants, the greatest concentration of which is presently in New Jersey.

Given the potential risks of irradiation on human health and its negative effects on food quality, it is best to avoid consuming irradiated food as much as possible.

NO GMOS
GMO is the acronym for Genetically Modified Organisms. Rivaling irradiation in questionable safety, genetically engineered foods pose a threat to the purity of our food supply. The genetic modification of food is changing the landscape of farming in a big way. Modern technology enables scientists to genetically engineer crops. This is simply gene splicing.

"The purpose of altering the genetic makeup of a food, in theory, is to improve its resistance to disease, decrease its ripening time (so food stays fresher longer), and in some cases, allow it to withstand stronger herbicides."[12] Proponents for genetic modification of foods cite less spoilage during processing, shipping, and storage (which will extend the shelf life of foods) and more productive, less disease prone plants and animals.

This all sounds good to the manufacturer and even appeals to the casually educated consumer, but trans-genetic foods are born in laboratories. Genetic engineering differs drastically from traditional breeding and botanical methods of growing food and raising animals. This is still a relatively new procedure, and it is unclear exactly how the final product is affected. It is possible that a genetically engineered tomato or bushel of corn might actually be toxic and allergenic to human beings.

Cloning animals for human consumption is still not an idea that many Americans are comfortable with, although cloned cows are "alive" right now and advocates are doing all they can to ensure that cloned meat enters our food supply – without special labeling to inform consumers that they are purchasing meat from cloned animals.

The genetic modification of our food and the cloning of animals is a precursor to human cloning. The cloning of animals will desensitize people to the moral implications of human cloning until, in the name of medicine and science, it is acceptable.

As much as possible, choose God-created foods that have not been tampered with by mankind. If you want to avoid the guinea pig syndrome while the food industry experiments with our food supply's genes, buy foods that are organic and labeled "Non-genetically modified organisms (No GMOs)."

READ, READ, READ

Your greatest weapon against unmasking the truth behind brash marketing claims is your ability to read. Read labels. Read ingredients lists. Read nutrition lists. My dad stopped eating the little round compressed "sausages" in a can after he read the ingredients: "Mechanically separated chicken parts." Yum...I wonder what that entails.

Did you know that those raspberry danishes for sale at the supermarket might not have even one raspberry in them? It seems that marketing methods can be as deceptive as is deemed necessary to sell goods. Think Cheez Whiz is cheddar cheese in a can? Think again. There is not a minute trace of real cheese in Cheez Whiz. A product that says "real strawberry flavor" doesn't mean that the strawberries are real; it means that the simulated strawberry flavoring is real. That product probably never saw a strawberry; it just contains chemicals produced in laboratories. Its flavors closely mimic the real thing. My husband and I once bought a bag of chocolate covered blueberries. What the label called blueberries was a chewy lump of unidentifiable who-knows-what.

It's rather scary when a company has to advertise their product by saying "Made with Real Cheese." That means that they are contrasting their product to others that look like cheese, taste like cheese, but aren't actually cheese. "Buttery flavor" is a dead giveaway that there is most likely no butter at all in that product. Everybody knows that butter tastes like butter. If a manufacturer advertises a product as having "buttery flavor" and tells us we should buy and eat it, their advertising is nothing more than an appeal to consumer gullibility and a subtle insult to our intelligence.

Have you ever wondered why a tomato purchased at the supermarket is bland and tasteless compared to those you get from the farmers market or your very own garden? Conventional tomatoes are grown for marketing, not nutrition. They are picked unripe, which is part of the reason they taste so different from fresh-from-the-vine juicy, flavorful tomatoes. Also, garden fresh tomatoes have all kinds of shapes. People have become conditioned to think that a tomato has to be perfectly round and a certain shade of red to be good. The opposite is actually true. Some of the best tomatoes I've ever eaten wouldn't make it to the grocery store shelves because people would think that they were misshapen. Have you ever eaten a purple tomato? How about a yellow tomato? Yum! We have become conditioned to believe that tomatoes should be shiny, too, without realizing that a wax has been applied to them to achieve that look.

Companies have traded the old methods of food production for a quicker yield and a more lucrative profit. What they lose in flavor and nutrition seems to be incidental; they make up the loss in profits.

Manufacturers spend a lot of money on advertising and packaging. Cosmetic appearances and catchy words on a package make the product visually appealing to the consumer. "Imitation," "Artificially Flavored," and "New and Improved" are all signs that tell you that you are about to enter the Fabricated Food Zone.

If you read something that sounds fishy, do some studying and find out what is really in that bag, box, or can. Make it part of your grocery shopping mission to put real foods in your cart, leaving fake foods on the shelves. (If you don't buy those fake foods, don't worry. They won't go bad if they sit on store shelves for the next few years. There is plenty of time for some unsuspecting shopper to buy them.)

Manufacturers market their products to catch the attention of people who want to be healthy but are uninformed consumers. Phrasing can lead a customer to believe that something is healthy when in reality it is detrimental. Don't blindly accept package advertising. Engage your brain and make wise choices. Don't let mega grocery companies whose chief concern is helping you transfer your hard earned money from your pocket to theirs determine the state of your health.

God did not design us to eat chemicals and laboratory produced imitation foods. Many food additives have negative repercussions in our bodies. Our bodies can filter out some of these additives but most of us overdose on them through our indiscriminate and disproportionate use of processed foods, and our health suffers as a result. We can choose to shun fake foods – the foods that are capable of producing headaches, contributing to obesity, aggravating heart problems, and creating other health problems. In their place, we can eat foods in the state closest to which God created them. These are whole foods.

REAL OR FAKE

It doesn't take the brain of a rocket scientist to make a correlation between food additives and foods that have little nutritional value; where you find one, you'll probably find the other. Only an ostrich with his head buried deep in the sand would fail to admit that the combination of artificial color, artificial flavor, artificial preservatives, and refined sugar is a recipe for health derailment.

Why are we surprised when kids can't sit still in school? Perhaps because it's easier to label them ADHD or reprimand them for being hyperactive than it is to take a look at the fake food they are eating that maybe, just *maybe*, is contributing to their behavioral disturbances.

We are not placing the blame for all behavioral disorders on food additives. Many kids with social and behavioral challenges also come from dysfunctional families with poor parental guidance and lives that are not centered on God, who can bring peace and balance to their lives. Food additives are just one spoke in the wheel of juvenile health. But it is one that needs to be addressed if we want our children to be a step closer to reaching their God-appointed destination of vibrant health. It is unrealistic to expect kids to thrive on chemicals. Chemicals don't supply nutrition; a diet that contains a lot of them can result in malnutrition.

It is strange that food manufacturers try so hard to improve the things that God created and put His stamp of approval on. "God saw every thing that he had made, and, behold, it was very good" (Genesis 1:31). God created healing foods, simple foods that are delicious and nourishing. Whenever man tries to improve on God's best, he will always fail.

A STICKY SITUATION

Fake flavors, colors, and textures are so commonly used that those who have been eating processed foods for long periods of time may actually think that the artificial tastes like the real thing. Some additives, such as high fructose corn syrup, sugar, and MSG have addictive tendencies, which keep consumers buying the products that contain them time after time.

Sugar is added to almost everything, being the cheapest food additive that will make food taste good. In the process, it has created sugar addicts and diabetics. A senator recently found out just how vehemently people will defend the foods they love, foods that are truly fake foods but in their minds are real.

"Kids in Massachusetts really like their Marshmallow Fluff, a silky white marshmallow spread and a popular lunch box staple. So, when Senator Jarrett Barrios tried to ban the stuff, he found himself in a sticky situation. Barrios was upset when he learned his third-grade son had been given a Fluffernutter – a peanut butter and Marshmallow Fluff sandwich – at school. He didn't think it was a very healthy option for growing kids and proposed a ban as part of the state's school nutrition bill. Barrios' spokesperson Colin Durrant said the proposal caused such an uproar that the idea was dropped."[13]

Just for fun, let's examine the ingredients lists of peanut butter and Fluff to see if Senator Barrios' proposal was legitimate.

- Peanut Butter: Peanuts, sugar, molasses, partially hydrogenated vegetable oil (soybean), fully hydrogenated vegetable oils (canola and soybean), mono-and diglycerides, salt.

After the peanuts, we get sugar, more sugar in the form of refined molasses, potentially carcinogenic trans fats, emulsifiers, and refined salt. Where did parents get the idea that peanut butter is good for their kids? If they were feeding them natural, fresh ground peanut butter with no additives, they might be doing the right thing. But commercial peanut butter is far from healthy.

- Fluff: Corn syrup, sugar, dried egg whites, vanillin.

Here we have sugar in the form of corn syrup, sugar, egg whites, and vanillin. For your information, vanillin might sound okay, but it is nothing more than artificial flavoring made either from eugenol (liquid compound derived from tropical trees) or the leftovers from wood pulp manufacturing.

If you prefer flavored Fluff, you can choose from strawberry or raspberry. There are pictures of strawberries and raspberries on the labels, so surely it must be healthy, right? In reality, these marshmallow crèmes are much worse than the plain Fluff. They contain absolutely no fruit of any kind; they are entirely artificially flavored and colored, and overloaded with sugar.

- Raspberry Fluff: Corn syrup, sugar, egg albumen, artificial flavor, Red 3, Red 40, Blue 1.
- Strawberry Fluff: Corn syrup, sugar, egg white, artificial flavor, Red 40, caramel color.

I propose that Senator Barrios had legitimate concerns about Fluffernutter sandwiches being fed to school age children. This is just one example of how passionately people defend the foods they love, the very foods that leach health from their bodies.

CHOOSE ORGANIC

When available, choose organic foods. These are foods that are grown the way God intended them to be grown – without toxic chemical sprays and tainted seeds. They are void of dangerous additives. They are uncontaminated. Studies prove time and again that organic foods contain many more vitamins, minerals, and antioxidants than conventionally grown foods. ("Conventional" means that those foods have been unnaturally grown with the use of pesticides, chemicals, and have undergone extensive processing.) Also, choosing seasonal and locally grown organic foods will ensure a fresher and higher quality product than can be purchased at the typical supermarket.

Many grocery stores are beginning to stock natural and organic produce, meat, dairy, and grocery items. If your store does not, let them know that you are interested in organics. If they do not carry a specific healthy product that you want, ask them to order it. Most stores are more than happy to assist you.

Become familiar with your local health food store, provided that it is a spiritually safe environment. (My husband and I have walked into health food stores and walked right back out because we could sense that there was spiritual activity that was directly opposed to the One we represent. Our personal choice is to not support such stores.)

Most health food stores emphasize organics and locally grown food. But read labels even at health food stores. Some are more uncompromising than others. Some of them give in to the desire to diversify in order to gain a broader customer base. By doing so they allow tainted foods on their shelves.

Also, don't make the mistake of thinking that processed ethnic foods are necessarily healthy. It is fun to try new ethnic foods, but they are not necessarily any better than typical American cuisine, especially if they have been "Americanized." Before purchasing products, read and educate yourself about ethnic foods and the most healthful ways to prepare them. The labels may be in a language unknown to you, preventing you from knowing what you are really buying.

KEEPERS AT HOME

According to God's plan, women are chiefly responsible for grocery shopping and meal preparation. This is not a book about marriage, but it is a pretty good guarantee that there will be tension in a marriage if the wife is unwilling to prepare meals for her husband. Why? Because the old adage is still true: "The way to a man's heart is through his stomach."

Aside from that nugget of homespun truth, it is simply part of God's order and plan that women be "keepers at home" (Titus 2:5). The interlinear translation of this term is a "stayer at home," one who is domestically inclined. When the wife refuses to do what God has told her to do, she is confusing the God designed order that makes a home operate smoothly.

This flies in the face of modern philosophy, but God dwells in eternity, not 21st century America. For those of us in the Kingdom of God, the ever-changing ideas that swirl around us should not influence us in the least. We should change our schedules and priorities to accommodate the Word, not excuse ourselves from certain portions of it for our own convenience, to accommodate our own desires, or because of society's norms.

Whenever God's plan is disregarded for convenience's sake or to build a bigger house and bank account, disarray and chaos usually result. Obviously, in some cases it is necessary for a woman to work outside her home but this is not what God prefers.

If you are a woman who absolutely must work outside your home to make ends meet, pray and ask the Lord to help you keep your priorities straight in the midst of all of your responsibilities. He understands the challenges you face.

If you are a woman who works when you don't really have to, re-evaluate your priorities in prayer. Maybe you are a rare woman with unlimited energy that can juggle a lot of things and you never seem to drop the ball. However, it's likely that something prompts you to divert your attention away from home. Be honest with yourself.

What is motivating you to work when there is so much to do for your family? Are your reasons really valid? Could you live with a little less money and a little less "stuff" if you were able to focus your time on meeting the needs of your husband and children? Do you have marital issues that need to be addressed, issues that make you want to be independent of your wifely role? Do you equate money with security and you work to make sure you have plenty of it? Have you bought into the feministic American lie that housewives and stay-at-home moms are unskilled and old-fashioned while career women are successful achievers and world changers?

Didn't someone really famous once say, "The hand that rocks the cradle rules the world"? The influence a mother has on her children and her ability to create the atmosphere of the home should not be underestimated. The biblical Mothers Hall of Fame includes such women as the unnamed mother of Moses, Hannah (Samuel's mother), and Eunice (Timothy's mother). These women placed a high priority on their responsibility to instill proper values into their children.

God created the woman to be a nurturer – to create a pleasant environment where her husband can find solace and her children can be loved and instructed. Part of being a keeper at home is planning and preparing healthy meals for the family. Though a few men enjoy cooking and baking and don't mind if their wives are not great cooks, most men really appreciate home-cooked meals. There is still an old fashioned instinct in most men that causes them to enjoy sitting down at their own table and being pleasantly served a delicious meal that their wives have prepared for them.

A friend of ours cooks for her husband about once a week. The rest of the time they go out to eat or make do with whatever may be handy and quick in the refrigerator and cupboard. This is a sore spot in their marriage. The man has a few health problems. He feels that if his wife really cared about him, then she would put forth more effort to prepare him healthy meals. She does work but only part-time and they do not have children.

Eating out at restaurants and throwing together dinner from a box should be the exception, not the norm. It is up to the lady of the house to carefully monitor what she feeds her family. The responsibility for meals falls first on the mother, not the government, school system, or other family members. The good nutrition children receive during their formative years will benefit them the rest of their lives.

Plan meals that call for fresh ingredients. Shop carefully, reading labels. Don't buy something just because it is cheap. Remember, when you invest in the health of your family you are investing in the temples of the Lord. As a wife and mother, the quality of what they eat depends primarily on your choices. Don't develop chemical kids, addicted to sugar and artificial flavors. Help them build healthy, strong bodies by eating God given foods – real foods. God created milk but not Milk Duds, potatoes but not potato chips, and fruit but not Fruit Loops.

Dr. Daniel Segraves' exposition on the Proverbs 31 woman lets us know that she invested thought and time into meal preparation. "Like the merchants' ships that sail to far ports and return with valuable cargo, so the virtuous wife ventures forth, conducts the business of shopping, and returns home with her purchases. If necessary, she brings her food from afar. That is, she shops wisely, not buying a product simply because it is convenient. She will search until she finds what she actually needs."[14] The virtuous woman was the picture of industriousness. She shunned the toss-it-from-a-box-to-the-microwave meal preparation routine. Healthy meals require planning, a lot more than opening a can of chemical laden soup or popping a synthetic meal into the microwave oven. Healthy meals do not have to be elaborate, but they do require some careful thought and planning and should be prepared with love and care.

MOTIVATED BY LOVE

While writing this book, I spoke with a Jewish rabbi about its contents. Unfortunately, like many modern Jews, he viewed the Bible as a book that could be objectively analyzed from a purely secular perspective. (And of course as soon as I mentioned the New Testament, he was ready to conclude the conversation.) In spite of proof from scientific studies, he thought that it was only an assumption that the foods in the Bible were healthier than the favorite foods of Americans – processed, fake foods. He disagreed that God knew what was best for His people when He established the dietary law. Instead of believing that God was trying to protect His people by placing parameters around acceptable foods, he believed that God only instituted those parameters to teach His people self-control.

Later, while pondering my conversation with this rabbi, I concluded that his ideology stemmed from a belief system that excludes God as the Creator who desires to be closely involved with the daily affairs of individual human beings. As a result, God becomes whatever objective thought deems Him to be, at least in their minds. And if God can be shaped by human thought and intellect, then there is no need to answer to Him – no accountability. When the Bible is not accepted at face value and studied by a mind and heart convinced of God's great love and deep interest in every human being, it becomes merely just another "sacred" book in the mind of the student. Objective analysis alone destroys the possibility of the Bible becoming alive to that person.

On the other hand, those of us that accept the Bible at face value accept the fact that God loves us as no one else ever could love us. He loves us more than we can comprehend. We don't view the Bible as a book to be tampered with by the finite human mind, but a book to love, a book to base our lives on, and a book to place our faith in. When God places parameters around us, He does so because He loves us and wants to keep us safe. Just as a loving parent wants his children to eat vegetables instead of candy bars for health's sake, so God created healthy foods to be consumed in their natural state so we can gain the energy and strength we need.

So we have a response to the accusation that it is merely an assumption that the whole foods of the Bible are healthier than the foods that have been tampered with by human beings for the sake of profit, shelf life, and mass production. We respond with a simple, childlike belief that *God* knows what is best for us – not men that can manipulate technology and operate machinery to create man-made imitations of wonderful whole foods. This belief is what motivates us to embrace the same foods that Abraham, Moses, Ruth, David, and many other biblical people enjoyed.

God's love motivated Him to carefully plant a garden for one man's benefit. His love motivated Him to make a difference between clean and unclean animals for the Israelites. His love still motivates Him to make available to us delicious and healthy foods for our enjoyment. Choose His foods over man's foods; He really does know what is best for us.

BETTER SAFE THAN SORRY

I've heard people flippantly say, "I don't want to know what is in the food I'm eating. I just want to enjoy it." To that I would like to once again quote Jeff Arnold: "Ignorance is not bliss; ignorance is bondage." Education gives us the opportunity to make wise choices. Without it, we are at the mercy of others who do not care about our health. Don't be satisfied with fake foods. Read before you make a purchase and think before you eat.

No doubt some people think that expressing concern over food additives, irradiation, and genetically engineered food is like making a mountain out of a molehill. The individual that is sounding the warning and trying to help people is often the person that is ridiculed and has his words demeaned. This is because people resist change. In the face of blatant facts and first-hand experience, people will choose to reject truth rather than change. Change requires humility; we must admit that we are wrong, that our previous ideas were incorrect, and that we have been making choices that have been harming us and our families. That is something few people are willing to do. It's much easier to scoff at truth, minimize the evidence, or invent excuses why we are exempt from change.

Over the last 100 years, many food additives have been pulled off the market after more conclusive studies have shown their potential to negatively affect human health. I'm sure that the officials and chemists that work for the FDA are well intentioned and hardworking individuals, but they operate on limited human understanding. Why does it have to take an expensive study or a citizen suffering sickness or death for the government and manufacturers to realize that our bodies were not designed to thrive on chemicals and fake foods?

Irradiation and modern genetically engineered foods are still in their prototype stages, yet they are being sold in grocery stores from coast to coast. Every person has to make their own choices, but when I have the opportunity I would rather be safe than sorry. If I were going to err (what some people might label over-the-edge extremism or unnecessary caution), I would rather err on the side of safety than the side of the unknown.

Though a meal now and then that is chemical in nature may not present much long-term harm, eating foods of that nature over extended periods of time might be. God's whole foods and simple methods of obtaining them are still best. Though it's not feasible for all of us to own our own cow, raise our own chickens, or even grow a family garden, we all can seek out fresh, untainted food that is free of additives and chemicals.

SIXTEEN

DON'T DIET – DO IT RIGHT FOR LIFE

G o to your local library or bookstore in search of the "perfect diet" book and you will find yourself in quite a quandary. It is overwhelming how many different diets there are for us to choose from. All diets claim to be the best diet on the planet. Each one is advertised as the long awaited answer to our health and weight problems.

The problem is that, in spite of their claims, few of these diets seem to be working for the vast majority of Americans. Statistics show that most people who go on a diet with losing weight as their main objective do lose some weight; however, after one year 66% of them have gained it all back. After five years, 97% have gained it all back.

Every few years a new diet comes on the scene. Its books are bestsellers and the "before" and "after" pictures are convincing. It seems like everyone talks about how wonderful this popular new diet is, not realizing that soon it will cycle off the diet scene to be replaced by the next new fad diet. If all of these diets really worked, then America would be getting thinner and healthier. Instead, America is getting heavier and sicker.

DIET DEFINED

Look up the word "diet" in your dictionary. You will find "diet" defined as a prescribed plan for eating which requires limiting or eliminating certain foods, usually for the purpose of losing weight. This is precisely what comes to most of our minds when we hear the word "diet." (Other things that come to mind might be "painful self denial," "misery," "drudgery," and even "torture.") We also think of diets as temporary.

However, the *first* definition listed in most dictionaries is the original meaning of the word "diet": a "way or manner of living." This is vastly different from our concepts of dieting today. We erroneously expect to go on a diet, lose weight, get healthy, go off the diet once we have achieved our goals, and live happily ever after. We are only interested in *temporarily* changing our diets. We want our temporary dietary changes to yield lasting, permanent results. So diets fail because we have unrealistic expectations.

And that is the primary reason why yo-yo dieting has sent America into a tailspin of disappointment and frustration. The very statement "I'm going on a diet" implies that sooner or later we will be saying, "I'm going off the diet." Self-indulgent Americans want to be healthy and fit without compromising their comfort zones.

If we want lifelong health, then we have to make a lifelong commitment to achieve and maintain it. We have to be willing to discontinue poor eating and lifestyle habits and implement new habits that are good for us. This requires change, and we must be willing to change if we want to improve the condition of our temples.

Jehoiachin was a king of Judah who was captured and placed in Babylonian captivity. After a time, a new Babylonian king took the throne and treated Jehoiachin kindly. The king provided Jehoiachin a daily allowance or ration of food, what Jeremiah 52:34 calls a "diet." In other words, Jehoiachin's diet was his daily provision of food.

The Hebrew word for "diet" used in this passage is "aruchah." It is used a few other times in the Bible but nowhere does it translate to mean "a quick fix method to remedy long standing problems." It is interesting that the word "diet" has its origin in the word "day." A diet was simply defined as a daily manner of living, a lifestyle, a cradle-to-grave approach to eating. There were no variations to accommodate quick weight loss through special food restrictions for a specified amount of time. The biblical meaning of the word "diet" implies that how we eat should simply be a way of life – making healthy choices day in and day out.

If we want to have healthy temples, we must stop "going on diets." On a daily basis, we must make wise choices about our food selections and lifestyle habits. We must commit to a way of life that will benefit us every day of our lives.

DRIVING THE POINT HOME

The following excerpts are from an article by Barb Jarmoska entitled "When Will the Weight Be Over?" Her statements serve to reinforce the importance of ditching "dieting" in favor of lifestyle changes.

"More than 400,000 Americans die annually due to poor diet and inactivity. 65 percent of all American adults are overweight and 31 percent are clinically obese, a term which is defined as a body-fat percentage greater than 35 percent of total weight. According to statistics from the CDC, the problem is getting worse. Thus, the way people are dieting today is not only ineffective; it's less effective than ever before.

"It's a strange paradox. In the United States the weight-loss industry is estimated at $33 billion a year. This astounding figure includes over-the-counter diet supplements, drugs, diet books, weight-loss programs and services, obesity surgery, and special diet foods. Why are so many people fat in spite of enormous spending and intense efforts to lose weight?"

As Barb's article progresses, she answers that billion dollar question with a simple explanation: "When you reduce the amount of food you eat, your body protects its fat stores by burning energy at a slower rate, even if you have plenty of spare fat. The body does this through changes in your 'basal metabolic rate,' the amount of energy used when you are at rest. You may lose weight, but a lot of it will be muscle and water, not fat. When you return to your old eating habits, you put on weight faster than ever before because your body's metabolic rate is still operating slowly.

"Therefore, the answer lies not in a diet, but in a commitment to a lifestyle. I would urge anyone who wants to permanently lose weight to give up dieting in favor of eating wholesome food and becoming more active. In other words, make a change for life with no intention of ever returning to your old habits.

"Rather than seeking the answer from a book or other resource, I suggest you first ask yourself, 'What should I eat?' What healthy foods do you like? Eat more! What unhealthy foods are you eating now? Eat less! Make the change gradually, and your cravings for [unhealthy foods] will decrease. As you (and your family) make a gradual change to a whole-foods diet, your tastes and cravings change with you. You reach the point where you actually prefer the apple to the danish. You also prefer flourless, multigrain bread to bagels, brown rice to white, natural peanut butter to Skippy, leaf lettuce to iceberg...green tea to coffee, stevia to Equal, and broiled chicken to fried.

"When you start to feel the effect of your new eating plan, your energy level will increase, often dramatically. Exercise is no longer a chore or obligation. You'll want to learn more about food. You'll read labels, and try new recipes. You'll explore the produce department for a vegetable you've never tasted and expect to like it. You'll drink more water, and feel the positive effects it has on your energy and your joints. You'll sleep better, you (and your kids) will need fewer doctor visits, and after six months or so, you'll begin donating your too-big clothes to the church rummage sale.

"After a year of gradual change, you'll look back and be amazed. You've lost weight, you have energy, some of the health challenges you've had are gone or significantly diminished...and best of all: it's no longer an issue of willpower. You truly don't want to eat another French fry or donut ever again."[1]

DISBANDING DIETS' DECEPTIONS

Perhaps you are emotionally attached to the idea of dieting, so you are still not convinced that dieting is futile and a waste of your efforts. Or maybe you simply want to believe that diet creators know what is best for your health. Maybe you are sure that the perfect, miracle diet is out there somewhere; if you can just find it, then you will be thin, trim, and happy as a clam.

The myriad of popular diet options is absolutely mind-boggling. How can they *all* epitomize perfect health, as they claim? Some of them are as different as night and day. For example, some people enthusiastically laud the benefits of dairy while others shun dairy products in any form. There are as many different slants on nutrition as there are doctors, nutritionists, research scientists, and opinionists.

In order to divorce ourselves from the diet doldrums, we must first acknowledge that nearly all diets have some advantages. This is because most diets restrict fattening foods or total calorie intake, which means that most people will experience some positive results.

The problem is that most Americans are unwilling to commit to a *lifetime* of eating certain foods and doing without others. After a time, willpower wimps out and the glamour of the diet loses its shimmer. In some cases this disillusionment is entirely warranted because most diets are unrealistic for the average person. Restriction for the sole sake of being on a diet requires much more willpower and focus than embracing a lifestyle of healthy eating.

Though space does not permit thorough evaluation of all diets, it will be advantageous to briefly analyze some of the current popular diet trends. Other books explain technically and medically why diets don't work; *Food for Thought* appeals to biblical principles and plain old common sense. Sooner or later, the diet world will probably catch on to the futility of some of its attempts. Dr. Clower believes this too. In *The Fat Fallacy* he writes, "If science knocks around long enough it eventually bumps into the hokey traditions of provincial common sense and hails them as remarkable discoveries."[2]

THE LOW FAT DIET

My husband and I were sitting in the recovery room of a 44-year-old woman who had just finished getting a heart catheterization. She had been fatigued and was sometimes on the verge of passing out. The doctors thought she might be having serious heart problems. As it turned out, she had no blockage and her complete blood count was normal. She had a very slight amount of plaque buildup but it was not enough to even assign a percentage to.

In came the lunch tray specially prepared for heart patients. A little later a nurse came by to tell our friend to eat a low fat diet to avoid heart problems in the future. She was also given a prescription for cholesterol medication, which she was told she would have to take for *the rest of her life*, despite the fact that the test she had just taken revealed virtually no heart problems. This is what was on her tray: Slices of processed turkey on "whole wheat" bread with Miracle Whip, baby carrots with lite ranch dressing, Dole mixed fruit in light syrup, Nabisco graham crackers, angel food cake, carton of 2% homogenized, pasteurized reduced-fat milk, Canada Dry ginger ale, and coffee. *Every single item* on the tray was a processed food filled with sugar and preservatives.

This is why we should always be skittish of marketing words such as "light," "low-fat," and "no-fat." Before you purchase a product, see what is being used in place of fat. You might prefer a little naturally occurring fat to what you find.

Is it too naïve to wonder if fake foods such as these might be the source of heart attacks? Maybe I'm being just a little too simplistic, but if hospitals put a little more emphasis on heart-friendly *whole* foods, they would have a lot less patients. With no differentiation between naturally occurring fats and chemical fats, it is no wonder America is mystified by the failure of the fat free diet. It is touted as being so healthy yet it doesn't seem to work.

I find it amazing that the low fat diet continues to prevail in America. Doctors encourage low fat diets but how many of them help their patients distinguish between "low fat and healthy" and "low fat and non-nutritious"?

The following quotes are from *The Fat Fallacy.*

"Cheese is normal. Milk is normal. We have become so indoctrinated into believing that low-fat products are healthy and slimming that our concept of "normal" has warped into something strange.

"Look at the big picture. Low-fat products are only prominent in this country, and only in the last 30 years! Remember, this is when our obesity epidemic really got rolling. Before that, our weight and the levels of fat in our diet were more like everyone else's in the world."[3]

"What happens when you deprive your body of fat? It's well known that fat-deprivation semistarvation diets lower the metabolic rate, resulting in the body burning less of its energy stores than before. Dr. Wadden and his colleagues have shown that basal metabolic rates can plummet as much as 15 percent after these types of intense caloric restrictions. Besides the fact that this is not good for you, it effectively retards the point of the diet in the first place. You metabolize energy slower. But it's even worse than that. The second result is that the body adapts to fat deprivation by *conserving fat,* not burning it. Once you return to a normal diet – or, all too commonly, binge – the body's adaptive response preferentially turns the food to fat first. Bottom line: Your body needs fat on board and responds to fat-deprivation diets by hoarding fat. It thinks you're starving.

"The point is that low-fat products are not normal, and neither is the low-fat mentality toward health and weight. Forget the fact that it simply doesn't work; it's a ridiculous and deviant change in our diets, compared with every other culture on the planet."[4]

THE LOW CARBOHYDRATE DIET

The low carbohydrate diet replaces carbohydrates with protein and fat. Dieters are encouraged to eat very few carbohydrates and emphasize meat, fish, eggs, dairy products, and fatty sauces instead. People will quickly lose weight on this diet, because the body goes into a state of ketosis. When the body is in ketosis the body burns up stored fat.

However, while the body is burning up fat it is also "burning up" electrolytes, potassium in particular. This places the person who is in ketosis at risk for heart arrhythmia or heart attack. Some experts believe that a low carbohydrate diet harms the body in a way similar to how an outright starvation diet harms the body. Both diets have the potential to harm vital internal organs.

Because people are given carte blanche to eat all the fat they want as long as they stay away from carbohydrates, their diets teeter dangerously on the edge of being disproportionately high fat diets, which are no better than high carbohydrate diets. Most low carbohydrate diets are not whole food diets; you can consume about anything you want as long as it is low in carbohydrates, whether it is a fake food or a real food. Quality and purity of food are not adequately addressed.

One reason low carbohydrate diets work is because by eliminating all carbohydrates, refined carbohydrates are invariably eliminated. Refined carbohydrates are a major contributor to waist expansion. And, while it is true that some people consume inordinate amounts of refined carbohydrates, not all carbohydrates are bad. Whole grains, beans, fruits, and vegetables are carbohydrates that the body thrives on.

Eliminating refined carbohydrates and correcting the imbalance in our diets is a much safer and healthier route than indiscriminately eliminating all carbohydrates, without considering if they are carbohydrates that detract from or contribute to good health.

VEGETARIAN AND VEGAN DIETS

Many people think that vegetarianism is the apex of healthful living. They think that vegetarians are *really healthy.* While there is little doubt that a vegetarian is much, much healthier than the average American on the Standard American Diet, the vegetarian diet is not necessarily the ultimate way to live, nor does it have biblical backing. The fact that a diet is stricter and eliminates more foods does not automatically make it superior to a whole foods diet that includes animal foods.

A few definitions are in order to clarify the terms "vegetarian" and "vegan." All true vegetarians and all vegans do not eat meat, fish, fowl, or products made from them. Lacto-ovo-vegetarians will eat dairy and eggs. Lacto-vegetarians eat all dairy products except eggs. Vegans will not eat any product of any animal whatsoever. Their food choices are guided by the belief that they should not eat anything that has a face. This excludes even honey from their diet, since honey comes from bees, which have faces.

For the born again believer, the first reason a vegetarian diet is not the ultimate way to eat is because the Bible does not support it. I have seen vegetarians grasp at straws and misconstrue Scriptures in an attempt to prove that biblical people were vegetarian. The patriarchs, prophets, and apostles did not advocate such a diet. Jesus, our greatest example, was not vegetarian or vegan. Lamb, fish, honey, and dairy products were all common foods of Bible days. Though there are literally hundreds of Scriptures that verify this, listing just a few should be sufficient.

- "And Solomon's provision for one day was…Ten fat oxen, and twenty oxen out of the pastures, and an hundred sheep, beside harts, and roebucks, and fallowdeer, and fatted fowl" (I Kings 4:22-23).
- "But the father said to his servants…bring hither the fatted calf, and kill it; and let us eat, and be merry: For this my son was dead, and is alive

again; he was lost, and is found" (Luke 15:22-24).

- "And they gave him [Jesus] a piece of a broiled fish, and of an honeycomb. And he took it, and did eat before them" (Luke 24:42-43).

Most Christian vegetarians base their beliefs on Genesis 1:29, which is the record of God telling Adam that he could eat "every green herb." Only three chapters later, Adam's son Abel is a "keeper of sheep" (Genesis 4:2). It is highly unlikely that Abel raised sheep for pets or even that they used the sheep for clothing alone. And by the time Noah got out of the ark, God had expanded man's diet to include "every beast of the earth," "every fowl of the air," and "all the fishes of the sea" (Genesis 9:2-3).

A vegetarian diet was suitable and God-ordained for Adam and Eve during their life in the Garden of Eden. But nowhere else in the Bible did God commend it as appropriate or superior to a diet that includes meat. Vegetarians assert that a meat-free diet is healthier. By referencing Genesis 1:29, they relay the impression that since life in the Garden of Eden was like living in Paradise, vegetarianism is one way to achieve Eden's purity. But God has never expected us to try to replicate the Garden of Eden. Vegetarianism was only ideal for that time and place.

We don't live in the Garden of Eden. Vegetarian diet proponents that base their diet on the foods that Adam and Eve ate in the Garden of Eden forget that a lot of things other than diet changed after the Fall. Women now have pain in childbearing. Men have to work hard to make a living (Genesis 3:16-19). A new diet was just one more dramatic, irrevocable change.

When we are baptized in Jesus' name and receive the gift of the Holy Ghost, we can commune with God freely. If we sin after we have been baptized in Jesus' name and filled with His Spirit, all we have to do is turn to God, confess and turn from our sins (I John 1:9). This restores us to communion with Him. In this regard I propose that the time in which we now live has the potential to be superior to the time of the Garden of Eden: Adam did not have that option. Sin severed his relationship with God with no possibility of restoring that relationship as it once was; he could never return to the Garden of Eden (Genesis 3:24).

In addition to the potentially superior spiritual benefits of our present age, the great variety of foods unavailable for Adam and Eve are available for us to eat. Instead of trying to roll back the curtain of time, why not take advantage of them, especially since there is not a single scriptural admonition that tells New Testament believers to not eat meat?

Creating any doctrine from just a single verse of Scripture is poor hermeneutics. Yet this is what so-called biblical vegetarians do when they base their diet upon a solitary reference – Genesis 1:29. A popular vegetarian diet called the Hallelujah Diet claims no other Scriptural basis than this one verse. George Malkmus, who offers only personal opinions and speculations as to why God allowed meat, dairy, fish, and fowl to be consumed throughout the Bible, founded this diet.[5] II Timothy 3:16 tells us that God inspired *all* Scripture, not just one verse out of thousands.

Daniel and his three friends' diet while in Babylonian captivity is often cited in an attempt to fortify vegetarianism as a biblical way of eating. "Daniel purposed in his heart that he would not defile himself with the portion of the king's meat...therefore he requested of the prince of the eunuchs that he might not defile himself" (Daniel 1:8). Daniel was granted his request and his diet of pulse (vegetables, grains, and beans) and water improved his health and complexion.

But why did Daniel refuse the food of the king? After all, the normal Jewish diet was not vegetarian. The Babylonians were a heathen people. They did not revere or serve Jehovah. As a result, they did not follow the Mosaic dietary laws, which were in place at that time. Daniel did not want to transgress God's laws by eating unclean foods. Also, Daniel did not want to endorse idol worship by eating meat that had been offered to idols, a common practice of the polytheistic Babylonians. It is highly likely that Daniel's special diet was a deviation from what he would normally have eaten if he had not been in captivity.

Daniel's special diet is erroneously called "Daniel's fast." Technically, Daniel was not fasting; he changed his diet. A fast has a beginning and ending. There is no record that Daniel and his friends ever stopped eating just pulse and water. Daniel died while in Babylonian captivity.

Shortly after Daniel's death, the Jews returned to Jerusalem under the leadership of Ezra, Zerubbabel, and Nehemiah. After the temple had been rebuilt, they reinstituted the Feast of the Passover (Ezra 6:19-21). This commemorative feast entailed eating lamb.

Nehemiah served 150 rulers at his table on a daily basis. In Nehemiah 5:18 he cites the foods that comprised their regular menu: "Now that which was prepared for me daily was one ox and six choice sheep; also fowls were prepared for me."

It is plainly evident that once the Jews were in their own land and no longer under the rule and law of a foreign nation, they reverted to their normal diet. While God certainly blessed him as a result, Daniel's special diet was a departure from the norm, an act of separation from heathen practices and dedication unto God.

The plus of modern day vegetarian and vegan diets is that they eliminate processed, refined foods. This in itself will make anybody healthier but can also be achieved without shunning meats. Vegetarians have to be careful to not substitute disproportionate amounts of fruit or sugar for meat when they need energy. The protein in meat is an excellent source of long-term energy.

While the vegetarian diet is useful for a short-term cleanse, its superiority to a well-rounded whole foods diet is debatable. It is possible for vegetarians to develop nutritional deficiencies – particularly vitamin D, vitamin B12, calcium, essential fatty acids, and possibly protein as well.

Vegetarians claim that they can get important vitamins, such as vitamin D, from plant foods and sunlight. However, some nutritionists say that the forms of the vitamins obtained from those sources are not the same nor are they as beneficial as the vitamins available from animal foods. Also, many nutritionists claim that it is impossible for vegans to get vitamin B12 from their diet. Vitamin B12 deficiency leads to anemia, can cause fatigue, and contributes to neurological disorders. Vitamin B12 is found in animal products, especially eggs. Long-term vegans may have gaunt and hollow appearances, which is a sign of missing nutrients. Though both sides fervently debate the nutritional deficiency issue, the bottom line is that vegetarianism is not biblically required nor is it necessary to achieve great health.

Vegetarians believe that animal foods are unhealthy. Yet even though animal products have been consumed for thousands of years, it is only in the last few decades that heart attacks and obesity have become as ordinary as the common cold. If animal food and the saturated fat some of them contain (which is said to be so harmful) were what make people sick, then why did God allow His people to eat it? Why did Jesus eat animal foods?

In closing, some people adopt vegetarian and vegan diets for social and religious reasons. Born again believers should not assume the mentality that being a vegetarian makes them more spiritual or superior to non-vegetarians. If that were so, then Abraham, Moses, and Jesus were not very spiritual.

THE SUGAR-FREE DIET

The number of people in the United States with sugar diabetes is staggering. Thus, sugar free and low sugar diets are coming to the "rescue" of our citizens. All sorts of sugar imitations are being marketed as ideal for diabetics so that they can have their cake and eat it too. The fact that these man-made sweeteners will probably cause other problems for the diabetic is not disclosed. If you are a diabetic, ask a naturopathic doctor to guide your sugar replacement decisions. There are several natural alternatives that may suit your health situation.

At the time of this writing, one of the newest diet trends is limiting sugar intake by following the glycemic index. The glycemic index is a gauge of how rapidly carbohydrates turn to glucose. Once again, however, this diet can interfere with God's natural provisions. I recently spoke with a non-diabetic who thought she should not eat watermelon because it was high on the glycemic index. While we certainly need to monitor our sugar intake, we must differentiate between imitation foods and whole foods. Some candy bars actually have a lower number on the glycemic index than some vegetables like carrots. If we buy into the glycemic index diet plan, we will be casting aside God's best in favor of man's much-less-than-best. The glycemic index may be used as a guide, but each food should first be examined for its general wholesomeness.

One popular low-sugar diet replaces white sugar with artificial sweeteners, while molasses, honey, maple syrup, and brown rice syrup are forbidden. This diet also allows for the use of margarine, store bought Italian dressing, and food coloring. This particular diet is mostly good but is still not a whole foods diet. While decreasing our sugar intake is needful, artificial replacements only create other problems. In itself, the sugar-free diet is not the complete answer. Overall nutrition and health must be addressed.

THE BLOOD TYPE DIET

The Blood Type Diet is cemented in the belief that human beings are the product of evolution, not divine creation. The premise of this diet is that as human beings evolved over millions of years, new blood types appeared when living conditions and environments changed, necessitating new food requirements. Depending on where your ancestors fell in the chronology of evolution determines your blood type and what kind of food you should eat.

This diet was developed by Peter D'Adamo, who was strongly influenced by his father. In order to accept the tenets of the blood-type diet, you must first accept that you are the product of human evolution. That is the foundational belief of this diet. D'Adamo claims that "human prehistory began in Africa, where we evolved from humanlike creatures."[6]

Type O people (the hunters) are from the "earliest humans, who were physically active and ate a diet composed mostly of the meat of large herbivorous mammals with little or no grain. As descendants, you require large amounts of meat and lots of exercise." Type A people (the cultivators) "descended from agrarian humans, are more docile, thrive on vegetables and fruit, and should avoid meat and dairy products, and require only moderate exercise." Type B people (the nomads) are the result of "the merging and migration of the races from the African homeland to Europe, Asia, and the Americas." Type AB people (the enigma) originated from "the modern intermingling of disparate groups" If you have type AB blood, you should avoid meat and eat fish, grains, and soy-based foods.[7]

According to D'Adamo, your blood type is the key to great health. He gives little thought to the benefits of whole foods. In fact, eating a balanced, individualized diet of whole foods is dwarfed by his blood type philosophies. For instance, if you are type A, you must avoid beef, lamb, haddock, butter, pistachios, lima beans, whole wheat bread, green peppers, sauerkraut, tomatoes, oranges, apple cider vinegar, and pepper. D'Adamo claims that honey is "just as empty of nutrients as white sugar," which makes one wonder if he reads comic books instead of nutritional manuals.

Most scientists consider the blood type diet a fad diet lacking substantial support. Instead of being a proven method of health maintenance, it sounds like the product of the imagination of a four-year-old who has been playing too long with plastic dinosaurs.

THE MACROBIOTIC DIET

In the early 1900s a Japanese man by the name of Yukikazu Sakurazawa became ill by eating too many refined foods. He recovered when he began eating traditional Japanese foods such as brown rice, miso soup, vegetables, and fish. He developed a diet based on his philosophies about food, assuming the pen name of George Ohsawa.

Ohsawa introduced the macrobiotic diet to America. Based upon an ancient Chinese medical manual, it has its foundation in the belief that everything in the universe falls into two categories: yin (female) and yang (male). Examples of yin foods are sugar, fruit juices, honey, tropical fruits, dairy products, vegetables, and legumes. Yang foods include pork, beef, game, poultry, eggs, fish, and grains.

Ohsawa's instructions were somewhat imprecise about acceptable and unacceptable foods. What he did make clear was the importance of brown rice. He believed that brown rice is the perfect balance of yin and yang energies.

Ohsawa had a student named Michio Kushi who popularized his teachings. Kushi developed the "standard macrobiotic diet" which gave clearer instructions than Ohsawa had provided. Kushi's diet was more vegetarian in nature, with the allowance of white fish. His instructions were directly opposed to the original ancient diet which considers "the five meats" essential.

The standard macrobiotic diet consisted of 50-60% whole grain products, 20-30% locally grown, mostly cooked vegetables, 5-10% soups, 5-10% sea vegetables, fermented soy products, and beans. Small amounts of fruit, fish, beverages, and naturally sweetened desserts were allowed. All dairy products, including eggs, and meat were disallowed.

The new leaders of the macrobiotic diet have acknowledged that Kushi may have been extreme and are giving some leeway for the consumption of oily fish and dairy products. Plainly, the macrobiotic diet is a diet that has evolved as new proponents have added their own unique twists and ideas.

Nutritionally speaking, the macrobiotic diet has some serious flaws. While brown rice is a very healthful food, the typical Asian has a larger pancreas than the average Westerner, making large quantities of rice easier for Asians to process. Such emphasis on brown rice and other whole grains can lead to imbalances. Mineral, vitamin, and protein deficiencies can result from strict adherence to such a limited diet.

On the other hand, there are a lot of good points to the macrobiotic diet. It essentially eliminates all processed foods. Daikon radish often accompanies macrobiotic foods. Daikon is high in lactobacilli, is used as a diuretic decongestant, and is a great source of vitamin C. In addition to Ohsawa, other people have recovered from chronic and terminal illnesses by following the macrobiotic diet. It may not be ideal for everyone, however.

The traditional diet that Ohsawa adopted was simply foods of his native culture. The Japanese ate those foods because they were the ones most readily available to them for hundreds of years. We accept that other natural, ethnic foods then unknown to the Japanese are healthful as well.

The word "macrobiotic" means "long or great life." It is a term that has been used for years to define living simply and naturally to achieve a long and satisfying life. The standard macrobiotic diet appeals to the health conscious. However, beneath the veneer of its healthy appearances lie some philosophies that are diametrically opposed to biblical concepts. The principles of the macrobiotic diet go beyond food and into spiritualism.

The underlying philosophy that supplies the foundation for the macrobiotic diet is the promotion of world unity and peace. Kushi purported that "a strict brown rice diet confers spiritual enlightment, and that diets based entirely on local foods brings peace to the planet."[8]

In many cases, this philosophy is simply impossible to implement, as Sally Fallon in her book *Nourishing*

Traditions, explains: "In many parts of the world, the two principles are impossible to implement jointly. Rice-eating macrobiotic disciples living in Montana must rely on foods imported from distant lands in order to practice their search for enlightenment, but in order to achieve world peace they would need to give up rice-eating for a diet of local beef."[9]

I was amused when an acquaintance of mine walked out of a New England convenience store with bottled water from Fiji. She was a fan of macrobiotics. Though Fiji water is purportedly very pure, my friend lived in close proximity to cold, clear, unpolluted mountain streams. In fact, it was not uncommon for us to be traveling along secondary roads and see people filling bottles at small waterfalls that supplied refreshing, pristine water to the locals. For my friend, though, convenience conflicted with her macrobiotic principles. And if the truth is told, eating locally 100% of the time is just not possible for most people who live in 21st century America.

In addition to being unrealistic, Kushi's philosophies propagated the formation of a one-world government. He believed that using whole grains as the main food of people around the world will promote equal distribution of wealth. He believed that grains make people less aggressive toward other nations. The potential sociological and political effects of a widely accepted macrobiotic diet have devious goals masked just beneath supposed goodwill toward all men.

While God tells us to give to the poor, the Bible never endorses equal distribution of wealth. And the formation of a one-world government and social system is the work of man, not God. From the time of the Tower of Babel until now, a unified world will only yield humanistic, anti-God results. As with the blood type diet, we must keep in mind that when we embrace the macrobiotic diet we are identifying ourselves with spiritual principles that most Christians oppose.

OTHER DIETS

In addition to those discussed above, a few other prominent diets are the raw foods diet, the acid-alkaline diet, the food combining diet, and the starvation diet.

The Raw Foods Diet

The raw foods diet has its foundation in the idea that heating food destroys enzymes and decreases vitamin and mineral availability. (Some adherents, albeit extremists, even eat raw meat, including blood. For Scriptural admonitions against raw meat and blood, see Exodus 12:8-9, Leviticus 17:10-14, and Acts 15:20.)

A diet of raw foods is excellent for short term cleansing. Raw foods support weight loss, provide energy, and clear the skin of impurities. It is true that heating foods to over 110° begins to destroy its enzymes. And generally speaking, most raw foods take less time to digest than cooked foods.

However, the human body is marvelously designed and a healthy person should have no problems assimilating cooked foods. The enzymes present in humans' digestive systems are equipped to break down food. When necessary, the pancreas can produce additional enzymes to aid the digestive process.

The bottom line is that an exclusive diet of raw foods has no biblical basis for lifelong application. Some foods such as tomatoes actually benefit from cooking; cooked tomatoes have more lycopene (a carotenoid) than fresh tomatoes. Some foods are easier to digest cooked than when they are in their raw state. Rather than shunning cooked foods altogether, a better path to follow would be enjoying both raw and cooked foods in proportions that your body is comfortable with.

The Acid-Alkaline Diet

The aim of the acid-alkaline diet is to balance the pH of the blood. Some foods are acidic and others are alkaline. Some proponents of this diet believe that people's diets should be comprised of 80% alkaline foods and 20% acidic foods. Because the Standard American

Diet creates excessive acidity, eating more plant-based alkaline foods helps bring a balance to our bodies. We are told that the reason we should have such a high percentage of alkaline foods is because human beings evolved from the ocean, which is alkaline. Before blindly diving into this diet, purchase a pH testing kit at the health food store. If you are overly acidic, altering your diet to include more alkaline foods may benefit you enormously. On the other hand, if your pH is normal, making unnecessary drastic alterations to your diet can be detrimental.

The Food Combining Diet

Proponents of this diet say that protein and starch should not be consumed during the same meal. The food combining diet dictates which foods should not be eaten together.

It seems to make sense that since fruit takes less time to digest than meat that fruit should be eaten prior to the meat or well after the meat has been eaten. If you notice that eating certain foods at the same time hampers your digestion, then it is time to "listen" to your body. You may need to put space between your consumption of certain foods.

However, food enzymes are equipped to break down both protein and starch in the stomach at the same time. A properly functioning body should not have difficulty processing both protein and starch.

There is no biblical precedent for the food combining diet. Jesus distributed bread (starch) and fish (protein) to thousands of people at the same event (Mark 8:6-7). Abigail brought David and his men bread, fruit, and meat (I Samuel 25:18). The original Passover meal consisted of meat, unleavened bread, and bitter herbs (Exodus 12:8). In none of these, as well as many other meals recorded in the Bible, did God tell people that they could not eat several different types of food at the same time.

A wonderful Sicilian lady we know prepared a true Sicilian meal for us. It was delicious and, because we did not understand how many courses she had prepared, we were quite satiated. The very last dish she served was a salad. She told us that in Sicily it is customary to serve the salad at the end of the meal, not the beginning, because it helps digest the meal. This is the case in some other countries as well.

The Starvation Diet

This diet needs no definition. When a person goes without food or drastically reduces his caloric intake, he does not give his body the nutrition it needs. This creates electrolyte deficiencies, potassium in particular. This is a very grave condition that seriously endangers the heart.

Anorexia nervosa is a condition that affects mostly girls and women. Though chemical imbalances and zinc deficiency may play a role in anorexia, it is usually the result of a poor self-image and distorted, unrealistic expectations. These psychological problems can be remedied when we attain a proper perspective of ourselves and trade in self-esteem for God-esteem. Anorexia is only a self-destructive symptom of inner issues that can be resolved when the Word of God is applied to a life.

Aside from fasting, if you skip meals or go for days without eating because you are obsessed with being thin, you need to remember that Barbie is plastic. Everybody has a flaw or two. Movie stars and models have the help of plastic surgery, special lighting, and flattering photography techniques.

If you over-eat one day, don't starve yourself the next day to compensate. Realize that each day is a new one; enjoy it, and ask the Lord to help you to be temperate and wise in your food choices.

Make creating a healthier habitat for the Lord your aim and losing weight or staying thin will be a by-product of your efforts. We should not desire to lose weight for aesthetic purposes alone; rather, any changes we make should benefit us in a complete, balanced way.

MIRACLE FOODS AND MODERATION

From time to time a new food will be "discovered" and lauded for its cure-all benefits. These "miracle" foods receive a lot of publicity and suddenly all sorts of products containing this food show up on grocery store shelves. People sometimes get the mistaken impression that an abundance of these foods or eating them to the exclusion of other foods is the secret to health. Ah, the power of the press and marketing!

At the time of this writing, for example, the soy craze has been in swing for several years. Studies are cited and women especially are encouraged to eat a lot of tofu and other soy products. Soy proponents laud the ability of soy to control cholesterol, regulate insulin and blood sugar levels, improve bowel function, treat osteoporosis, and help prevent certain cancers, especially stomach cancers.

What the media does not tell us is that most Americans already have an overabundance of soy in their diet because soy is used as a filler in many products. (Read labels.) TVP (textured vegetable/soy protein) is highly processed soybean meal. It is a hidden ingredient in many foods, including foods created for vegetarians. Soy is used to make soy cheese, soy milk, and soy protein powders. It is a key ingredient in margarine, shortening, sauces, lunch meats, hard candy, cooking oil, and salad dressings. Though unrefined, expeller pressed soybean oil is available, commonly used soybean oil is the product of high temperatures, chemical solvents (usually hexane), bleach, and hydrogenation.

Additionally, soy contains phytates and enzyme inhibitors which may contribute to intestinal disorders, prevent proper absorption of protein, minerals, and nutrients and hinder glucose uptake in the brain. Unfermented soybeans are difficult to digest.

Phytoestrogens (plant estrogens) are purported to make soy the miracle food for breast cancer prevention. However, one naturopathic doctor I spoke with thinks that too much soy actually *causes* breast cancer. Phytoestrogens have also been implicated in depressed thyroid function.

One thing that researchers seem to agree on is that popular soy products are not appropriate for infants and small children. "Besides the toxic levels of aluminum and manganese in soy formula, soy itself is an inappropriate food for children. Soy foods and soy formulas depress thyroid function. They can induce a hypothyroid state in infants. Soy formula feeding is associated with hormone disruption and premature sexual development in small children. A soy-fed baby receives the equivalent of five birth control pills' worth of estrogen every day. Soy feeding in infancy has also been linked to diabetes. Soy interferes with the absorption of calcium, magnesium, zinc and iron. Soy formula should never be given to infants."[10]

Given all of the potential dangers of soy, some naturopathic physicians discourage people from consuming too many popular soy products. While soy proponents point to Asia as leading the way in the use of soybeans, they rarely mention that Asians have traditionally employed soy in its fermented forms – miso, natto, tempeh, and cultured, naturally brewed soy sauce. When unpasteurized, these foods contain live microorganisms and beneficial enzymes, which make them very easy to digest. These foods are natural antibiotics and promote an alkaline environment in the body. In addition to their staple use as condiments, Oriental people add miso, natto, tempeh, and naturally brewed soy sauce to soups, rice, grains, noodles, sauces, gravies, marinades, dressings, dips, and spreads.

While the jury is still out, I think I'll stand on the sidelines of caution and let the soy bandwagon pass me by until the controversy is resolved. Clearly, God created the soybean, but to overemphasize it to the extreme violates the balancing principle of moderation.

We should not use one healthy food to the exclusion of other healthy foods. For example, when choosing a type of oil for a recipe, don't use *just* butter or *just* coconut oil. Use both and glean the beneficial properties of

both and use other oils besides. When choosing a sweetener, don't use *just* honey. Though I use honey more
than any other sweetener, I also use brown rice syrup,
molasses, maple syrup, agave nectar, and other natural
sweeteners. This method of variety gives us a balance.
You will, in time, create your own balance of healthy
foods, depending on your individual health needs, taste
preferences, and cooking styles.

When I was a teenager, I stayed with a lady for a
week. For that entire week I saw her eat only one food:
popcorn. Every day she planted herself in front of her TV
with a big bowl of popcorn beside her. Her goal was to
lose weight. I didn't stay around long enough to know if
it worked. But that is a perfect example of eating one
food to the exclusion of others, hoping that it will make
you healthy. If I did what she did, it would only make
me sick of popcorn!

The cabbage soup diet is another good example of
moderation gone south. Cabbage soup is healthful and
delicious the first time. Leftovers a time or two are also
okay. But cabbage soup for weeks on end?!?! No thanks.

I love fresh grapefruit and could easily eat them
several days in a row. They are so refreshing. The Grapefruit Diet is superb for a short term cleansing diet and
a terrific weight loss aid, but eating nothing but grapefruit for extended periods of time could cause diarrhea,
boils, and other problems.

In her book *The Front Row*, Gwyn Oakes tells a
comical story about an evangelist and his wife who came
to minister to the church her husband pastored: "One
young couple that came for a revival drank nothing but
hot Jello. That was a relatively easy request and also inexpensive. They liked all flavors, so that wasn't bad.
Just mix as directed and drink while hot. Try it you
might like it! I've often wondered if it set up inside or exactly what did happen. They sure had nice hair and
nails."[11]

Educate yourself about food but don't naively buy
into all the propaganda of the media. It shifts like Flori-

dian sands in the midst of a hurricane. Use your own brain and think for yourself.

It is true that periodically eliminating certain foods and emphasizing others for a certain period of time is highly beneficial for detoxification and cleansing. And because of allergies, individual health issues, and food intolerances, some people find avoiding certain foods or food groups (i.e. grain, dairy) benefits them. Generally speaking, however, making proper choices and using discipline on a day-to-day basis is the best way to maintain good health. While some diets that veer away from the Standard American Diet (fake, processed foods) are an improvement and most diets have their merits, they should not be chosen as the path we follow for life. You must evaluate your specific needs and create a lifestyle of food choices that will create optimum health for you as an individual.

INTUITIVE EATING

To the credit of many diet inventors, most of them are sincere people who want people to invest in their idea of the perfect diet and commit to it as a way of life. They have spent years of study and effort to create a diet that they believe will help people. Some of them have wonderful testimonies about how the diet they created restored their health and changed their lives. Many of them include "lifetime maintenance plans" in their diet strategies. They hope that people will make permanent lifestyle changes for long-term results.

In reality, however, most people just don't do that. And all diets are not good for all people. We are all individuals with different needs. Health history, age, and even ethnicity determine the type and quantity of food we need.

I personally know people who, though they lost weight, experienced frightening adverse effects from the low carbohydrate diet. Many mainstream diets encourage the use of synthetic foods (i.e. artificial sweeteners, processed foods) and discourage the use of whole foods (i.e. some fruits, vegetables, and meat). This violates the principles of purity and balance that create healthy, normally functioning human beings.

Once you have made some changes and are on the road to better temple maintenance, if you will "listen" to your body, it will tell you what it needs. There may be specific foods that you personally should avoid and others that you should integrate into your lifestyle diet.

A healthy body will tell you what kind of and how much food it needs. It will communicate normally, not out of pain, as an unhealthy body does. There is no "perfect diet" that is good for every human being on the planet. Our dietary needs are determined by varying specifications. What one person can eat a lot of another person must avoid. That is why this book presents a principles-based approach to eating, not a stringent diet that claims to be the best diet for every person on the planet. You may need a salad for dinner and your spouse wants a steak. You are two different people and your nutritional needs are different. Eating intuitively and sensibly eliminates the need to follow fad diets.

GO GOD'S WAY

The avocado is high in fat, the potato is high in carbohydrates, and the apple is high in sugar. These all would be shunned by those riding the diet trend train. Yet the avocado, potato, and apple are all God-created whole foods rich in health and energy enhancing properties. The fat, carbohydrates, and sugar in these natural foods are what your body craves and recognizes as real food. Most diet fans would replace the avocado with a low fat refined white bagel, the potato with low carbohydrate preservative laced bacon, and the apple with a packaged diet bar sweetened with a man-made chemical.

Again, we must differentiate between types of fat, carbohydrate, and sugar. Not all fats, carbohydrates, and sugars are bad. Lumping all carbohydrates into the same category is like saying that all Germans are evil because Adolf Hitler was evil and he was German. It so happens that I married into a German family. They happen to be wonderful people, responsible and respectable citizens.

Some people laud the supposed benefits of traditional and primitive cultures to such an extent that we are led to believe that such societies never experienced sickness and disease. Be cautious of diets that promote certain foods that some remote African tribe eats. The statements some people make about primitive cultures and their diets lead us to believe that we would all be better off if we moved into the jungle, ate roots, and drank the blood of animals. (I'm not exaggerating. There are some far-out philosophies and their ideologies are alive and well.)

It is common knowledge that many native cultures are void of the serious diseases that plague America, but that does not mean that they are completely sickness-free, nor does it mean that it is the right diet for every person in the world. Don't buy into everything you hear. Run it past the measure of the Word of God and you will save yourself time, money, and energy.

Some people are lured into weight loss drug advertisements, attracted by catchy phrases and attractive pictures. Some of these drugs have potential side effects, many of which are serious, and are best left alone.

Who knows what will be next, but some new Miracle Diet will come on the scene soon. While all diets have merits, most people will not find long-term success with them. The answer lies in life application of a balanced whole foods diet personalized for specific health needs.

The Bible does not endorse or mention modern diets. Current diets are not the first to come on the diet scene, nor will they be the last. As long as people are alive they will be searching for the Miracle Diet. Unfortunately, their searches usually exclude God and His Word.

The principles of the Bible have been around for thousands of years. Why do we think that a few modern-day scientists know more than the Creator of this entire universe? Many Americans think that the world revolves around them. Though Americans are pacesetters in some things, the rest of the world does not share the egocentric view we have of ourselves. We think that we know what is best and ideal in regards to nutrition and wonder why the rest of the world doesn't get in line with our perfect programs. The first reason they don't jump on our diet bandwagons is because most of them are not as unhealthy and overweight as Americans. The second is because they understand that common sense approaches to eating are the best way to go.

That the ideal diet should be based upon simple biblical principles such as portion control and balance is ludicrous to the mind that demands scientific explanations for proof. Yet, God's ways are simple, easy to understand, and best of all – they work.

DO IT RIGHT FOR LIFE

Instead of counting calories, points, fat grams, or carbohydrates, popping pills, measuring food, drinking meal-replacement powdered shakes, or eating diet program frozen meals, focus on moderately eating whole, minimally processed foods that are full of nutrients. Be skeptical of all fad diets and get-thin-quick schemes. The only thing that will get thin is your bankroll. An instant society wants instant results, but a responsible person acknowledges that lifestyle modification is a better choice. The best diet is a well ordered life.

Avoid discouragement by avoiding diets. A wise man learns from his own mistakes; a wiser man learns from the mistakes of others and does not repeat them in his own life. Diets have failed millions of people, but God's lifelong plan for eating whole foods in moderation will never fail. Diets were created by man but healthy foods were created by God. Diets come and diets go, but God's principles never change.

Choose God's definition of the best diet – a way of life that will bring Him glory.

PART III

WHOLE FOODS

Following the Blueprints

SEVENTEEN

GREAT GRAINS

Take thou also unto thee wheat, and barley, and beans, and lentiles, and millet, and fitches, and put them in one vessel, and make thee bread thereof.
Ezekiel 4:9

In light of the recent overrated low-carbohydrate diet craze in America, carbohydrates have been deemed the villain of poor health and obesity. In a style reminiscent of the low-fat fad, in which all fat was bad, the low-carb craze proclaims that all carbohydrates are bad. Strangely enough however, neither the low-fat nor low-carb theories have made Americans skinnier or healthier.

The low-carb proponents have inflicted extensive damage upon the minds of many trusting Americans. Believing the low-carb propaganda, they shun grains like rice and wheat and some fruits and vegetables such as corn and potatoes – all foods that God created for us to eat.

If God wanted us to live a low-carbohydrate life, then why did He create such foods in the first place? Why did Jesus allow his disciples to pluck wheat or barley from a wayside farm, rub it in their hands to separate the chaff from the grain, and eat it (Matthew 12:1)? Why did He break bread and give it to His disciples to eat, using it as a symbol of how His body would be broken for them (Matthew 26:26)? Why did He place His stamp of approval on these foods if He knew that His disciples were going to get fat and sick from eating them?

Could it be that, just as all fats are not equal, so all carbohydrates are not equal? Could it be that it is not the God-created substance that is bad, but that man's meddling has produced something unhealthy out of that which was nourishing in its original state? Could it be that man has "refined" the health right out of delicious, wholesome foods?

Instead of blindly believing every statement of the media, we must examine their claims by the light of the Word of God. If we indiscriminately label all carbohydrates as bad, we will rob ourselves of the very nutrition that God knows our bodies need. After all, He is the One who designed and created us, so if anyone knows what foods are good for us and what foods are bad for us, it is God.

SIMPLY COMPLEX

One basic principle some people fail to consider when making food choices is that there are two distinct forms of carbohydrates: simple and complex.

Simple carbohydrates are "quick energy" foods. Usually high in sugar, they are quickly digested and enter the bloodstream rapidly. This creates a dangerous spike in blood sugar levels. A simple rule is that, the more "refined" a food, the more likely it is to be a simple carbohydrate. Simple carbohydrates have limited nutritional benefit and should be consumed sparingly.

Complex carbohydrates are the kind of carbohydrates our bodies need for long lasting energy. They are digested slower than simple carbohydrates, helping us feel fuller longer. These carbohydrates are found in whole grains, fruits, and vegetables.

Complex carbohydrates are a great source of fiber. Fiber deficiency contributes to a host of health problems such as constipation, which in itself is the root cause of many painful conditions such as diverticulitis, appendicitis, hemorrhoids, hiatal hernia, and colon cancer. Proper fiber intake lessens the risk of heart disease, diabetes, obesity, and gallstones. The fiber in complex carbohydrates also stabilizes blood sugar by regulating the absorption of nutrients and sugar in the digestive tract.

WHOLE GRAINS

In this chapter, we will explore the benefits of whole grains, one of nature's superb sources of healthy carbohydrates. It is important to clearly define whole grains (complex carbohydrates) and explain how they differ from refined grains (simple carbohydrates). Quite simply, whole grains are the entire grain. Another way of understanding this is to say that *com*plex carbohydrates are the *com*plete grain. The grain suffers no separation of its three main components: bran, germ, and endosperm. It is free of pesticide and harmful chemical processing. Simply, man has tampered with it very little, providing us with all of the nutrition innate to the grain.

The bran of the grain contains fiber, minerals, B vitamins, and protein.

The germ, or embryo, is also a source of protein, minerals, and vitamins. In particular, the germ contains antioxidant vitamin E, which aids circulation, promotes healthy skin, and contributes to reproductive health.

The endosperm is the starch of the grain.

The hull is the protective outer coating of the grain. It is hard, tough, and inedible, has no nutritional value, and is almost always removed.

All of the protein, vitamins, and minerals in whole grains combine to provide a balanced source of good nutrition.

THIEVES AND ROBBERS

God created whole grains and the Old Testament patriarchs, prophets, and spiritual leaders ate them. The Israelites were given many dietary restrictions for their health's sake but never once did God prohibit them from eating grains. He placed His sanction upon bread and used it to illustrate spiritual lessons.

Bread was a common food during Bible times, so common, in fact, that the words for "bread" and "grain"

(Hebrew: lechem/Greek: sitos) were synonymous with the word "food."

The two chief grains used in Bible lands were barley and wheat. Barley was the food of the poor masses and wheat was the food of the rich.

Egyptians may have been the first people to bake bread. Archaeologists have found Egyptian stone grain grinding mills that date to the third millennium B.C.

"Biblical people took their grain boiled and parched, soaked and roasted, and, at times, even ate it green from the stalk. It was pounded, dried or crushed to be baked into casseroles, porridges, soups, parched grain salads and desserts such as puddings and flans."[1]

Sowing and reaping was a labor intensive process but was completely void of the harsh chemicals and processing that we consider normal today.

The fields were plowed and the seed was sown by hand. When it was time for harvest, the grain was cut by hand, then threshed and winnowed. The grain was then stored until ready for use, when it would be ground at home using a small hand mill or a mortar. This ensured fresh bread, which was usually prepared daily. It was a blessing until mankind decided to try to improve upon what God created.

Though from time to time various civilizations have attempted to "refine" bread, desiring to make it whiter and lighter, it did not become a common practice until relatively recently. Before, only the wealthiest ate refined bread and, in some cultures, the color of one's bread actually indicated his economic place in society. The darker his bread, the lower he was! Ironically, history reveals that the upper echelon of some of these societies, such as England's, actually suffered inferior health as a result of their "refinement."

Once ground, whole grain flour goes bad quickly because the germ contains oil and the bran contains fiber, both of which contribute to rancidity. The germ and bran are "alive," in the sense that they contain 26 naturally occurring vitamins, minerals, and proteins. Once the whole grain is opened and the germ and bran are exposed, the potency of these vitamins, minerals, and proteins begins to diminish, similar to how an apple oxidizes as soon as its skin is removed. The longer the apple is exposed to air, the more nutrition is lost. That is why, throughout history, grain was ground only as needed.

In the early days of America, mills were located in nearly every town of size, usually beside a river or stream to utilize waterpower. Local farmers brought their corn or wheat to the mill to be ground. The *entire* grain was ground between two stones, providing complete nourishment. Wheat flour was light brown in color.

As America's population mushroomed, its lifestyle changed. Replacing small towns and independent farms, large cities, big industry, and mass production began to alter the landscape of food production. In 1874 steel rolling mills replaced the traditional stone ground method. The grain, primarily wheat, was now crushed rather than ground. The germ and the bran were flattened and separated from the endosperm, leaving behind a starchy, white substance. The germ and bran were thrown away and the remaining "food" was refined into a simple carbohydrate which "turns" into sugar upon entry into our bodies. Because the life was thrown away, this flour promised a long shelf life and loaves and loaves of fluffy, white bread. This was good for the bread manufacturers' bank ledgers but bad for the consumers' health.

Whole grains are divine gifts of nutritional life. A powerhouse of balanced vitality, they contain 26 essential vitamins and minerals. Modern processing eliminates nearly all of these vitamins and minerals. By law, modern flour manufacturers are required to replace a small percentage of the vitamins that are lost in processing. That these replacement vitamins are synthetic in nature is overlooked. They're just happy that they can now advertise their flour and bread as "enriched" and "fortified," convincing us that they are doing us a big favor.

If you entrusted someone with $26.00 and they handed you back $6.00 as they pocketed the other $20.00, would you feel en*rich*ed? Not hardly. You would probably feel cheated instead. To add insult to injury, they did not return to you the same $6.00 that you gave them; instead, they handed you foreign currency that was of significantly less value than yours.

That is exactly what is done to our bread. We entrust our health to massive food corporations who, despite what they advertise on their marketing labels, care much more about turning a profit than they do about our health. "The very notion that such a useless product builds strong bodies is an insult to the health and intelligence of every person. It's a wonder that such products can legally be sold as food."[2]

BACK TO REAL FOOD

In light of the nearly absolute depravity of commercially available flour, it is time to question our dependence on modern day food manufacturers to determine our food choices – and the state of our present and future health. There are so many natural alternatives that, by God's design, give our bodies the energy and fuel they need. These alternatives are tried and proven sources of a superior quality of life.

Grains are the seeds and fruits of cereal grasses, though the term "grain" encompasses plant sourced foods as well. There is such a wonderful variety of grains that you'll never again need to buy a loaf of white bread made from grains robbed of their life. Here is a discussion of these grains. Included are some grain byproducts that have been partially processed or refined, such as pearled barley. They are listed in our discussion for clarity, to provide a simple but thorough understanding of the various grain forms available. Cooking instructions provided are for preparation of the whole grains for use in porridge, side dishes, etc. Consult the notes about individual flours for proper whole grain flour usage.

Amaranth

Amaranth does not come from a grass, but from a plant. As such, it is technically not a grain but is usually classified as such. It was a staple food of the Aztecs because it thrived on the climate of Central and South America. It has also been familiar to India, Pakistan, and China for centuries. It is now grown throughout the world, including the United States.

Amaranth is a veritable gold mine of nutrition. It is higher in fiber than wheat, corn, or rice, has more calcium than milk, and contains four times the iron of brown rice. Amaranth is high in protein; in fact, it contains more protein than corn or beans. Most of the protein is from the germ, which is rich in lysine and methionine, two essential amino acids. It also contains potassium, phosphorus, linoleic acid, and vitamins A, C, and E.

~ Place 1 cup amaranth grains and 3 cups cold water or vegetable broth in a pan and bring to a boil. Simmer, uncovered, for 25 minutes. Add spices, herbs, vegetables, or other grains. (Amaranth is relatively unappetizing by itself.)

Amaranth flour is at its best when used in conjunction with other flours, rather than as the primary flour. In place of refined white flour, use 1 part amaranth and 3 parts whole wheat or other flour. If you do attempt to substitute just amaranth for white flour, use 7/8 cup amaranth in place of 1 cup white flour. Also, do not use amaranth in recipes that require baking yeast.

Barley

Barley, of indefinite origin, was the primary grain of the Middle East for years. Barley (Hebrew: seorah/Greek: krithinos) is mentioned 37 times in the Bible. It was one of the foods of the Promised Land (Deuteronomy 8:8). One of Israel's judges, Gideon, overheard an Amalekite tell of his dream in which "a cake of barley bread" tumbled into the enemy camp and conquered it (Judges 7:13). Ruth worked for Boaz during the wheat and barley harvests (Ruth 2:23). Jesus used a lad's two small fish and five barley loaves to feed five thousand men.

Barley was the principal grain in Europe for several centuries until it was replaced by wheat. There are winter and spring barley varieties.

Whole grain barley is easily digested and is soothing for those with sensitive stomachs. Convalescents benefit from barley's soothing nature. The water used to cook barley can be used to treat sore throats. Cooked barley can be made into a poultice and applied to sores and abrasions.

Barley is loaded with dietary fiber, vitamins and minerals such as B2, B6, folic acid, and pantothenic acids. The tocotrienols in barley are family members to tocopherols (vitamin E) but some nutritionists consider them superior. Barley is known as heart medicine in the Middle East.

Barley has a malty sweetness that is great in soups, stews, salads, and casseroles. It may also be used in the place of potatoes, pasta, or rice. By itself, it is not preferred for bread making but has traditionally been combined with millet, spelt, or pea meal.

Barley has not just one, but two, inedible outer hulls. After they have been removed, the barley is still nutritionally intact.

~ Add 1 cup whole grain barley to 3 cups water. Simmer, uncovered, for about 1 hour.

Pearled barley is a nutritionally depleted form of whole grain barley. It is the victim of pearling, an abrasive process that removes the aleurone, a third edible hull which is rich in protein, B vitamins, and fiber. Almost all of the fiber and more than half of the protein, fat, and minerals of the whole barley kernel are lost when this third layer is removed. Its one saving grace is that it is mild and easy on the stomach and can be used during times of sickness. Quick barley is the instant form of pearled barley.

Rolled barley (barley flakes) is processed the same way as oatmeal. It takes less time to cook than the whole grain and can be used to make a hot breakfast porridge or muesli.

Barley grits are barley grains that have been toasted, then cracked or coarsely ground. They cook quickly and may be used in salads, casseroles, and baking. Some people use them for a breakfast cereal or in place of rice.

Barley flour is excellent for baking but is best used in conjunction with wheat or other high gluten flours. Use one part barley flour with five parts other flour(s). You may substitute 1-3/8 cup barley flour for 1 cup white flour; however, expect overly moist baked goods if you use barley as the primary flour for a recipe. Barley can also be used as a thickening agent.

Buckwheat

Said to have originated in Manchuria and Siberia, buckwheat was first cultivated in China. It is technically not a cereal grain, but an edible fruit seed that is harvested from a plant that resembles a wild bush rather than a grass.

Buckwheat contains all eight essential amino acids, containing more lysine than any other grain. It is fairly high in protein and is a good source of B vitamins, vitamin E, potassium, magnesium, calcium, iron, and dietary fiber. It aids in circulation and even protects against the harmful effects of radiation.

Once the hull is removed, the result is white or light green three-cornered seeds, called groats. Buckwheat groats may be used in place of rice. Some usage ideas are mixing it into a cold pasta salad, serving it with cooked winter squash, adding it to stuffing, pilafs, or soups, or cooking it as a cereal. Some people recommend combining uncooked buckwheat with egg before it is cooked in water. This purportedly binds the buckwheat and keeps its shape intact.

Try soba noodles, made from buckwheat – a Japanese favorite!

~ Add 1 cup whole buckwheat to 2 cups boiling water; cover, and simmer for 15 to 20 minutes.

Kasha is toasted buckwheat, a longtime Russian staple. The inedible outer hull of the buckwheat groat is removed and the raw groat is lightly toasted. This brown, hearty food is a more complete protein than any other grain. Toasting buckwheat makes the iron content more available.

~ Mix one part kasha into one part hot or boiling water; let it stand for a few minutes. Add a little butter.

Buckwheat grits are buckwheat groats that have been coarsely cracked and finely ground. They have a creamy and soft texture. They are easy to digest but they lack the freshness of whole buckwheat groats. People use them in pudding-type desserts and soufflés.

Buckwheat flour has a hearty flavor that can be used in baking. Because it is low in gluten, you may find it more satisfying to mix it with wheat flour when making bread. However, my husband loves all-buckwheat pancakes. Use 3/4 to 7/8 cups buckwheat flour in place of 1 cup white flour.

Corn

Corn is the only cereal grain native to the American continents, cultivated by Native Americans such as the Peruvian Incas. Though most of us think of corn as being yellow or white, some types common to these peoples were actually blue, red, pink, and even black. Central and South Americans have many uses for corn, grinding it into tortillas, tamales, and other unleavened breads. In the Southern United States, corn is eaten as grits and hominy.

There are many varieties of corn. The sweet vegetable, corn on the cob, is softer, moister, and sweeter than grain varieties. Popcorn, a high fiber, low calorie snack food, is another variety. Dent corn is a variety that is mostly used for animal feed; the rest is processed into corn oil, corn syrup, cornstarch, and breakfast foods. Flour corn is used to make corn flour and cornstarch as well. Flint corn (Indian corn) is the variety from which corn chips and tortillas are made. Atole (blue corn) is a type of flint corn. It is sweet and contains more protein, manganese, potassium, lysine, and iron than yellow corn.

Corn is a balanced starch. Most corn types are low in the essential amino acids lysine and tryptophan but high in oleic, linolenic, and arachidonic acids. It is also high in thiamine, pantothenic acid (vitamin B5), folate, vitamin C, phosphorus, manganese, and fiber. Whole grain corn is the only grain that contains vitamin A. When corn is combined with beans it becomes a more complete protein food.

~ Soak 1 cup of yellow corn grains in water overnight to reconstitute. Simmer in 3 cups water about 35 minutes, or until tender. Try it mixed with other whole cooked grains or rice. Season with cumin, garlic, green onions, cilantro, or parsley. Try adding it to soup.

Cornstarch and corn flour are used as thickening agents and to make tortillas. Corn flour may be added to breads. Commercial cornstarch and corn flour are void of nutritional value because the nutrition has been "refined" away. 1 cup corn flour may be substituted for 1 cup white flour.

Cornmeal is coarsely ground corn grain. Look for stone ground, whole grain cornmeal. It can be used in tamales, pancakes, tortillas, and muffins. 1 cup cornmeal may be substituted for 1 cup white flour in recipes.

Masa is produced from whole kernel corn that has been soaked or boiled, drained, washed, and ground into a paste. This paste can be shaped into balls, flattened and cooked like a pancake.

Polenta is coarsely ground, cooked cornmeal. Again, look for whole grain polenta for optimal nutrition.

~ Bring 3 cups salted water to a boil. Add 1 cup polenta. Cover, reduce heat, and simmer 25 minutes. It can be fried or grilled and served with vegetables or topped with marinara sauce, pesto, or cheese.

The versatility of corn yields many more uses than these listed here. Don't be afraid to eat corn and corn products because of its high carbohydrate content; just enjoy it in moderation!

Kamut

Kamut is an ancient Egyptian wheat. Interestingly, in the language of ancient Egyptians, the word "kamut" translates to "wheat."

Kamut is purer than the wheat most commonly used today. Superior to wheat in many ways, it has more protein, magnesium, zinc, and vitamin E. Kamut is easy to digest and is a great source of energy. Though it contains gluten, many wheat sensitive people can eat it without adverse reactions.

~ Add 1 cup whole grain kamut to 3 cups boiling water. Reduce heat to low and simmer for about 2 hours. Mix it with rice, black beans, garlic, red pepper, cilantro and tamari. It can also be eaten hot or cold. Add it to salads or soups.

Kamut flakes are made in a similar way as rolled oats. They can be added to cookies, meat loaf, or used anywhere you would use oats.

~ To use kamut flakes to make hot cereal, add 1 cup kamut flakes to 2 cups boiling water. Cover, reduce heat and simmer until soft, about 15-20 minutes. Add vanilla extract, dried fruit, cinnamon, or nuts. Sweeten with honey or maple syrup.

Kamut flour is a delicious substitute for white flour. Use 7/8 to 1 cup kamut flour in place of 1 cup white flour for general purpose needs. Some people find it unsuitable for high-rise baking but excellent for pizza crusts, pasta, and the like.

Millet

One of the ingredients in Ezekiel's bread, millet (Hebrew: dochan) is an ancient grain that Asians and Middle Easterners are well acquainted with (Ezekiel 4:9). It has a distinctive flavor and is highly nutritious. It is gluten free and easy to digest. It is the only alkaline grain and is one of the least allergenic. It has the most complete protein of any of the true cereal grains. It is rich in fiber and silica, which help detoxify the liver. It is also an excellent source of niacin, thiamine, riboflavin, methionine, lecithin, vitamin E, iron, magnesium, manganese, phosphorus, and potassium.

~ Combine 1 cup millet and 3 cups water. Bring to a boil, reduce heat and simmer, uncovered, for about 30 minutes. Remove from heat and let stand about 15 minutes before serving. Try serving it with curry flavored vegetables.

Cracked millet, millet meal, and puffed millet are all forms of millet which will add versatility and flavor to your traditional meals.

Millet flour is best when used in conjunction with other flours when making a high-rise baked product. For non-leavening baking needs, use 3/4 cup millet flour in place of 1 cup white flour.

Oats

Oats are thought to be of western European origin. Today we often think of the Scots when we think of oats, as oats have been integral to their diets for many years. There are both winter and spring varieties of oats. Outside of oatmeal, where most of us get our ration of oats, there are many uses for oats.

Oats are an antioxidant and are warming on a cold winter's day. They are high in fiber and possibly helpful for those with under active thyroid glands.

Whole oats are entirely unprocessed and yield all the benefits of the bran and germ of the oat. They may be used in porridge, combined with other grains, and, after precooking, used for baking.

Oat groats are hulled, cleaned, dried, and slightly roasted whole oat kernels. Most of the nutrition of the whole oat is retained. Use them in baking or cereal.

~ Simmer 1 cup oat groats in 3 cups water for about 2 hours.

Rolled oats are made by slicing and steaming the groats and then rolling them flat. The amount of pressure used in the rolling process determines how much the groats are flattened. Rolled oats are used to make oatmeal.

~ To cook rolled oats, add 1 cup rolled oats to 3 cups boiling water; cover, reduce heat and simmer for 20 minutes.

Quick (instant) oats are finely rolled oat groats. They cook faster than the thicker rolled oats. Quick oats are generally used in bread products and to make toppings for fruit crisps. Both rolled and quick oats that are made from the whole grain should be stored in the refrigerator to prevent rancidity.

~ To cook quick oats, add 1 cup quick oats to 2-1/2 cups boiling water; cover, and simmer for 5-10 minutes.

Steel cut oats are whole oats that have been sliced, not rolled. This creates small oat chips. These are sometimes called Scotch or Irish oats. Soak before cooking.

~ Add 1 cup steel cut oats to 3 cups water; cover and simmer about 30 minutes.

Oat bran is a source of soluble fiber and helps lower blood cholesterol. Store whole grain oat bran in the refrigerator to prevent rancidity.

Oat flour can be used in place of white or whole wheat pastry flour. It adds a light flavor to breads and pastries. Use 3/4 to 1 cup oat flour in place of 1 cup white or whole wheat pastry flour. Adding oat flour to baked goods helps preserve freshness, on account of its antioxidant content. When making leavened bread, oat flour needs to be used in conjunction with high gluten flour in order for the bread to sufficiently rise.

Quinoa

Quinoa is the fruit of an annual herb, not actually a cereal grain. There are hundreds of different strains of quinoa that vary in shape, flavor, and color. The colors of quinoa may be yellow, orange, red, pink, purple, black, and white though the ones most available in the United States are pale yellow. These small, flat, disk shaped seeds have been farmed in the mountain regions of Peru and Bolivia for thousands of years. They use quinoa in soups and stews, boil it like rice, and grind it into flour for tortillas, breads, and biscuits.

About twice the protein of barley, corn, and rice, quinoa is a good source of calcium, iron, vitamin E, phosphorus, and some B vitamins, making it a high energy food. Quinoa contains all the essential amino acids. It cooks quickly, and its delicious flavor nicely complements vegetables, beans, and meat. Quinoa may be substituted for bulgur in tabouli.

~ Rinse the quinoa thoroughly. Add 1 cup quinoa to 2 cups boiling water; cover, reduce heat and simmer for about 15 minutes, or until all the water is absorbed.

Quinoa flour adds moisture to baking recipes. Its light texture makes nice pastry products. Combine it with gluten containing flours when making leavened bread.

Rice

Rice is the most widely consumed staple food in the world. Half of the world's population uses rice as a main part of their diet. Rice is especially common to Asians. In fact, the Chinese word for "rice" translates to "good grain of life." A moist, subtropical climate is necessary for the cultivation of rice and ninety percent of all rice is grown in India, China, and Japan.

There are thousands of strains of rice. Rice is an incomplete protein and should be combined with beans or meat.

Refined white rice is the rice most familiar to Americans and it is the one that should be most avoided. Processing removes the vitamins, minerals, and protein from the grain. Because refined white rice is almost all starch - a simple carbohydrate - low-carb fanatics do their best to defame rice. While refined white rice will promote obesity, rice in its natural state is a healthful whole food that has been sustaining societies for thousands of years. Low-carb contenders fail to distinguish between refined white rice and whole grain rice. By doing so, they deprive the public of a host of exciting and delicious healthy rice varieties.

Arborio rice is often used to make traditional Italian foods such as risotto, paella, and rice pudding. It is nearly round and naturally white.

Brown rice is a great source of B vitamins, calcium, phosphorous, vitamin E, iron, and dietary fiber. Brown rice is available in short, medium, and long grain varieties. The nutrition is similar no matter the size. Short grain brown rice is chewier than medium or long grain brown rice. It is sweeter, starchier, and stickier than long grain brown rice. Medium grain brown rice cooks into a fluffier rice than short grain brown rice. The texture of long grain brown rice resembles that of white rice when cooked and is the preferred rice for salads. Instant brown rice has been cooked and dried. It is fast cooking and most of the nutrients are still intact.

~ To cook non-instant brown rice, combine 2 cups water and 1 cup rice. Bring to a boil, lower heat, and simmer, uncovered, for about 45 minutes.

Basmati rice originated in Asia. It is usually brown but is sometimes polished white. It has a nutty flavor and is lower in starch than other long-grain rice varieties. It is often used in Indian cuisine. Wehini (or, Wehani) and Calmati rice varieties are grown in California. Texmati rice is grown mostly in Texas.

Jasmine rice is a long-grain white rice grown in Thailand. Soft and a little sticky, it is similar to basmati. Both are a pleasant departure from refined white rice.

Sweet brown rice is a sticky short grain variety that is used in Asian desserts, and is mixed with regular brown rice to make sushi.

Other types of rice that you might want to try are Golden Rose, red rice (also known as Christmas rice, similar to Wehini), Japonica (Thai black rice), and wild pecan rice (grown in southern Lousiana).

Rice flour is usually made from brown rice. It may be used in pancakes, baked goods, and gravies. To substitute, use 7/8 to 1 cup rice flour in place of 1 cup white flour. This may create a drier product than desired; if so, blend with other whole grain flours.

Rye

Rye is high in essential amino acid lysine. It contains B vitamins, iron, vitamin E, and protein, making it a powerhouse tool for artery cleansing and liver support. It is a great source of energy and strengthens the muscular system.

Rye berries are whole rye kernels that are often sprouted, then added to breakfast cereals, breads, soups, or salads.

~ To cook, add 1 cup rye berries to 4 cups water; cover, and simmer for 1-1/2 hours.

Cracked rye is whole rye berries that are broken or ground into pieces. Though most rye is used for bread baking, it can be used in this form to enjoy as a hot breakfast cereal. Some people add cracked rye to soups.

Rye flakes are whole grain rye berries that are processed similarly to rolled oats. They can also be used as a breakfast cereal and added to bread products. Try using rye flakes in place of oatmeal when making meat loaf and use them as a soup thickener.

~ To cook, add 1 cup rye flakes to 3 cups boiling water. Cover, and simmer for 30 minutes.

Rye flour gives bread a dark brown color. Using rye flour exclusively will yield dense, moist bread. Try combining it with other flours. Rye is the main ingredient in pumpernickel bread. Rye bread is very filling. The hearty signature flavor of rye is exactly why it is probably the grain I like the least and why others like it a lot.

Spelt

Along with barley and wheat, spelt is also specifically mentioned in the Bible. It is called rie (Hebrew: kuccemeth) and should not be confused with the rye that is more common to many of us. Because it was not grown up, rie, as well as wheat, escaped the plague of hail that came upon the Egyptians (Exodus 9:32). Isaiah 28:25 and Ezekiel 4:9 also mention rie – or spelt, as it is called today.

Spelt is highly water soluble; thus, it is relatively easy to digest, much more so than wheat flour. Though spelt does contain gluten, some people who are gluten sensitive can tolerate it. Spelt is similar to wheat in many ways and can be used almost anywhere traditional wheat would be used.

Spelt flour creates breads with a pleasant texture. It is excellent when used to make sourdough bread. Substitute 1 to 1 for white flour and reduce the liquid in the recipe by 25%. Take care to not over knead the bread dough.

Teff

Teff originated as a wild growing grass of northern Africa. Ethiopians in particular found teff a source of energy and health. Still today they ferment teff for several days before making injera, their common bread. When I was a kid, I tasted injera at an Ethiopian restaurant in St. Louis. It was shaped similarly to a tortilla but thicker. In true Ethiopian style, we used it to dip into sauces and scoop up accompanying foods.

Teff is the tiniest grain in the world and its color ranges from white to reddish-purple to brown. Soups, stews, cereals, and porridges all benefit from the addition of teff. Teff is loaded with calcium, copper, zinc, and protein. It is an excellent source of iron. Your specific health needs will determine the color of teff you choose: The darker the teff, the more iron it contains. The lighter the teff, the more protein it has.

~ To cook, add one cup teff berries to 4 cups boiling water. Cover and simmer for 15 minutes.

Teff flour is great in unleavened recipes for muffins, pancakes, cookies, and quick breads. Do not use just teff flour in traditional yeast recipes. Instead, use 1 part teff and 5 parts whole wheat flour. Teff is unique in that it makes naturally leavened bread and can be used in place of sourdough starter. Simply mix one cup of teff flour with one and a half cups water; cover, and allow to stand at room temperature for 24 hours.

Triticale

Triticale is the product of the marriage of wheat (*Triticum*) and rye (*Secale*). Triticale is higher in lysine and lower in gluten than wheat, and higher in protein than either wheat or rye. Triticale has a richer flavor than wheat but does not have the heavy flavor of rye.

~ To cook, add 1 cup triticale berries to 3 cups boiling water. Simmer, covered, for two hours. (If the berries have soaked overnight, cooking time will be only 50-60 minutes.)

Cracked triticale serves the same purposes as cracked wheat. Make your own by putting whole kernel triticale in a blender and processing until coarse.

Triticale flour has a sweet, nutty flavor and can be used in baking. Though it is best when combined with other flours, 1 cup of triticale flour can be used in place of 1 cup white flour.

Wheat

For thousands of years many societies have cultivated wheat. Wheat (Hebrew: chittah/Greek: sitos) is mentioned 51 times in the Bible. There are many, many varieties of wheat and it is still a staple food worldwide.

Wheat is not native to the United States but was introduced by American colonists who brought it with them from across the seas. Now the United States produces more wheat than any other nation in the world and it consumes far more wheat than any other grain. Unfortunately, that consumption is a genetically altered, highly refined, nutrient deficient form of wheat.

Wheat is high in B vitamins, vitamin E, chromium, iron, magnesium, manganese, zinc, and fiber. The insoluble fiber in wheat protects against and cures constipation, prevents intestinal infections, hemorrhoids, varicose veins, and colon cancer.

~ Wheat berries can be cooked as a cereal. Combine 2 cups water and 1 cup wheat berries. Simmer, uncovered, about 45 minutes.

Here is a simple breakdown of common wheat varieties:

Hard wheat has a higher gluten content than soft wheat, making it ideal for baking that requires leavening.

Hard spring wheat is planted in the spring and harvested in the fall. It is the best choice for bread baking because it has a little more gluten than hard winter wheat.

Hard winter wheat is planted in the fall and harvested in late spring or early summer. It lies dormant in the winter and its longer growing season provides it with a higher vitamin and mineral content than hard spring wheat.

Soft, or white, wheat (also available in spring and winter varieties) is ideal for making cakes and pastries.

Now for a discussion of wheat products. Throughout history, wheat's versatility has made it a source of many uses to people in varying cultures. These listed here are only some of the more common.

Bulgur is whole wheat berries that have been steamed, dried, and cracked. As bulgur is being processed, the bran is usually removed, destroying many of the nutrients; in this form, it is not a whole food. Try to find bulgur that says that it is "whole grain" bulgur. Dark colored bulgur is from hard red wheat. White bulgur is from soft white wheat. Dark bulgur has a stronger flavor than white bulgur. Tabouli (tabbouleh) is a popular Lebanese dish that uses bulgur as its main ingredient.

~ Add 1 cup bulgur to 2 cups water, and simmer for 15-25 minutes. Let stand, covered, for 10 minutes before serving.

Couscous is usually made from semolina. Semolina is the endosperm of durum wheat. The germ and bran are removed. After the endosperm is ground, it is mixed with water. This substance is then cracked into small pieces, steamed, and dried. The end product is quick-cooking tiny round granules. Unfortunately, this process also removes most of the fiber, protein, fat, and minerals native to the wheat berry. Couscous in this nutritionally depleted state is not exceptionally healthy. Look for a non-refined, whole grain couscous that has retained the bran and germ. Couscous is a traditional food of North Africans, who often serve it with meat.

~ Add 1-1/2 cups boiling water to 1 cup couscous, and let stand for 15 minutes.

Cracked wheat is just what it sounds like it is: whole-wheat berries that have been cracked into small pieces. It is very similar to bulgur. It is used in cereals and breads and can be used in place of either bulgur or rice. Cracked wheat cooks more quickly than whole-wheat berries, which are actually rarely eaten because of the jaw action required.

Cream of wheat (farina) is sometimes made from the whole grain and sometimes made from just the endosperm. Again, examine labels to see what you are really buying. Cream of wheat is mostly used as a hot breakfast cereal.

Durum wheat is hard spring wheat. It is, in fact, the hardest of all wheat species. It has a high protein and gluten content. When durum wheat is ground, the endosperm is milled into a product called semolina, which is often used to make pasta. Unfortunately, since it is refined, widely used semolina is not necessarily the healthiest choice for flour and pasta needs.

Whole wheat flour is easily substituted for white flour. Simply use 3/4 to 1-1/4 cup whole wheat flour in place of white flour. The uses of this flour are endless and can be used anywhere you would normally use white flour. It is light brown in color and denser than white flour. Regular whole wheat flour is made from hard wheat. Whole wheat pastry flour is made from soft wheat.

The health benefits of whole wheat are many. Whole wheat contains protein, iron, and calcium as well as traces of barium and vanadium, which are essential for heart health. Wheat stimulates the liver, which cleanses the body of toxins. The germ of wheat is one of few foods that contain the complete vitamin B complex.

Like rice, wheat is most frequently consumed in its most nutrient deficient state, especially in the United States. When wheat is stripped of its "life" – the bran and the germ – it loses up to 80% of its vitamins and minerals and as much as 93% of its fiber. The synthetic B vitamins that are added to enriched bread are difficult to digest because they are not in the proper proportions necessary for assimilation.

To make white flour, the bran and germ are removed and the endosperm is pulverized into a fine starchy powder. The powder is bleached and manipulated with "dough conditioners." Carcinogenic preservatives are the final insult before synthetic vitamins are added for any nutrition to be present at all. That white flour hurts more than it helps is a moot point. For example, alloxan, one of the bleaching agents that makes refined flour so white, destroys the beta cells of the pancreas. The little saying that circulates among the health conscious - "The whiter the bread, the sooner you're dead" - may be a little brash but contains a measure of truth, considering the un-debatable facts.

Wild Rice

Neither a rice nor cereal grain, wild rice is the fruit seed of tall marshland grass. Native to the United States and Canada, it grows in shallow ponds, lakes and wetland areas.

Some packages that say "wild rice" are not really wild at all. Using hybrid seeds, this rice is commercially grown and cultivated with the use of agricultural chemicals and mechanically harvested. This type of rice is usually a shiny dark color.

True "wild rice" is still harvested by hand and parched over open fires. Its color will range from a red-brown to a gray-green.

Wild rice is a rich source of protein, iron, and B vitamins. It has a nutty, smoky flavor and is often mixed with other rice. There are three grades of wild rice: 1) "Select" – short, broken grains, 2) most common "extra fancy" – ½ inch long grains and 3) most expensive "giant" – 1 inch long grains.

~ Add 1 cup wild rice to 4 cups boiling water; reduce heat and simmer, uncovered, for 45 to 60 minutes.

Wild rice flour is a nice departure from white flour when baking muffins, pancakes, and waffles.

SHOP SMART

In the world of marketing, packaging and labeling is everything. Train yourself to look beyond blatant claims to the fine print. Become a savvy reader of ingredients lists. Some advertisers use phrases like "Great Source of Fiber," "Multigrain," Whole-grain Bread," "Wheat Flour," and "Made with Whole Grains" in an attempt to appeal to your desire to eat healthily. Their claims may or may not be true and it is up to you to find out the truth by reading beyond the bold, splashy front label.

The following terms refer to flours that are highly refined and not recommended: all purpose flour, enriched flour, bleached flour, bread flour, gluten flour, self rising flour, unbleached wheat flour, and white flour. These are all nutritionally inferior wheat products that are the result of ultra refinement. They are depleted of innate vitamins, minerals, and necessary fiber when the bran and germ are milled away and contribute little or nothing to our good health, but rather detract from it.

The first ingredient on the ingredients list of a true whole-grain flour product should be "whole grain" or "whole wheat." Look for bread products that are truly whole grain. Just as it is wise to read the fine print when purchasing a vehicle or house, it is important to read about what you are committing yourself to when you purchase food that you will eat. After all, you are making an investment in the health of your body - the house of the Lord.

GRINDING AT THE MILL

You can avoid the label confusion at the supermarket altogether by grinding your own flour at home. A small kitchen mill is relatively inexpensive and enables you to grind flour as needed. This will ensure you fresh, whole grain flour. Most mills allow you to grind the grain as coarse or fine as you need. There are several types of kitchen mills available, all of them easy to use.

Be sure to store extra flour in the refrigerator for up to one week or in the freezer for up to one month, as it will otherwise quickly become rancid. Each day after grinding, the flour loses a percentage of its enzymes and vitamins when left at room temperature and the chances of rancidity increase. Remember, such flour still contains all of the "life" of the whole grain. When exposed to air, it begins to oxidize.

WHOLE GRAIN FLOUR

Adjustments will need to be made when cooking or baking with whole grain flour in place of refined white flour. The notes above for individual flours are provided as a primer for your natural-flour experimentation. Keep in mind that baking with whole grains is not a fine science. Different grains behave differently according to their individual gluten and protein content and other unique properties. Use the tips and suggestions as a guide and tweak them in as necessary to compensate for variables such as your oven temperature, altitude, fineness of flour, and personal taste.

Also, substitutions are not provided for all gluten-free flours. They are best when combined with other flours, instead of being the only flour used for a recipe. When baking with gluten-free flour, it is necessary to add gluten to bind it together and help the bread rise. In the case of gluten intolerance, plant based xanthan gum or guar gum may be added to yield satisfactory results.

GLUTEN INTOLERANCE

Gluten is a protein found in wheat and similar grains. It is what creates elasticity when making leavened bread. Celiac disease is gluten intolerance. Gluten intolerant people cannot eat foods that contain gluten because their immune systems cannot process it appropriately and the gluten damages the lining of their small intestines.

Gluten is found in many products and masquerades under many names such as hydrolyzed vegetable protein, textured vegetable protein, and hydrolyzed plant protein. Grain vinegars, malt vinegars, some soy sauces, and modified cornstarch all contain gluten and must be avoided by gluten intolerant individuals.

However, the most obvious and prevalent gluten-containing-foods are grains and their byproducts. Some high gluten grains are barley, kamut, spelt, rye, triticale, and wheat. Some gluten-free and low gluten grains are amaranth, buckwheat, corn, millet, quinoa, rice, teff, and wild rice.

Note: There seems to be some debate about the link between oats and gluten sensitivity. If in doubt, do without. Also, there are other low gluten grains, like sorghum, that are not discussed in this book. Those with celiac disease are encouraged to further investigate their gluten-free options.

It is interesting to note that some researchers have suggested that wheat allergies may be due to the genetic modification of wheat, not the wheat itself. If you have a wheat allergy, perhaps you should attempt to grind, soak, and bake your own organic wheat products before shunning them altogether. It is possible that consuming wheat and other grains as God created them might be more acceptable to your body than modern man's "new and improved" varieties.

THE PHYTIC ACID FACTOR

Phytic acids are compounds located in the outer layer and bran of grains that interfere with nutrient absorption. Because untreated phytic acid inhibits proper assimilation of calcium, magnesium, copper, iron, and zinc, people who consume great amounts of unfermented grains may experience bone loss and mineral deficiencies. Phytic acid has been linked to anemia, rickets, and nervous disorders.

Soaking whole grains and freshly ground flour overnight enables the enzymes in the grain to break down, thereby neutralizing the negative effects of phytic acid. This aids digestion and allows your body to retain and utilize the inherent healthful properties of the grain. Soaking is simple and yields tremendous nutritional benefits by creating an environment for beneficial enzymes to increase the availability of many vitamins, particularly B vitamins.

Grains that contain high levels of gluten are generally more difficult to digest because they contain higher levels of phytic acid. Thus, it is more essential to soak gluten-containing-grains than gluten-free grains. The soaking process breaks down the gluten, aiding digestion. Whole rice and whole millet have less phytate content than other grains.

Soaking is a process that has been intrinsically used by a variety of cultures and societies throughout time. For example, sourdough bread, the absolute staple bread of England and colonial America, was fermented. Some of the foods that create a good environment for the soaking of grains are yogurt, kefir, and buttermilk. A little whey, lemon juice, or vinegar added to water will produce the same effects.

Also, soaking and sprouting whole grains increases vitamin, mineral, and enzyme availability. When grains are sprouted and then made into loaves of bread they are less subject to oxidation than ground grains.

Though space does not permit thorough directions for soaking, fermenting, and sprouting whole grains and other whole foods such as beans, nuts, and seeds, your local health food store should be able to direct you to some additional resources on this subject.

BALANCE AND CREATIVITY

Though whole grains are much preferred to their refined counterparts, they should not be eaten exclusively. We should strive to achieve a nutritional balance and glean from the entire spectrum of God's bounty, from fats to dairy to grains. Traditionally, grains were eaten with beans, meat, or dairy products. Though most grains provide most of the essential amino acids, the protein found in some grains may be low in one or more of them. (Amino acids are the building blocks of protein.) Other foods contain the amino acids that grains lack and sufficiently complement them.

Eating whole grains for breakfast will provide long lasting energy and keep you from getting listless and hungry, as is often the case with the consumption of simple carbohydrate, high sugar breakfast cereals, breads, and pastries. Soak the grains overnight and then cook them in the soaking water or drain that water and cook the grains in milk or fruit juice for flavor variation. Be creative and mix in your favorite additions. Some ideas are raisins, fruits (fresh or dried) such as apples, bananas, and peaches, and nuts such as walnuts and pecans. Use hearty spices like cinnamon and ginger. Sweeten your nutritious concoction with something light like honey or agave nectar. With just a little forethought, you will have a breakfast that is easy to prepare and requires little clean-up.

A little butter or cream helps the minerals in grains to be better absorbed.

Since most pasta is made from grains, the same principles that apply to grains apply to pasta. Wholegrain, even sprouted pasta is far superior to enriched pasta.

THE STAFF OF LIFE

In Jesus' lesson to His disciples, He used bread as an object lesson to teach them about prayer. "Give us this day our daily bread" (Matthew 6:11). Hearing about bread that was baked daily was something they could relate to.

In the Bible, the term "staff of bread" referred to the nourishing staple of the times. Bread was such a common, wholesome food that the phrase "staff of bread" evolved into "staff of life" because people equated bread with life. A staff was a multi-purpose object, one of its uses being a support. Thus, bread was considered life support for our biblical forefathers.

Man's tampering with the staff of life has resulted in the nourishing qualities of bread being broken. We eat, and are not satisfied, because the God-placed nutrition in the grains He created has been removed and replaced with chemicals and laboratory produced substances (Leviticus 26:26).

Bread of Bible days had very few additions. Depending on the purpose of the bread, oil might be added (Exodus 29:2). It is possible that honey was sometimes used as a sweetener (Exodus 16:31). And, depending on the purpose of the bread, leaven might be added (Matthew 13:33). Compare these simple ingredients to the ingredients list on the label of the loaf of "enriched" bread in your kitchen. Most of them are difficult to pronounce, let alone define.

By destroying the germ and bran of the grain, the life is removed. Bread is no longer a sustaining food to be enjoyed fresh daily, but a product void of life that serves to deliver a profit to the manufacturer but rob the consumer of the benefits of the whole grain.

It is time to return to enjoying grains the way God designed them to be enjoyed: in their wholesome state, complete and untainted. Try your hand at grinding your own flour, baking your own bread, and eating grains whole. It is fun, and creating healthful "staff of life" recipes for your family will be intensely satisfying.

EIGHTEEN

SIMPLY SWEET

My son, eat thou honey, because it is good;
and the honeycomb, which is sweet to thy taste:
Proverbs 24:13

Refined white sugar, the most common type of sweetener found in America's homes and present in the majority of packaged commercial foods, is made from sugar cane or sugar beets. White sugar, or sucrose, is a disaccharide (double sugar). It is made from glucose and fructose. It is highly processed and bleached. During production, any beneficial properties of the original sugar product are eliminated.

SUGAR'S HISTORY
The date of sugar's initial "discovery" is unknown. We do know that around 500 B.C. India became the first country to make sugar from the cane. Shortly thereafter sugar was imported from Asia to the Middle East. Europeans were not exposed to sugar until the 8th century, when the Arabs planted cane in Spain. It was then called "the honey-bearing reed" and was a luxury item for only the wealthy. It was not available for common use in European households until the 17th century.

Early American housewives used honey, sorghum, molasses, native New England maple sugar, or no sweetener at all until the late 1700s. Even though sugar became more accessible, only relatively recently has it gained widespread acceptance.

Americans led the way in sugar consumption. "The U.S. has consumed one-fifth of the world's production of sugar every year but one since the Civil War. By

1893, America was consuming more sugar than the whole world had produced in 1865."[1]

Early sugar processing was a fairly harmless procedure. People would grind or pound the cane to extract the juice. The cane juice was boiled and, as the water evaporated, sugar crystals formed. These crystals contained fiber, vitamins, and minerals. To people years ago, these crystals resembled gravel. The Sanskrit word for sugar (sharkara) also means "gravel" or "pebble."

MODERN SUGAR PROCESSING

Today, sugar processing is a fine art, striving to supply a high demand. Manufacturers employ every technological, chemical, and mechanical means available to ensure that they can produce a huge volume of sugar with limited expense. In their efforts to make sugar production as efficient and cost effective as possible, the simple archaic process of obtaining sugar from the cane or beet has been discarded.

Contrast the following complicated modern steps of sugar cane production to the original simple method.

"Sugar cane is harvested by hand or by machine. The cut cane is taken to a factory, where the stalks are washed and shredded. They are then placed in a crushing machine or into vats of hot water that dissolve the sugar. Crushing machines burst the cane, squeezing out the sugary liquid from the stalks. Sprays of water dissolve more sugar from the shredded stalks.

"The mixture of sugar and water, called cane juice, is then taken away for purifying. The cane juice, still diluted with water, is heated. Lime (calcium hydroxide) is added to the juice to settle out impurities, and carbon dioxide is used to remove the excess lime.

"Workers then put the clarified juice in huge evaporator tanks, where most of the water is evaporated and the juice becomes thick and syrupy. However, more water must be removed from the syrup so that sugar crystals will form. The syrup is heated in large, dome-shaped vacuum pans to remove excess water.

"After large sugar crystals form in the thick syrup, workers put the mixture in a centrifuge. This machine spins at extremely high speeds and separates most of the syrup from the crystals.

"To obtain pure white sugar for table use, the yellowish-brown raw sugar must go through several more steps. The film that gives raw sugar its yellow-brown color is rinsed off. Next, the sugar crystals are dissolved in water, and the solution is poured through filters until it becomes a clear, colorless liquid. The liquid is then evaporated until crystals form again. The crystals are again spun in the centrifuge, and pure white sugar flows from the machine into drying drums. Heated air in the drums absorbs any remaining moisture. The sugar is then packaged for market."[2]

Somewhere during this procedure, sulfur dioxide is added as a bleaching agent. By the time the entire sugar production process is complete, any nutrients that were original to the cane are gone. They have been heated, treated, washed, and bleached away. The pristine white sugar that we have grown accustomed to using has absolutely no nutritional benefits.

NOT-SO-SWEET FACTS ABOUT SUGAR

Sugar has no healthful properties. As a matter of fact, rather than providing a service to our bodies, it actually *robs* our bodies of nutrients. Ponder the following detrimental health hazards (just a few of many) of sugar.

- Sugar diabetes is a relatively new disease, one that developed as people began to eat more sugar. It has been said, "There would be no diabetes if everyone ate the way a diabetic is *supposed* to eat," i.e. do without sugar.
- Sugar consumption depletes calcium from the bones.
- Long-term sugar use weakens the health of our adrenal glands.
- Refined sugar decreases immune response by as much as 30% for four hours after ingesting sugar.

It stands to reason that those who subsist primarily on sugar-based foods are susceptible to infections, viruses, and colds.

- Tooth decay is the outward sign of sugar's inner workings.
- Refined sugar lacks chromium, present in raw sugar cane, and a mineral that is needed to regulate blood sugar.
- Sugar, a simple carbohydrate, serves as a quick pick-me-up. But it causes blood sugar to rise and fall rapidly. As the body quickly digests it, abnormally large amounts of sugar (or glucose) enter the bloodstream. This sugar surge requires the liver and pancreas to work overtime to withdraw the excess in order to balance blood sugar. The liver converts this excess glucose into starch and stores it in the cells as glycogen, which in turn changes to fat. As blood sugar levels drop, a person feels a craving for more synthetic energy food – sugar - creating a vicious cycle. This is the simple explanation of how we gain weight.
- Eating too much sugar can lower good cholesterol (HDL) and elevate triglycerides.
- Heart disease has been linked to excess sugar consumption.
- One of the key contributors to gastrointestinal cancer is the over consumption of sugar based products.

Again, sugar provides zero nutritional benefits. Sugar does contain calories, however: empty ones. Not a single beneficial vitamin, mineral, or enzyme can be found in sugar. There is *nothing* good in refined sugar. It actually *depletes* our bodies of good stuff and lowers our immune systems. When we eat sugar, our bodies don't identify it as real food because it does not actually nutritionally feed us. So shortly after we eat sugar, our bodies are unsatisfied and tell us they need something more. And what do we do then? Usually, we reach for more sugar, creating a sugar addiction cycle.

SUGAR, SUGAR EVERYWHERE

"The Sugar Association of the United States of America insists that...a quarter of our food and drink intake can safely consist of sugar."[3] Most Americans would rejoice with that assumption because most people do get about 25% of their daily intake of calories from sugar.

The average American consumes half a cup of refined, bleached sugar a day, well over *150 pounds* a year! Take a measuring cup and measure out half a cup of sugar. Look at it. Think, "I eat this every day." You might respond, "I don't eat a lot of sweets. I don't eat half a cup of sugar a day." Though you may not eat a box of candy bars or an entire pie in one day, you probably *are* eating more sugar than you think.

That's because sugar comes in many guises. Other than being called sugar, it is most frequently called high fructose corn syrup. The ingredients lists on products sometimes name dextrose as a sweetener. Dextrose is made by boiling cornstarch with acid. Other sugar derivatives and names for sugar are cane juice, caramel, dextran, fructose (also called levulose), glucose, invert sugar, maltodextrin, maltose, refiner's syrup, and yellow sugar. The ending "-ose" usually refers to some type of sugar.

Also, some people mistakenly conclude brown sugar to be relatively harmless and better than white sugar. Most brown sugar, however, is produced by adding molasses back into completely refined white sugar. The darker the brown sugar, the more molasses has been added. Chemicals and dyes are sometimes used in brown sugar processing.

In one form or another, sugar has made its way into nearly every commercially available food product. Canned soups, crackers, frozen entrees, sauces, salad dressings, juice, hamburger buns, bagels, and boxed dinner mixes all contain added sugar. Manufacturers add sugar to these and many, many more products to cheaply improve the flavor of food. Sugar is America's most commonly used food additive.

Sorbitol, mannitol, maltitol, and xylitol are called sugar alcohols. Strangely enough, they are neither sugar nor alcohol. They are carbohydrates that resemble sugar and alcohol. They are about half as sweet as sugar.

Excessive intake of sugar alcohols has been known to produce diarrhea, gas, cramping, and bloating. They are not metabolized well by all people. Xylitol is discussed later in this chapter because it does have some beneficial characteristics. But, along with these other sugar alcohols, it should be used with caution.

SOME INTERESTING OBSERVATIONS

~ The Kellogg Report – Joseph D. Beasley, MD and
Jerry J. Swift, MA *~*

One of the earliest warnings about the rising tide of sugar in our diet came from that 1942 AMA report: "The consumption of sugar and of other relatively pure carbohydrates has become so great during recent years that it presents a serious obstacle to the improved nutrition of the general public." In the strongest terms possible, the report called for "all practical means to be taken to limit consumption of sugar in any form" in which significant nutrients are not present (AMA 1942: 763, 765).

It was a call unheeded. From the end of war-time rationing to the present, the food industry has known no limit, beyond the technical, in using sugar to cheaply enhance the appeal of its processed and fabricated foods. In these last 40 years industry has more than doubled the sugar it adds to our diet. But protests are no longer heard – the watchdogs of the public's welfare appear to have been pacified.

In the mid 1970's the blue ribbon FASEB (Federation of American Societies for Experimental Biology), on contract to the FDA, wholeheartedly recommended the agency again approve sugar as a food additive, saying that with the possible exception of dental caries sucrose presents *no* risk to human health (FASEB 1976).[4]

~ *Sugar Blues* – William Dufty ~

In the summer of 1965, I met a wise man from the East, a Japanese philosopher who had just returned from several weeks in Saigon. "If you really expect to conquer the North Vietnamese," he told me, "you must drop Army PX's on them – sugar, candy, and Coca-Cola. That will destroy them faster than bombs."[5]

SWEET KIDS

The group being robbed the most by the ravages of sugar is our future generation of leaders.

While most adults get 25% of their calorie intake from nutrient-free sugar, sugar fills about half of the calorie intake of some children and adolescents. This translates into malnourishment that manifests itself into behavior disorders and impaired concentration in school. During their formative and adolescent years, when their bodies are still growing and changing, these children are disadvantaged as they attempt to flourish with only half of the nutrients they need.

The reduction of refined sugars, along with chemical food colorings, artificial flavorings, and processed foods can dramatically better a child's mood and behavior and increase his comprehension and concentration. The elimination of sugar and fake foods has been known to successfully alleviate allergies and even increase children's IQ's.

NATURAL SUGAR SUBSTITUTES

In the face of all the negative reports about sugar, there is hope. Learning to enjoy the natural sweetness of fruits and trading in refined, simple carbohydrate foods for whole foods is the beginning of a brand new way of living. Ceasing to rely on manmade, artificial, imitation nutrition is liberating. A return to foods as God made them is delicious and healthful.

When it comes to sweeteners, there are many, many wonderful natural substitutes for refined sugar. Most of them have nutritional benefits along with providing a rich variety of naturally sweet flavors.

Because of individual health needs and the varying properties of natural sweeteners, there is no hard-and-fast rule about which sweetener is the best. Educate yourself about them all, try them and see how your body responds to them, and then choose the ones that are best for you.

Natural sweeteners are extracted from a variety of sources, including grain and fruit. Some are liquid; others are dry. In addition to the natural sweeteners listed here, try cooking and baking with applesauce, bananas, and dates.

Raw honey – unfiltered and unprocessed - is our top pick. I use raw honey when baking and cooking and to sweeten tea. The flavor of honey just can't be beat. Its flavor will vary depending on the nectar source. Generally speaking, the lighter the honey the milder its flavor. Raw honey is available in varying degrees of sweetness. Honey is a natural combination of fructose, glucose, and water.

In order to produce one pound of honey, bees must visit two million flowers and fly more than 55,000 miles! In spite of all that effort, the average worker bee makes only one-twelfth of a teaspoon of honey during the course of its 6-week life.

Honey is mentioned 56 times in the Bible and honeycomb is mentioned nine times. While one admonition warns of the dangers of consuming too much of it, honey is almost always used in a positive connotation (Psalm 25:16). It is frequently used to describe the sweetness of the Lord and His Word (Psalm 19:7-10; 119:103). Honey was one of the foods that Joseph's brothers took to him in Egypt (Genesis 43:11). Honey sustained David in the wilderness and was what "enlightened" Jonathan's eyes (II Samuel 17:29; I Samuel 14:27). Proverbs 16:24 says, "Pleasant words are as an honeycomb, sweet to the soul, and health to the bones."

The most common honey of Bible days was wild honey from bees, found in such places as hollowed out trees or rock crevices. Interestingly, some of the mentions of honey referred to the syrup produced from boiling down dates or grapes. Only during the times of Roman rule were bees colonized into hives and maintained by humans.

Amylases are enzymes that aid carbohydrate digestion. They are present in honey that has not been heated over 118 degrees. This means, for example, that raw unheated honey spread on a piece of whole-grain bread will assist you as your body digests the carbohydrates.

Because the enzymes in honey are destroyed by heat, baking with it will cause it to lose some of its nutritional properties. Compared to sugar, though, it is much preferred for baking purposes.

Raw honey contains antioxidants. The darker the honey, like buckwheat, the more antioxidant power. There are two exceptions to this rule: 1) Light, sweet clover honey is high in antioxidants and 2) dark, mesquite honey is relatively low in antioxidants.

Honey is very versatile and its benefits are many. Honey, mixed with a little lemon, has long been the standby remedy for sore throats. It has antimicrobial and anti-inflammatory properties and may be used to treat wounds, cuts, and burns. It does not have the same tissue aging properties as fructose and it does not raise triglycerides. Honey contains trace amounts of vitamins and minerals including C, E, some B vitamins, calcium, copper, iron, magnesium, manganese, phosphorus, potassium, and zinc. Eating local honey on a regular basis provides allergy relief. Many people like raw honey because they find that it does not affect their blood sugar in the same way that sugar does.

Purchase honey that is truly raw – unfiltered, unheated, and unrefined. Pure honey is loaded with live enzymes, many of which are destroyed by commercial processing. Enzymes activate the vitamins and minerals natural to the honey. For the best product, look for labels that say the honey contains bee pollen, propolis, and enzymes.

When substituting honey for sugar, reduce the liquid in the recipe by 1/4 cup or add 1/3 cup flour for each cup of honey used. Add about 1/2 teaspoon baking soda for each cup of honey used and reduce the oven temperature by 25°.

Notes: Never feed honey to a child under a year old. Honey is high in calories, so enjoy it in moderation.

Pure maple syrup was used by Native Americans long before colonial times. It is obtained by tapping maple trees for its sap and boiling the sap into syrup. 35 to 50 gallons of sap are needed to produce one gallon of maple syrup. Pure maple syrup is a great source of calcium, potassium, vitamin E, and trace amounts of B vitamins. Pure maple syrup is far superior in taste and nutrition to commercial table syrup. We make our own yogurt and sweeten it with pure maple syrup, sometimes adding homemade granola and/or sliced fruit. It's delicious.

The result of the first tapping, Grade A Light Amber maple syrup is lightest in color and flavor and is best used as a food topping. The syrup becomes darker-colored and stronger-flavored as the season progresses and the sap changes, producing Grade A Medium Amber, Grade A Dark Amber, Grade A Extra Dark Amber, and Grade B. Darker-flavored maple syrup is better for use in baking and cooking than the lighter varieties. Grade B is more nutritious than Grade A.

There's another grade that should be avoided at all costs. Grade C is commercially produced maple syrup made at the very end of the season. Formaldehyde pellets are sometimes used during the tapping process and chemicals are added throughout the entire procedure.

Don't fall for the misleading label that says "Maple Flavored." This is commercial syrup that probably contains only 3% real maple syrup. Whatever the other 97% is, you can rest assured that it's not natural.

Look for syrup that has been minimally processed. Organic maple syrup production seeks to preserve purity. Always refrigerate pure maple syrup after opening. Freeze maple syrup that will not be used within a few months of opening. When using maple syrup in place of refined sugar, reduce the liquid by 1/4 cup.

Agave nectar is juice extracted from the wild agave plant. 25 to 40% sweeter than sugar, it has a thinner consistency than honey, is amber in color, and has a light flavor. Agave nectar is a delightful sweetener for herbal teas. Agave nectar has a low glycemic index and metabolizes slower than sugar.

The glycemic index (GI) is the rate at which carbohydrates turn into glucose. A lower number indicates a slower change and a little more control over blood sugar. However, along with checking a sweetener's glycemic index, it is important to examine the *type* of sugar it is. How natural is it? Is it partially or completely a chemical?

Agave nectar passes both tests. It is very low on the glycemic index and how much more natural can you get than a wild cactus plant?

When using agave nectar instead of sugar, you may need to reduce other liquids in the recipe.

Molasses is the byproduct of sugar cane and sugar beets. This was the most common sweetener in America until World War I, when refined sugar became cheaper. The flavor of molasses is quite strong but it is not overly sweet. It contains iron, calcium, zinc, copper, and chromium. When baking with molasses instead of sugar, reduce the liquid in the recipe by 1/4 cup.

Blackstrap molasses has a lower sugar content than refined sugar. It is a great source of iron and also contains calcium, magnesium, potassium, and B vitamins. Blackstrap molasses has a very heavy flavor.

Barbados molasses, or light molasses, differs slightly from blackstrap molasses. It has a higher concentration of sucrose. It is useful when blackstrap molasses is too strong or not sweet enough.

Sorghum molasses is similar to the molasses listed above but has a milder flavor. It is made from the sweet sorghum plant. It is less sweet than honey. It contains many antioxidants and minerals. Sorghum can be used instead of maple syrup.

Brown rice syrup, as its name implies, is made from brown rice that has been sprouted. It is one of the first refined sugar alternatives I ever bought. Brown rice syrup metabolizes slowly and steadily, providing consistent energy without spikes in blood sugar levels. It is thick, golden in color, and has a unique, mild flavor. It contains antioxidants. Brown rice syrup may be substituted for equal amounts of honey. It is sometimes called rice malt. When substituting for sugar, reduce liquid by 1/4 cup per cup of syrup used and add 1/4 teaspoon baking soda.

Barley malt syrup is made from sprouted barley grains. It contains complex carbohydrates and has a slower insulin response than sugar. It contains B vitamins, iron, magnesium, and vitamin E. It has a hearty flavor. It contains dextrin and maltose. Try adding barley malt to foods such as squash, baked beans, and savory baked goods like gingerbread. When substituting barley malt syrup for sugar, reduce the liquid 1/4 cup per cup of brown rice syrup. Barley malt syrup can be used in the place of molasses or brown sugar.

Fruit juice concentrates are fruits that have been cooked down at low temperatures until they form thick syrup. Fruits commonly used to make these sweeteners are grapes, apples, peaches, pears, and pineapples. They can be used to flavor and sweeten beverages. Being very sweet, you may not need a lot. The fructose in fruit concentrates may negatively affect insulin metabolism. Reduce liquid by 1/3 cup.

Date Sugar is simply dehydrated, ground up dates. Dates are a great source of fiber, potassium and other vitamins and minerals. Date sugar metabolizes more slowly than sugar. Though it doesn't dissolve well in beverages, it can be equally substituted for brown sugar. Try it on oatmeal or porridge.

Evaporated sugar cane, most commonly known by the brand name Rapadura, has been used for thousands of years by the native people of India. It is simply unrefined cane juice that has been evaporated. It yields pleasant baking results and is loaded with minerals, among them chromium, which is a diabetic deficiency.

Raw sugar is a combination of molasses and crystallized white sugar. From this blend you gain the nutrition of molasses and the baking properties of white sugar. However, since it is somewhat refined, much of the nutrition has been removed.

Sucanat (sugar cane natural) and turbinado are forms of "raw" sugar. Sucanat is freshly squeezed sugar cane juice that is dehydrated, then evaporated and milled. It has a lower sucrose level than sugar. No chemicals are added to sucanat. Turbinado is created by spinning sugar cane in a cylinder or turbine. It is a pale brown color. Sucanat and turbinado are definitely a step up from refined, bleached white sugar but they should still be used sparingly.

Natural brown sugar, sometimes classified as raw sugar, is the unrefined product of incomplete sugar cane processing. It contains minerals that are absent from conventional brown sugar and is also free of chemicals and dyes. It can be found in most health food stores under the names Demerara and Muscovado.

It is easy to make your own brown sugar. Simply add molasses to natural cane sugar and mix together. For dark brown sugar, add one tablespoon molasses to one cup of sugar. For light brown sugar, add one to two teaspoons molasses to one cup of sugar.

Stevia is technically an herb, not a form of natural sugar. Relatively new to the United States, it has been used in Japan and South America for decades. It is calorie-free and is about 300 times sweeter than sugar so you only need to use a small amount. It is available in powdered and liquid forms. Stevia is a very safe sweetener for diabetic-prone people because it does not alter blood sugar levels and may actually assist in regulating blood sugar. If you have a hard time acclimating to stevia's unique taste, substitute it for half of the sugar in a recipe. Use another natural sweetener for the other half. Carmel Capotosto, a friend of ours, served us a blueberry cake. It was half stevia and half maple syrup. We couldn't even taste the stevia. Yet her technique substantially decreased the calorie and sugar content of the cake.

Xylitol is a sugar alcohol that was discovered in Germany in the late 1800s and came into commercial use in Finland in the 1940s due to sugar shortages. Originally it was made from hardwood trees such as birch or beech. Xylitol is the alcohol form of xylose. Along with being found in hardwood trees, xylose naturally occurs in straw, corncobs, many fruits and vegetables, cereal grains, mushrooms, and some forms of seaweed. Xylitol's flavor varies depending on its source. Most xylitol available in stores is made from corncobs but if you look hard enough you can find xylitol made from hardwoods.

Xylitol helps reduce tooth decay and promotes good bone health. Some diabetics find it useful in regulating blood sugar.   It is found in some chewing gum and toothpaste. It has the same sweetness as sugar and can be used in the place of sugar when cooking and baking.

SUGAR EQUIVALENCY CHART

This chart will help you replace white sugar with healthier alternatives. The amounts listed are equal to 1 cup of refined, white sugar. These equivalency amounts are not exact due to personal preferences. Experiment until you find an amount you like that works for your nutritional needs. (NOTE: Not all "natural" sweeteners are created equal. Though most have nutritional benefits, some are high in calories and raise blood sugar levels, though not usually as dramatically and quickly as white sugar. Diabetics especially should be cautious when experimenting with new sweeteners.)

SWEETENER	MEASURE
Raw Honey	1/2 to 3/4 cup
Maple Syrup	1/2 to 3/4 cup
Agave Nectar	3/4 to 1 cup
Molasses	1/2 to 3/4 cup
Blackstrap Molasses	3/4 to 1 cup
Sorghum	1-1/3 cups
Brown Rice Syrup	1 to 1-1/2 cups
Barley Malt Syrup	1 to 1-1/2 cups
Fresh Fruit Juice Concentrate	1 cup
Frozen Fruit Juice Concentrate	1/2 cup
Rapadura	1 cup
Date Sugar	2/3 to 1 cup
Maple Sugar	1/2 cup
Turbinado Sugar	1 cup
Stevia	1 tsp to 2 T
Xylitol	1 cup

THE IMITATORS

Whoever coined the adage "Those who don't learn from history are doomed to repeat it" knew what he was talking about. In 1969, cyclamates, artificial sweetening agents used in a variety of products ranging from chewing gum to soft drinks, were removed from the market because they were found to be detrimental to public health.

Since then a variety of artificial sweeteners has risen in their place. The United States currently has their stamp of approval on five of them: acesulfame K (K = potassium), aspartame, neotame, saccharin, and sucralose. These artificial substitutes are high intensity sweeteners. Most of them are hundreds of times sweeter than sugar. This means that less sweetener is needed to manufacture processed foods.

There have been many reports of side effects directly linked to these sweeteners, from headaches and heart palpitations to brain tumors and lymphatic cancers.

How long will it be before the FDA takes them off the market too, as they did cyclamates? Why do we participate in their experiments by purchasing products that contain chemical imitations? A chemical will never replace the wholesomeness found in God's natural foods. Our bodies were not designed to assimilate chemicals.

Acesulfame K has been the cause of thyroid damage and has been known to cause cancer in lab animals.

Aspartame is a chemical compound of two amino acids, aspartic acid and phenylalanine, and its use in NutraSweet and Equal is prevalent in products labeled sugar-free. It is about 200 times sweeter than sugar by volume. The possible consequences of consuming aspartame include headaches, dizziness, seizures, tremors, memory loss, slurring of speech, confusion, fatigue, nausea, menstrual problems, high blood pressure, behavioral problems, visual problems, mood swings, ringing in the ears, and insomnia. Because aspartame alters the neurochemicals in the brain, it may cause neuronal damage in children's developing nervous systems.

G. D. Searle is the company that makes aspartame. One of their employees discovered it in 1965. At that time its suitability for food use was rejected because initial testing questioned its safety. It is interesting that while the company was doing its best to get approval to manufacture aspartame, "even the National Soft Drink Association lobbied the FDA not to approve NutraSweet. They opposed it because when aspartame gets above 86 degrees F, it breaks down into a common poison known as free methanol (wood alcohol). Your body, as you know, is normally 98.6 degrees F. Methanol is a problem because it breaks down into formic acid (normally used to strip off epoxy) and formaldehyde (the embalming fluid). This means that every time you boil up your sugar-free Jell-O or put that little blue packet in your hot tea or coffee, you could be getting more than you bargained for."[6]

When all else fails, employ the power of politics.

"In 1981, FDA Commissioner Arthur Hull Hayes approved aspartame as a food additive. He was closely associated with the artificial sweetener industry having several close friends, most notably Donald Rumsfeld, then CEO of G.D. Searle. Hayes cited data from a single Japanese study."[7]

Saccharin, the sweetener component of Sweet 'N Low, which is 300 to 500 times sweeter than sugar, may be the cause of tumor formation.

Sucralose, more commonly known by the brand name Splenda, is not sugar, as the company's marketing campaign alleges. Their slogan is "made from sugar so it tastes like sugar." This new kid on the artificial sweetener block takes sugar and processes it into a chemical. This is accomplished by replacing three hydroxyl groups of atoms found in natural sugar with three atoms of chlorine. This modified sugar compound is 600 times sweeter than sugar.

Splenda is not sugar. Already people are experiencing adverse effects such as headaches, memory problems, skin troubles, and gastrointestinal distress from its use. Testing of sucralose has shown that it promotes shrinkage of the thymus, a gland that is the foundation of the immune system. It also causes swelling of the liver and kidneys. Sucralose produces many kinds of problems in laboratory animals.

Apparently such evidence is considered inconclusive and so researchers must rely on the general population to participate in experimental research. Each time you buy a bag of Splenda, you are paying to be a part of their program.

Beware of advertising. Many artificially sweetened foods are advertised as "fat-free," "low-calorie," "sugar-free," "low-sugar," and "cholesterol-free." These claims and others are an attempt to divert us away from the true content and nature of the product (i.e. fake, chemical foods) to supposed benefits of the food. As we have seen above, not only do most artificial sweeteners leave an unpleasant aftertaste, they have adverse side effects. If in doubt, do without.

SOFT DRINK ADDICTION

Depending on what area of the nation you live in, this fizzing beverage may be called something other than a soft drink. Pop, soda, soda pop, or coke may be how you refer to America's favorite non-alcoholic beverage obsession. Regardless of its handle, the content is the same: empty calories. "Empty calories" means that you get calories, but no nutrition.

Coca-cola has a shady origin. In the 1880s John Pemberton, a medical chemist, created coca-cola. His original concoction consisted of Peruvian coca leaf extract (cocaine), wine, and the kola nut. Due to Prohibition, the wine was replaced with sugar. And though cocaine is no longer an ingredient in cola products, the sugar and caffeine they contain provide a stimulating "high" that many Americans can't imagine themselves living without.

Soda is one of the worst culprits of sugar. Each ounce of soda contains approximately a teaspoon of sugar. For example, one 12 ounce Coke contains 10-12 teaspoons of sugar. (Note: 1 teaspoon = 4 grams.) 10 teaspoons equals 150 calories. A person that stops at the convenience store, buys a big 32-ounce soft drink and sips it throughout the day consumes 450 nutrient-free calories that do nothing but leach health out of his body.

Normally, only about two teaspoons of sugar, or glucose, are present in your blood stream. One soda pours 10-12 teaspoons into you blood stream at one time, throwing your blood chemistry into chaos.

High fructose corn syrup is the "sugar" that many soft drink manufacturers use to cut costs. It is found in other products as well. High fructose corn syrup should be avoided. It changes the balance of minerals in the body, disrupting their distribution and excretion. High fructose corn syrup increases blood pressure, insulin levels, LDL, triglycerides, and total cholesterol.

The sugar in soft drinks affects metabolic rate which encourages fat storage. When I was 20 years old, I lost over 20 pounds by doing two simple things: 1) I had a change in the kind of food I was eating, due to a college transfer (This meant a slight decrease in fast food and Famous Amos cookie consumption and a minor improvement in cafeteria food quality.) and 2) I stopped drinking soda. Before, I was practically addicted to Dr. Pepper and drank several cans a day. I thought nothing of having it for breakfast!

I have been virtually soda-free for over ten years now and I can't stand the taste of soda. Only on rare occasions will I even take a drink of one and cannot imagine actually consuming an entire can of soda. If I would have been drinking soda, especially in the amounts I previously consumed it, I shudder to think what the scale would be telling me now!

When we begin to eat sugar and drink soda or coffee, we are "rewarded" with a sugar and/or caffeine high. As we ingest these substances, we build tolerance to them. In order to produce the same sugar or caffeine high, we need more of the substance than we needed before. If we don't get the established amount of sugar or caffeine, we experience withdrawal symptoms.

Inadequate calcium and impaired calcium metabolism contribute to osteoporosis. "Carbonated soft drinks contain high amounts of phosphates. These cause the body to eliminate calcium as the phosphates themselves are excreted, even if calcium must be taken from the bones to do this."[8]

The soft drink industry is a lucrative industry. "Americans told Datamonitor that they spend about $31 per month on soft drinks."[9] That equates to $372.00 a year. Its easy to see how we are making the soft drink companies rich: If a family of four eats out once a week and they all order soda, they will spend at least $5.00 a week, $20.00 a month, on just soda, and that is if the restaurant gives free refills. Throw in a few cases bought at the grocery store every month, a soda purchase made at the soda machine or convenience store now and then, and you're talking about spending *a lot* of money – on sugar!! If you think you can't afford to buy fresh fruits and vegetables because they are so expensive, drop the soda habit and you'll probably have money left over *after* you buy your produce.

SOFT DRINK ALTERNATIVES

Don't just switch from one soft drink to another, thinking that one is better because it contains less caffeine or is less addicting. Diet soda is actually worse than regular soda on account of artificial sweeteners.

Quit drinking soda altogether. If you have to, gradually wean yourself away from it and start drinking water, herbal teas, and fresh juices instead. You will be surprised at how good you feel when you are free from the bondage of sugary soft drinks.

Water

If you're concerned about the quality of your tap water, consider buying a water filter to purify your water. They are not all alike and there is probably not a single water purification system that is capable of removing all known contaminants. If you have your water tested, you will be better equipped to choose an appropriate filter, since you will then know specifically what harmful contaminants need to be filtered out of the water.

If you get your drinking water from a well, don't assume that it is contaminant-free, especially if you live in an agricultural or industrial area. Pesticide runoff affects groundwater. Toxic heavy metals may be in your well water. Deep artesian wells are usually purer than shallow wells but both should be tested to be on the safe side. Some companies will perform water testing at no charge.

If you buy water from the store, look for spring water. Read the labels carefully. Sometimes water labeled "spring water" is nothing but water from a "municipal water supply."

Keep in mind that exclusive, long-term use of distilled water may contribute to mineral deficiencies.

I love water. It is what I drink most of the time. Some people can't tolerate the taste of water. Try squeezing a little fresh lemon in your water if you need to.

Tea

In regard to teas, herbal teas are a good choice. Different herbal teas can actually help your body heal. Buy loose tea instead of bagged tea when possible. Black, green, red, and white teas all have different beneficial properties. It is good to drink a variety of teas, rather than just one type of tea, unless of course you are using a certain tea to treat a particular ailment. Some teas, green for example, contain high levels of wonderful antioxidants but also contain tannins, agents that reduce protein absorption, so one should not drink it exclusively.

Some people prefer teas that do not contain caffeine. On the other hand, if you are used to drinking soft drinks or coffee for the energy boost they provide, be careful that you do not look to caffeinated tea to give you the same temporary lift. But whatever you do, learn to enjoy drinking tea.

Fruit and Fruit Juice

Fruits are a good source of water too. By eating fruit you will get hydrated at the same time you are filling your body with the nutrition it needs.

Most people think that juice is good and that all juice is created equal. Not so. Most fruit juice available in the grocery store has very little juice and a lot of sugar. Check the ingredients list. 5% juice means that there is 95% other stuff.

If you want really good juice, buy a juicer and make your own juice. It will be fresh, non-pasteurized, and preservative free. Fresh juice supplies you with a high concentration of nutrients. For example, a large glass of freshly squeezed carrot juice will have the juice of about eight carrots in it.

If juicing is unfeasible and you still want to drink

juice, at least read the labels first. Check in the health food store for bottles of juice that are just juice. Don't assume that since it is juice, that it is healthy. Juice that is labeled "not from concentrate" is superior to juice that has been concentrated. If you purchase orange juice from the store, be sure to buy that which contains the pulp; the pulp is where much of the nutrition of the orange is found.

COFFEE CAUTION

A word about coffee is in order here. Most people are aware that caffeinated coffee can be detrimental to their health. It wreaks havoc on the user's central nervous system. Those who consume a lot of caffeinated coffee get addicted to the energy "high" that gets them through the day. No doubt many people are so accustomed to coffee's effect on their bodies that they cannot differentiate between natural energy and the manufactured energy created by caffeine. This manufactured energy overrides the body's voice that tells us when we need a rest. Instead of resting or feeding our bodies some nutritious, natural energy-producing food, caffeine enables us to bulldoze our way through the day, ignoring our body's needs.

Aside from the obvious dangers of caffeine, coffee itself – even decaffeinated coffee – is not a healthy beverage. Research has shown a definite link between coffee consumption – either regular or decaffeinated – and pancreatic cancer, a cancer which has an alarmingly low survival rate.

In her book *Life Without Caffeine*, Marina Kushner writes about the only selling factors of coffee, which do not include any nutritional benefits: "In true Madison Avenue method, the ads sell consumers the sizzle and not the steak. They talk in glowing terms about the taste, aroma and even appearance of coffee. What you'll see in those commercials are folks practically caressing their coffee cups, deeply inhaling the aromatic vapors. Or you'll see some thirty-something guy who is actually awakened by the smell of a distant percolating. It's all smell and taste. But NEVER a word about any good that coffee can do for you. And it's easy to see why. Coffee doesn't do anything good for you."[10]

Kushner also states that both coffee and caffeine affect "the cardiovascular and respiratory systems, and foul the gastrointestinal tract."[11] Caffeine over stimulates the heart muscles and dilates blood vessels.

Many people compare coffee and caffeine to drugs because of their withdrawal symptoms: headaches, "lethargy, lightheadedness, sleeplessness, nervousness, tremulousness, depression, severe upset stomach, excitability, dizziness, diarrhea, grouchiness, irritability, tenseness, nausea, fever, chills, and weakness."[12]

Add a spoonful of sugar and scary non-dairy creamer to that cup of coffee and you have created an even more unhealthy beverage. Given coffee and caffeine's addictive and harmful potential, we will benefit from abstaining or at least limiting our use of them.

HELPFUL HINTS

- When you want sweets, try brushing your teeth. That simple act has been known to defer many a sweet tooth.
- Eat a handful of nuts such as raw cashews, raw almonds, or pecans. You might be amazed at the natural sweetness in nuts.
- Instead of sweets filled with refined sugar, enjoy fresh or dried fruit. Try some fruits you have never tried before. Many fresh fruits are naturally sweet. Along with their sweetness, they have vitamins and minerals that our bodies need. Many fruits that are sweet contain fiber. Fiber helps offset the effects of the sugar in the fruit. There is a wide variety of fruit to choose from. When purchasing dried fruit, look for fruits that do not have added sugar or sulfur dioxide. Dried mango, papaya, and pineapple are all great sweet tooth satisfiers. (Remember to always brush your teeth

after eating dried fruit.) Dried fruit contains a much higher percentage of nutrients than fresh fruit, but also a lot more calories. This is due to the concentrated nature of dried fruit. Fresh fruit has a much higher proportion of water than dried fruit does. (See I Samuel 25:18 and 30:12 for examples of dried fruit.)

- If you recognize the dangers of excess sugar consumption and want to decrease your intake, don't buy sweets at the grocery store. Pass by the doughnuts, cookies, candy bars, cakes, sweet rolls – the list is endless. If you buy sweets and they are accessible in your home, somebody will eat them.

MODERATION

Caution! Eat a *little* honey (Proverbs 25:16). We sometimes make the mistake of thinking that since a food is good and God-given, we can eat as much of it as we want. Just because a sweetener is somewhat natural, don't go "hog wild" with it.

Keep in mind that many natural sweeteners also affect immune response just as sugar does. The upside of using them over sugar is that they have vitamins, minerals, fiber, and enzymes to help offset negative effects. Also, many of them do not produce the drastic blood sugar changes of refined sugar.

Many times we struggle with guilt because we want to eat sweets. God created us with the desire for a little sweetness in our lives. The human tongue has four types of taste buds, creating four basic taste desires: sweet, sour, salty, bitter.

Due to our overuse of sugar and salt, most of us give our sweet and salty taste buds a lot of attention and neglect the sour and bitter taste buds.

It is not wrong to desire to eat something sweet. What is wrong is when we become unbalanced because we allow our uncontained desires for sweets to override moderation.

NO MORE BLUES

Most Americans are obsessed with sugar, addicted to the temporary energy high it provides. Some people can't imagine life without the highs that sugar provides.

However, the less sugar you consume, the less you will crave it. Your taste buds will change. The things you once loved, you will find too sweet. You will start to genuinely enjoy and crave the very foods you once passed by in favor of sweet and heavy foods.

Dr. Will Clower offers some more wisdom on this subject: "If you increase your sensitivity to sugar, you decrease the amount your body asks for. You stop sooner. This makes it very easy to say no to sweets, snacks, and candies. You won't turn them down because you're one of those stoic people who bravely turn their backs on pleasure. You say no because your sweet tooth is satisfied. You just don't want it. People sometimes tell me that they eat sweets because they have a sweet tooth. But isn't it the other way around? They have a sweet tooth because they eat sweets. Your behavior creates your cravings, not the other way around. You are in control."[13]

Retrain your brain. Trade in your sugar blues for natural, simply sweet whole foods. The change will make your insides healthy and happy!

NINETEEN

THE DELIGHTS OF DAIRY

*And he hath brought us into this place,
and hath given us this land,
even a land that floweth with milk and honey.*
Deuteronomy 26:9

God likened the Promised Land to a place flowing with milk and honey, giving the children of Israel a vivid word picture of the prosperity they would enjoy. Milk was highly prized for its nourishment and diverse usefulness.

Milk (Hebrew: chalab/Greek: gala) and its byproducts are mentioned over fifty times in the Bible; the first mention is found in Genesis 18:8.

Throughout the Bible God used various food items – including dairy products – to illustrate spiritual and practical truths. For example, Job's emotional distress was apparent as he asked, "Hast thou not poured me out as milk, and curdled me like cheese?" (Job 10:10). Joel 3:18 describes the blessings of peace and prosperity that God would bring to His people by saying "the hills shall flow with milk." In I Peter 2:2, the phrase "sincere milk of the word" was used to represent the pure and untainted Word of God.

The Israelites used goat (Proverbs 27:27), sheep (Deuteronomy 32:14), camel (Genesis 32:15), and cow's milk (II Samuel 17:29).

Goat's milk especially was prized. Each milk goat produced about six pints a day. This milk was used to make yogurt and cheese. Goat's milk, rather than cow's milk, is sometimes given to infants and children because its composition more closely resembles human mothers' milk than cow's milk does.

It takes about 20 minutes to digest goat's milk and about four hours to digest cow's milk. When raw and organic, both are great for healthy digestion.

Many times the Bible describes milk as "flowing." This is probably a reference to new milk, or milk in its fresh state.

Refrigerators and freezers are relatively new inventions. Though few of us can imagine life without the convenience of modern refrigeration, people have enjoyed dairy products for thousands of years without it. Aside from fresh, free flowing milk, biblical people had simple methods for preserving milk in a hot, arid land.

In all likelihood, the nutrition they obtained was far superior to that which can be gleaned from the overly processed dairy products most commonly consumed today, despite so called "modern advances" in the production, storage, and preparation of dairy products.

Milk was fermented, or cultured, to produce yogurt, cheese, kefir, and butter. These foods were usually stored in skin bags. These natural preparation and preservation methods ensured vitamin retention and supplied an accessible energy source to so-called primitive people.

There is a wide array of dairy products available today. From ice cream to sour cream, cottage cheese to cheddar cheese, and whole milk to buttermilk, dairy products are a prominent part of the American diet. Aided by elaborate marketing and labeling strategies, many Americans consider these products "healthy," consuming them in abundance, not once pausing to consider that they are being fed foods that are far inferior to the dairy products that our Old and New Testament heroes consumed regularly.

FROM SKEPTIC TO ENTHUSIAST

A number of years ago, my husband and I were ministering at a church in southern Missouri. While there, the pastor mentioned that he was going to a local farm to purchase fresh milk. If he had told me that he was an alien from outer space, he might have gotten a similar response. I thought it was really, really weird for someone to drink milk that wasn't purchased at the grocery store. I was raised in a city and hadn't spent much time hanging out on farms. (My dad said that when I was a child I once mistook a cow for a horse.)

Aside from thinking that it was strange and primitive to drink milk that was not packaged in a plastic jug, I was skeptical about the cleanliness of milk "straight from the cow." Needless to say, I did not drink any of that pastor's farm milk, in spite of his enthusiasm about its supposed healthful properties and wonderful flavor.

No doubt some readers are now having a good laugh at my expense. Perhaps you are familiar with farm life so you instinctively and experientially know that fresh milk is great. Others are probably in the same boat I was – repulsed by the thought of what will hereafter be referred to as "raw milk," that is, milk that is obtained from pastured, grass-fed animals, milk that is fresh and completely unprocessed.

Once it is obtained from the cow, raw milk is rapidly cooled to 36°F to 38°F, and then bottled. That's it, plain and simple. Raw milk has not been filtered nor has anything been added to it. Because it has not been homogenized, once the milk has set for a while, a thick layer of pure cream rises to the top. Raw milk is unpasteurized, something that most of us can't imagine. After all, wasn't Louis Pasteur the hero of his time because of his discovery of the power of pasteurization?

You might object, "Isn't raw milk bad for you? Doesn't it make people sick?" "Considering raw milk's role throughout history, it's simple to see that it's not a deadly food. If it were, all those dairy-loving primitive cultures would have died out long ago, leaving their vegetarian cousins to mind the store. At the very least, people would have dropped it out of their diets entirely."[1]

Before the modern dairy plant, before refrigerated transport trucks, before synthetic vitamins – there were cows...and goats...and sheep...and other milk-producing animals. When our biblical forefathers began to obtain milk from these animals, they became recipients of liquid nutrition. What they drank was what we now call raw milk.

Jesus lived a couple of thousand years before pasteurized-homogenized milk was even thought of. Raw milk and raw milk products were common in His day. Jesus had every opportunity to warn His people to abstain from drinking raw milk if doing so would make them sick. He was not the least bit intimidated by people and did not hesitate to confront erroneous ideas even if they were the social norm. I believe that if He had thought raw milk was poisonous and the source of food borne illnesses – as is the general mindset in America today – He would have addressed the issue.

But He did not, because the society in which He lived knew how to properly use and preserve raw milk.

In fact, nomadic people in Israel and other biblical countries still enjoy and preserve milk products using the same methods that were employed 2,000 years ago.

My husband and I have been drinking organic raw milk for years now and not once has it made us sick. It is naturally sweet and absolutely delicious. After enjoying raw milk, commercial pasteurized-homogenized milk tastes bitter. Aside from its wonderful flavor, raw milk is a powerhouse of nutrition, as we will discover later in this chapter.

Raw milk is also the liquid source of many uses. We make yogurt, whey, cream cheese, and hard cheese from raw milk. There is absolutely no comparison between true homemade yogurt and store-bought yogurt. They are worlds apart in texture and taste, with the homemade yogurt being far superior, of course. Sour cream, buttermilk, cream, and kefir can also be made from raw milk.

Unlike supermarket milk, raw milk is still useful after it sours because raw milk is a real food.

As you may have guessed, I am now an enthusiastic advocate of raw milk. The tables are turned, and now people are questioning my sanity! If you are still skeptical, as I once was, and you think drinking farm fresh milk is really, really weird, read on. You never know; you too might just change from a skeptic to a raw milk enthusiast!

CREAM OF THE CROP

Raw milk naturally has a thick layer of cream that rises to the top. People today have become conditioned to think that milk without this "cream line" is normal. Because of this mental conditioning, some people are turned off by milk with cream in it, though that is the way milk naturally is.

Homogenization is the process that prevents the cream from rising to the top. The fat globules are broken down into small particles. The molecular restructuring of these fat globules causes them to be absorbed into the body, whereas the larger particles of unaltered milk-fat pass easily out of the body.

Once again falling prey to the "fat makes you fat" philosophy, people conclude that raw milk with a layer of cream is fattening. However, just the opposite is true. When milk is homogenized, because the body retains the smaller fat globules, weight gain can occur.

Because milk is a natural diuretic, it flushes excess fluid from the body and reduces swelling. Some of the thinnest and fittest people I have met are dairy farmers who regularly drink their own full-fat raw milk.

Homogenization is an industry norm that is utilized for aesthetic purposes only. Unless you have tasted milk with the cream intact, you have not tasted real milk. It is thick, creamy, sweet, and delicious!

THE WHOLE TRUTH ABOUT WHOLE MILK

Invariably people will ask, "What about 2% milk?" or "Is skim milk okay to drink?" Here again we find that the low-fat fad has taken its toll on Americans' minds, this time in relation to good, old-fashioned milk.

There's nothing wrong with the fat in milk. The fat in raw milk contains valuable vitamins. The fat in milk is necessary for your body to digest the proteins found in milk. The short-chain and medium-chain fatty acids in whole raw milk support your immune system and prevent disease.

To appease fat phobic America, manufacturers remove the fat from milk and use it to make butter, cream, cheese, and other products. Whole milk contains at least 3.25% butterfat, with most milk having 3.5%. Most organic raw milk contains 4% butterfat and some old-fashioned, non-genetically selected cows produce milk with over 5% butterfat.

2% (reduced fat) milk contains 2% butterfat and 1% (low-fat) milk contains 1% butterfat. Skim (fat-free) milk typically has 0.1% butterfat, a very negligible amount, which is apparent in its watery, boring flavor.

Because much of the nutrition is in the butterfat of the milk, manufacturers are required to replace the vitamins that they remove. Unfortunately, the vitamins with which they "fortify" the milk, such as vitamins A and D3, are synthetic and possibly toxic.

When the butterfat is removed from milk, the perfect synergistic balance of vitamins, fats, proteins, carbohydrates, enzymes, and bacteria is disrupted. Do yourself a favor: drink perfect, whole, real milk.

COOKED MILK

Pasteurization is the process used to heat milk. Producers employ several types of pasteurization, after which the milk is rapidly cooled.

Vat pasteurized milk is heated to 145° for 30 minutes. Vat pasteurization is the gentlest form of pasteurization. Mainstream milk manufacturers do not use this method. A few small-farm operations utilize vat pasteurization, as do some Amish groups.

Flash pasteurization heats milk while it is undergoing a continuous, controlled flow. It is heated to 150° and held at that temperature for 15 seconds.

High temperature short time pasteurization (HTST) heats milk to 161° for 15 seconds.

Ultra heat treated, or ultra high temperature (UHT) milk is heated to 280° for 2 seconds.

Ultra pasteurization (UP), or HHST (Higher Heat-Shorter Time) is another term used in the dairy industry. It's definition, however, seems to vary. To some manufacturers UP milk is synonymous with UHT milk and is heated to 280° for 2 seconds. Other companies define UP milk as milk that has been heated to 191° to 212°.

Raw milk lasts only about a week to ten days. It is a real, "live," food. Pasteurized milk lasts for several weeks. And, although UHT milk is placed in stores' refrigerators, it is not necessary. This cooked milk does not need to be refrigerated until it is open because essentially, it is a "dead" food. Most ultra heat treated milk can last for six months without refrigeration.

The shelf life contrast between raw milk and cooked milk is similar to the life of all other real foods. Cherries have a limited life but canned cherry pie filling can last for years. It has been packed with syrupy preservatives. Whole grain flour and bread will go rancid quicker than pasty, tasteless white flour and bread because the "life" is still in the whole grain products. Real foods have a natural expiration date.

Most uninformed consumers consider milk to be better if it is pasteurized. When UHT milk was first placed on store shelves, it was purchased without consideration. Customers thought, "If pasteurized milk is safe and healthy, then using higher heat must make it even better."

When milk is pasteurized, approximately 10% of vitamins A, B1, B6, B12, D, E, F, and folate are lost. About 25% of the vitamin C in milk is lost. Ultra heat treatment results in even greater vitamin loss. For instance, 10% of the whey protein in milk is lost during pasteurization, 70% during ultra heat treatment. Pasteurization destroys many of the minerals and enzymes in milk, alters the profile of important amino acids, and changes the metabolic availability of carbohydrates and fats.

One of commercial milk's claims to fame is calcium. However, pasteurization destroys milk's live enzymes, one being phosphatase. Phosphatase is crucial for the proper absorption of minerals, including calcium.

Amino acids are the building blocks for protein. While raw cow's milk has all 20 standard amino acids intact, pasteurization alters amino acids, thus prohibiting milk's protein from repairing the body's tissues.

The protein in milk helps minerals to be assimilated into the body. When pasteurization alters milk's protein structure, the absorption of more vitamins, such as folate, zinc, and vitamin B12, is compromised. Some nutritionists believe that this unnatural alteration of protein plays a role in dairy allergies.

There's no need to fret, we're told. Just as is done with denatured bread, producers will graciously add back in the nutritive properties that they removed from the milk during processing. So when we read labels that say, "Fortified with calcium" or "Vitamin D added" we think we are purchasing a really nutritious product.

However, the truth is that the body does not properly absorb synthetic vitamins that are not original to the milk. The balanced profile of raw milk ensures that all of its components naturally work together. Adding a single vitamin cannot compensate for the loss and alteration of many complex components that flawlessly intertwine to make milk such a wholesome food.

The core of the pasteurization argument lies in the discussion of bacteria. People get sick when they ingest bad bacterial "bugs." About a century ago, the logical solution seemed to be pasteurization, which kills harmful, disease-causing bacteria.

However, milk contains beneficial bacteria too. Pasteurization cannot differentiate between good and bad bacteria but indiscriminately destroys them both. The good bacteria in raw milk are equipped to fight the bad guys. Pasteurization removes the more than sixty enzymes and other infection-fighting agents that naturally defend milk from contamination.

Some people are unaware that pathogenic contamination can occur in store-bought milk. They think that pasteurization is a guarantee of forever-sterile milk. However, pasteurization is not a complete safeguard because post-pasteurization contamination allows bacteria to enter the milk after it has been heated. This can occur from bacteria transferred to the milk from filling machines, human hands, and even the air.

In raw milk, friendly bacteria are present to fight these bad guys. But pasteurized milk is nearly defenseless. As a result, bad bacteria can proliferate quicker than it would in raw milk. Glass for glass, raw milk is safer because of its built-in germicidal, antiviral, and antiseptic properties.

For thousands of years, cultures the world over drank milk. They knew how to care for their cattle and preserve their milk. When Europeans began to settle America, they brought dairy cattle with them. It was common for families to have their own dairy cow and personal supply of fresh milk. History is absent of the mention of health problems that occurred as a result of milk consumption.

But just over a century ago, a blip on the scale of time, real problems began to be connected with milk, particularly in large American cities with exploding populations. Tuberculosis, typhoid, scarlet fever, diphtheria, infant diarrhea, undulant fever, and other diseases began to be linked to milk. In large cities, the infant mortality rate skyrocketed.

Why did milk suddenly become the culprit of so many serious and deadly diseases, when for thousands of years it was a staple food? Did wholesome, healthful milk just suddenly become bad and harmful?

There was nothing inherently wrong with the milk that people consumed. Human handling of this precious commodity was the reason raw milk got a bad rap and undeservedly acquired a stigma that unfortunately continues to this day.

In the early 1800s, grain distilleries began to operate in cities and villages, providing citizens with a local supply of intoxicating beverages. The filthy wastes from this beverage making process were called swill. Distillery operators decided that it would make economic sense to feed this swill to their cattle. They discovered that the more swill a cow was fed, the more milk it would give. It also made the milk a pale blue color. To conceal its unnatural color, these renegade dairymen added ingredients to their milk to make it the color of real milk. Some even added chalk to this substandard food. Swill milk was so pathetic that making butter and cheese from it – common in those days – was out of the question. This polluted milk was then fed to adults and little babies alike.

As the cities began to grow, sanitation became a major issue also. City cattle were not cared for in the traditional small farm way. Contamination from careless workers contributed to the problem. There were no inspections and regulations to keep milk from being contaminated by filth during production and delivery.

Compounding the problem, few people had access to ice to keep milk cold, especially poor folks. As the population began to rapidly multiply and more people moved into cities to perform industrialized jobs, the demand for milk grew. Corresponding to the devaluation of grain, the need for more milk that would last longer made pasteurization seem like the golden key.

Well meaning individuals, led by a man by the name of Nathan Straus, viewed pasteurization as the solution to a big problem. The other option at the time was milk certification, which would have entailed the inspection and enforcement of stringent guidelines on tens of thousands of small dairies that supplied milk for urban populations. Killing the germs by heat treatment seemed much more feasible than trying to implement such an extensive monitoring system.

At the time, pasteurization no doubt saved many lives, including babies and small children. But a century later, things are a lot different. Routine inspections, careful maintenance of cattle health, modern milking machines, stainless steel milk tanks, and refrigerated trucks render pasteurization completely unnecessary.

The only roadblock is our mindsets. We can safely enjoy raw milk just as people have done for thousands of years but first we much realize that it is not the evil source of ill health that many people think it is. Milk began to be pasteurized because of human contamination, *not because there was anything inherently wrong with the milk.* In and of itself, when properly produced and delivered, milk is an incredibly healthy food.

MORE MILK

Conventional dairy cows are routinely subjected to selective breeding, scientific technology, and synthetic bovine growth hormones. Bovine somatotropin (bST), or bovine growth hormone (BGH) is naturally present in cattle's pituitary glands. The laboratory-created hormone that simulates this hormone is called recombinant bovine somatotropin (rbST) or recombinant bovine growth hormone (rBGH). Recombinant indicates that genetic engineering has been used. This hormone is only used with dairy cows.

When injected with these added stimulant hormones, cows produce more milk. Never mind that this leads to mastitis (a condition that pumps high numbers of white blood cells, or pus, into the milk) and antibiotics must be administered as a result. Never mind that these cows are more prone to lameness because of the nature of the hormones. What is important to large dairy corporations is that the production of milk stays high.

"Average annual yield per cow climbed from 3,050 pounds of milk in 1890 to 4,508 in 1950, 9,609 in 1970, and 18,204 in 2000."[2] Production continues to climb each year. The average annual yield for 2006 was 19,951 pounds.

Consider the following statistics from the state of Missouri: "Between 1975 and 2000 the number of farms with dairy cows in Missouri decreased from 11,000 to 3,900 (65% decline). During this period, the number of dairy cows decreased from 302,000 to 154,000 (49% decline). Milk production per cow increased from 9,404 pounds per cow to 14,662 pounds per cow (56% increase)."[3]

From the above stats we draw the following conclusions: 1) There are less small dairy farms. Large, commercial dairies are producing more of our country's milk. 2) There are about half as many dairy cows as there were in 1975. 3) Milk production has substantially increased.

With the aid of genetic engineering, growth hormones, and mechanical and computerized technology, cows produce more milk, which in turn stimulates profits. More milk means more money for milk manufacturers. These heavy hitters milk modern techniques for all their worth.

The overuse of recombinant bovine growth hormones receives little attention from manufacturers, the government, and the average consumer. Yet the idea that side effects from injected hormones are not passed on to humans is an example of the "ostrich with his head in the sand" mentality.

At the time of this writing, several countries, including Australia, Canada, the European Union, and New Zealand, do not allow the use of rBGH in their dairy cattle. Studies have created concern that rBGH may cause cancer, especially breast and gastrointestinal cancers. Because of their potential long-term dangers, consumers would be wise to avoid milk and milk products that contain recombinant bovine growth hormones.

FEED ME GREEN

Cows and other milk animals were designed to roam outdoors and eat grass. However, mass milk production demands that cows live their entire lives in confinement dairies. These money-making operations make the cow's home-on-the-range only a dream. Instead of roaming freely and eating the diet they were created to eat, confinement cows must settle for life in spaces so small that they are lucky if they have enough room to turn around. Instead of grass, they are fed grain. Grain-fed, confinement cows have a shorter lifespan than cows that are free to leisurely graze on fresh green grass.

Humans were designed to thrive when eating certain foods, just as birds, deer, and moose all have their own diet that is unique to them. Cows are not any different. They are in alignment with their Maker's plan when they are consuming grass.

What cows eat affects the quality of the milk they produce. Too many starchy grains in a cow's diet can alter the nutrient and fat content of milk. Milk from confinement cows contains less CLA (conjugated linoleic acid) – a very important fatty acid – than the milk from grass-fed cows. Milk from grain-fed cows also has a less percentage of natural antibiotics than milk from grass-fed cows.

In spite of all these facts, some people might think, "They're just cows. What does it matter what they eat?" Human beings who eat real foods instead of refined foods will agree that what they eat makes a world of difference in how they feel and the energy they have. It's the same with cows. Sure, they can exist on commercial feed, just as you and I can exist on candy bars, ice cream, donuts, potato chips, and soda. But we were not designed to eat fabricated foods and eating too many of them will catch up with us and most likely have a detrimental affect on our health and well-being. When cows are fed healthy foods, they generally stay healthy – and the milk they provide for our consumption is healthy as well.

Feeding cows a diet almost exclusively of grass substitutes like soybean meal and alfalfa causes them to produce more milk. This certainly benefits milk manufacturers' bottom line. It is not very good for the cows, though, and neither is it good for the people who drink the milk. The scenario has a familiar ring to it; in the name of convenience and profit, milk is denatured in the same way that grain is. While milk and flour manufacturers sing the praises of their refined products, the consumer gets the short end of the stick.

NO SOY PLEASE

Many people use soy milk in place of milk, believing that it is superior to dairy products. Most soy products have sugar added to them to enhance their bland flavor. Synthetic vitamins, especially B2, are added to soy milk. Synthetic vitamins are a poor imitation of the perfect balance of those found in raw milk.

Soy milk is faced with the same problems of other industrial soy products. Unless the soybeans used have been grown and fermented in a traditional way, it is likely that they have been genetically engineered and tampered with. When given the option, organic raw milk is far superior to soy milk.

MILK FOR BABES

If you have ever said, "Milk is only for babies" then you have, whether you knew it or not, repeated a statement that has its root in evolution. One resource, quite typical of "milk is only for babies" propaganda, proclaims: "Milk is not designed for adults. No adult animal drinks milk after weaning."[4] (Evidently, these people have never been around cats, which love nothing better than a bowlful of fresh milk.) This thinking is regurgitated over and over again by both anti-dairy, vegan enthusiasts and casual, uninformed citizens. "Milk is only for babies" proponents imply that human adults that drink milk are inferior to "other animals."

People inadvertently buy into the idea that we should not drink milk, never realizing that they have been placed in the same category as animals. Aside from this being personally insulting (apes are *not* my cousins), it directly contradicts Scripture.

The person or persons that first classified human beings as animals seems to have escaped the annals of historical record. This idea seems to go farther back than Darwin, perhaps originating with Greek philosophers who were forever spouting off all sorts of absurd nonsense in their efforts to avoid accountability to the one Creator of the universe.

Even before Aristotle (384-322 B.C.) defined humans as "speaking animals" a Greek philosopher by the name of Anaximander (611-546 B.C.) was paving the way for Darwin. He "is credited with the first written work in natural science, a classical poem entitled 'On Nature.' In this poem he presented what may be the first written theory of evolution. He wrote that animals arose from slime which had been evaporated by the sun. He thought that the first animals lived in the sea and had prickly, scaly coverings. As these fish-like creatures evolved, they moved onto land, shed their scaly coverings, and became humans."[5]

While we may not know who actually started the ball rolling with the "human beings are animals" gibberish, we can be assured that he and God do not agree on the subject.

First, the Bible *never* calls human beings "animals." I Corinthians 15:39 tells us that "all flesh is not the same flesh: but there is one kind of flesh of men, another flesh of beasts, another of fishes, and another of birds." Ecclesiastes 3:21 expounds on the different destinations of humans and animals: "Who knoweth the spirit of man that goeth upward, and the spirit of the beast that goeth downward to the earth?"

Secondly, God gave mankind dominion over animals. That fact alone should warrant him a category separate from animals. In Genesis 1:28, God told Adam and Eve that they had "dominion over the fish of the sea, and over the fowl of the air, and over every living thing that moveth upon the earth." Psalm 8:6-8 echoes God's decree: "Thou madest him to have dominion over the works of thy hands; thou hast put all things under his feet: All sheep and oxen, yea, and the beasts of the field; The fowl of the air, and the fish of the sea, and whatsoever passeth through the paths of the seas."

Thirdly, using sheep and birds as examples, Jesus very plainly declared mankind to be "better" than animals (Matthew 6:26; 12:12).

In a feeble attempt to prove that milk is only for babies – not adults – some refer to New Testament teaching on spiritual maturity. Spiritual foods that are necessary for healthy spiritual growth are compared to milk and meat. This analogy is referred to several times:

~ I Corinthians 3:2: I have fed you with milk, and not with meat: for hitherto ye were not able to bear it, neither yet now are ye able.

~ Hebrews 5:12-13: For when for the time ye ought to be teachers, ye have need that one teach you again which be the first principles of the oracles of God; and are become such as have need of milk, and not of strong meat. For every one that useth milk is unskilful in the word of righteousness: for he is a babe.

~ I Peter 2:2: As newborn babes, desire the sincere milk of the word, that ye may grow thereby:

The parallels are quite clear: Spiritual infants need to be fed the basics of the Word of God. They need to be taught ground-level fundamental doctrines. Just as a five-year old is incapable of understanding trigonometry because he has not yet mastered elementary mathematics, so newborns and infants need to be taught basic things that they can understand.

If it has been a long time since an individual has experienced the new birth, yet he still does not understand basic fundamental concepts of the Word, then it is obvious that his spiritual growth is stunted. An indication of spiritual maturity is that a person is eating "meat" instead of "milk."

But does this mean that a believer will never again need milk? Will he never again need to be reminded of the basic fundamental doctrines of the Bible?

Consider the following verses of Scripture that emphasize the importance of repetition:

~ I Corinthians 15:1-4: Moreover, brethren, I declare unto you the gospel which I preached unto you, which also ye have received, and wherein ye stand; By which also ye are saved, if ye keep in memory what I preached unto you, unless ye have believed in vain. For I delivered unto you first of all that which I also received, how that Christ died for our sins according to the scriptures; And that he was buried, and that he rose again the third day according to the scriptures:

~ II Peter 1:12: Wherefore I will not be negligent to put you always in remembrance of these things, though ye know them, and be established in the present truth.

~ I Timothy 4:6: If thou put the brethren in remembrance of these things, thou shalt be a good minister of Jesus Christ, nourished up in the words of faith and of good doctrine, whereunto thou hast attained.

The Shema was the most fundamental spiritual understanding of the Jewish people: "Hear, O Israel: The LORD our God is one LORD" (Deuteronomy 6:4). Among 600-plus laws and regulations, this was the most basic and foundational truth. Yet it was this basic truth, not some of the more obscure, complex laws that might tend to slip people's minds, that was to be in their hearts and minds at all times. When Jesus called the Shema the "first of all the commandments," He was telling His people that remembering and adhering to it was to be their highest priority (Mark 12:29).

If you remove fundamental biblical doctrines from people's lives, their entire structure will eventually fall.

Just as the Bible never advocates the abandonment of basic doctrines while pursuing deeper doctrines, it does not advocate the abandonment of milk products just because a person is capable of eating "meat." I Corinthians 3:2, Hebrews 5:12-13, and I Peter 2:2 do not say, "Adults should not drink milk." These passages simply state that babies are incapable of eating the foods that adults can eat.

By his analogy in I Corinthians 9:7, Paul makes it plain that it was normal for adults to eat dairy products: "Who goeth a warfare any time at his own charges? who planteth a vineyard, and eateth not of the fruit thereof? or who feedeth a flock, and eateth not of the milk of the flock?" Infants do not go to war or plant vineyards, nor are they shepherds. Just as adults, not infants, become soldiers and vineyard planters, so do adults, not infants, become shepherds. According to this passage of Scripture, one of the benefits of being a shepherd is enjoying the milk of your flock.

I believe that it is hermeneutically safe to conclude that believers were not forbidden to partake of milk products any more than they were forbidden to lay aside basic biblical doctrines. Nowhere in the Bible is milk prohibited from adult humans.

LACTOSE

Another reason that people insist that milk is only for babies is because of the lactose in milk. When babies are born, they have the lactase necessary to digest milk. In varying degrees, lactase production decreases after a child's early years. I believe that this is because the primary food is no longer milk, so not as much lactase is needed.

Adults that become particularly deficient in lactase are said to be "lactose intolerant." "Lactose, or milk sugar, is the carbohydrate in milk. Some people lack the ability to make adequate amounts of lactase, the enzyme that digests lactose by splitting it into the simple sugars galactose and glucose, and they may experience a variety of symptoms when consuming milk products. Unabsorbed lactose attracts water into the intestines and disrupts beneficial bacteria. The result may be intestinal cramps, flatulence and diarrhea."[6] However, "the belief in widespread lactose intolerance is a misconception; most people are simply intolerant to the pasteurized homogenized milk products commercially available. People who test positive for lactose intolerance and have problems with commercial milk often digest raw milk with no problems at all, especially raw milk from animals fed mostly grass."[7]

The reason for this is because raw milk contains lactase. Unfortunately, pasteurization destroys this enzyme. Once again, we see an example of the detrimental effects that occur when wholesome, real food is "refined." The bottom line is that, for many people who are labeled lactose intolerant, it is pasteurized, homogenized milk that they cannot tolerate. Raw milk products, with their inherent lactase fully intact, can be enjoyed instead.

In particular, those who are lactose intolerant more easily tolerate fermented milk products such as yogurt and kefir. As has already been discussed, fermented dairy foods have been key foods down through history. When milk is fermented, this souring process breaks down part of the lactose and converts it to lactic acid. This "predigests" the milk and makes it more digestible.

CHEESE

Several Hebrew words are used to define "cheese": chalab and chariyts (I Samuel 17:18), shaphah (II Samuel 17:29) and gebinah (Job 10:10). We cannot know for certain the taste, texture, smell, and consistency of these cheeses, but they were no doubt nourishing and strengthening if they were delivered to King David and the warriors of Israel.

Commercially, mass-produced cheeses such as American, Velveeta, and low-grade cheese spreads are poor substitutes for real cheese. Most processed cheeses contain additives and dyes and are usually high in sodium.

If you are new to artisan cheeses, you are in for a treat. Every homemade and small-scale production cheese is unique. There are literally thousands of varie ties of cheese, each one defined by its own unique flavor and texture. The distinctive, complex flavors of handcrafted cheeses are due to the type of milk used, the methods employed by individual cheesemakers, and the aging process.

Certainly a new concept to many, making cheese from raw milk is a millennia-old process. Raw milk cheeses contain enzymes, live cultures, and beneficial bacteria. Still concerned about the safety of raw milk products? Nina Planck, author of *Real Food*, has some reassuring words: "Raw milk cheese is very safe. The beneficial bacteria created by fermentation actually inhibit the pathogens everyone is so worried about. The acidity of cheese (a pH of four to five) kills harmful bacteria. Nor does pasteurization guarantee safety. Nearly all outbreaks of food poisoning from milk and cheese in recent decades involved pasteurized milk."[8]

There are several factors that contribute to the safety of raw milk cheeses and make it more resistant to the growth of harmful bacteria. These factors are a lower pH, longer aging time, less moisture, and greater salt content. These are all properties of hard cheeses. Soft cheeses tend to be more concerning, since they have a higher pH (about 7.0), they contain more moisture and less salt, and they are not aged as long. With that said, however, the beneficial bacteria in raw milk cheese is present just as it is in raw milk and it is usually successful at warding off the bad guys.

But almost all domestic cheeses are required to be pasteurized, unless they are aged for at least 60 days. "Much of the milk used in the United States for aged raw-milk cheesemaking is subjected to some form of heat treatment, generally thermization. As a rule this treatment consists of heat treatment at 131° for a period ranging from 2 to 16 seconds."[9]

While U.S. regulations prohibit the sale of soft, creamy raw milk cheeses such as chèvre, it is possible to legally purchase other inspected, certified organic raw milk cheeses in health food and specialty stores. In addition to raw domestic cheeses, imported raw cheeses – especially those from European countries – are worth seeking out. Cheesemaking is truly an art and purchasing quality handcrafted cheeses is a great delight.

WHEY

When cheese is made, the curds are separated from the whey. The curds are used to make cheese. The whey is a watery liquid that is a goldmine of vitamins (especially vitamin B2) and minerals (potassium, calcium, magnesium, phosphorus). It is a source of easily digestible proteins; it contains all eight essential amino acids.

It was a spider, not the curds and whey she was eating, that alarmed little Miss Muffet and with good reason, since whey is not only nutritive but healing as well. For centuries, whey has been recommended and prescribed for treating a wide range of ailments. It was known as a healing agent at least as far back as the fourth century, when Hippocrates placed his stamp of approval on it. Whey cures became extremely popular during the 18th and 19th centuries, when hundreds of spas in Europe based their treatment on its use.

"Whey's therapeutic activity is beneficial to the major organs of the body: heart, liver, kidneys, and intestines. Its action is cleansing, detoxifying, and regenerative. It has been – and still is – used with success for liver diseases (hepatic insufficiency, hepatitis, gallstones); kidney disorders (infections, kidney stones, edema); intestinal disorders (flatulence, constipation, chronic indigestion, bloating); joint diseases (rheumatism, arthritis, osteoarthritis, gout); and against the scourge of modern illnesses. Whey is also very effective in the fight against excess weight (obesity) and skin disorders (acne, eczema), and for improving general health and well-being."[10]

In addition to such an impressive repertoire as listed above, whey effectively fights pathogenic bacteria. The immunoglobulins lactoferrin and lysozyme boost the body's immunity. When harmful bacteria attempt to bind toxins to intestinal walls, whey fights to gently yet powerfully expel them from the body. The healthy intestinal environment that whey promotes enables the body to better assimilate minerals and vitamins.

Athletes and bodybuilders sometimes use whey protein powders to increase endurance during workouts. Whey promotes fat loss while it supports muscle development.

If at all possible, making and using your own whey from fresh, organic raw milk is preferred to whey protein powder. Liquid whey can be kept in the refrigerator for several months. Use it to soak grains, make lacto-fermented vegetables, and add it to soup stock. Regular consumption of whey may ease joint pain and a tablespoon eaten with meals may aid digestion. Whey can be added to homemade mayonnaise and other condiments.

BUTTER
Hebrew: chemah

"Surely the churning of milk bringeth forth butter" (Proverbs 30:33). The butter referred to in the Bible was probably not exactly like the butter we eat today. It was more similar to milk that was cultured to produce a form of yogurt.

However, butter as we know it is a good source of nutrition that, when eaten in moderate amounts, can benefit us much more than processed substitutes. In recent years, butter has been given a bad rap. Instead of butter, we are advised to use margarine or spreads that contain processed vegetable oils, soy protein isolate and a host of additives. Yet, butter has many beneficial substances.

First of all, butter contains cholesterol. One hundred years ago, people ate a lot more butter than we do and there were a lot less heart attacks. To make a blanket statement that the cholesterol in butter and other raw milk products causes heart attacks accuses butter of being a terrible villain when it might actually be our ally. Cholesterol is an antioxidant that fights free radicals.

Cholesterol is as normal to our bodies as the blood that flows through our veins. "Our bodies make most of what we need, that amount fluctuating by what we get from our food. Eat more, make less. Either way, we need it. Why not let raw milk be one source? Cholesterol is a protective/repair substance. Our body uses it as a form of water-proofing, and as a building block for a number of key hormones. It's natural, normal and essential to find it in our brain, liver, nerves, blood, bile, indeed every cell wall. The best analogy I've heard regarding cholesterol's supposed causative effects on clogging of our arteries is that blaming it is like blaming crime on the police because they're always at the scene."[11]

Since cholesterol to our bodies is as natural as breathing, wouldn't it make more sense to choose our cholesterol sources wisely, choosing real food such as raw milk products instead of processed non-foods?

Children that are placed on low fat diets and eat chemical butter substitutes would probably fare better using a moderate amount of butter and healthy oils instead. The first food of babies – mother's milk – is naturally high in cholesterol. Proper development of children's brains and nervous systems requires cholesterol, such as that found in butter.

Like eggs, butter is also equipped with lecithin, which helps break down any cholesterol that may be harmful. Butter contains vitamin D, iodine, and antioxidants selenium and vitamin E.

Antioxidant vitamin A is another substance that may actually protect *against* heart disease. Correctly functioning thyroid and adrenal glands assist the cardiovascular system; vitamin A contributes to the health of these important glands. Babies whose mothers are vitamin A deficient tend to have heart abnormalities. Butter is the best source of absorbable vitamin A.

Don't be afraid of butter. Instead, avoid butter imitations that are filled with chemicals and dyes. Eaten sensibly, in small amounts, butter can be a good and delicious addition to a healthy diet.

Of course, the best butter is homemade butter. It's easy: take a little raw milk, place it in a container with a lid, and shake it until butter forms. If this is unfeasible, search for fresh farm butter made from raw milk. If I, who will always be a city girl at heart, can grow to prefer fresh, homemade butter, so can you!

(See Genesis 18:8; Deuteronomy 32:14; Judges 5:25; II Samuel 17:29; Job 20:17; 29:6; Psalm 55:21; Isaiah 7:15, 22.)

YOGURT

I can vividly remember the first time I tasted yogurt. Our youth group had gathered at the church, preparing to depart for a youth convention. Someone brought a big cooler full of individual containers of yogurts. I sampled one of them and thought that it was one of the worst things I had ever tasted. I didn't try yogurt again until many years later.

Now, I think that homemade yogurt is one of the most delicious foods I have ever eaten. A far cry from pasteurized, artificially flavored, store-bought yogurt – both in taste and texture – homemade yogurt is smooth and tangy. Sweetened with pure maple syrup or fresh berries, it is perfect for breakfast, a snack, or dessert.

Yogurt – sometimes spelled yoghurt – is a food present in many societies. The flavor, consistency, and use of yogurt vary from culture to culture. Yogurt has long been made from the milk of goats, cows, sheep, and camels. It was the natural solution to milk preservation problems.

Yogurt is milk that has been cultured (i.e. fermented, or inoculated with bacteria). The beneficial bacteria that yogurt contains includes lactobacillus acidophilus and bifidobacterium, as well as vitamins A and B and calcium.

Lactobacillus fortifies the immune system. Like kefir, yogurt is beneficial for those who have had to use prescription antibiotics.

Yogurt restores intestinal balance, remedies both constipation and diarrhea, and slows the growth of cancer cells in the colon and gastrointestinal tract.

My husband makes yogurt as often as possible. If making your own yogurt is unfeasible, look in your local health food store for yogurt that contains live, active cultures. As I did, you will most likely find the taste difference absolutely amazing.

KEFIR

Kefir, another highly beneficial dairy product, is a slightly tart beverage. According to Dr. Steven Novil, "the drink we now call kefir originated in ancient times when Eastern nomadic shepherds discovered that fresh milk carried in leather pouches would occasionally ferment into a deliciously effervescent beverage. It is thought to originate from the Turkish word "Keif" meaning "good feeling," for the sense of well-being experienced after drinking it. In many parts of the Caucasus Mountains, the natives (many who are still active and live past 100 years of age) drink kefir."[12]

Kefir is a lactic acid fermented food. It is made when kefir grains are added to raw milk. The natural yeasts and bacteria in the grains are activated as the milk is permitted to sour, or ferment.

Kefir is a natural antibiotic. It creates an environment for beneficial bacteria to thrive. Its mild laxative properties make kefir ideal for anyone with intestinal disorders. People who are recovering from serious illnesses, intestinal operations, or are taking prescription antibiotics can benefit from kefir because it restores the health of intestinal flora.

EXCELLENT EGGS
Hebrew: beytsah/Greek: oon

Jesus taught that a loving earthly father would not give his son a scorpion if he asked for an egg. He then said, "How much more shall your heavenly Father give the Holy Spirit to them that ask him?" (Luke 11:12 13).

In recent years, eggs have received some bad blows. The low-fat fad claims that eggs raise cholesterol levels. As a result, anyone who is at risk for heart problems are encouraged to avoid eggs, especially the yolk.

Interestingly, egg yolks are a brilliant nutrition source. They contain lecithin, an emulsifier, which breaks down bad cholesterol and prevents most of it from being absorbed into the bloodstream. So instead of causing heart disease, eggs may actually help prevent heart disease. Egg yolks also contain choline, which is important for normal memory and brain function.

Additionally, eggs contain essential amino acids, folate, vitamins A, B6, B12, C, D, E, and K and minerals iron and zinc. They are an excellent source of protein. When one considers that eggs fight bad cholesterol, raise good (HDL) cholesterol, reduce triglycerides, and decrease insulin response, they don't seem like such a creepy culprit after all.

Eggs are fairly low in calories, with one medium egg providing 78 calories. There is no nutritional difference between white and brown eggs.

When at all possible, purchase organic eggs. Commercial eggs are from hens that are fed processed grains that contain antibiotics to promote growth. The free-range chickens that provide organic eggs are allowed access to the outdoors, unlike conventionally raised chickens, who live in crowded conditions and may never step foot outdoors. Organic eggs come from chickens that do not receive antibiotics. Their feed is organic, vegetarian, and antibiotic-free.

(See Deuteronomy 22:6 and Isaiah 10:14.)

BENEFITS OF REAL MILK

The controversy that rages over whether milk is helpful or harmful rarely includes real milk. Raw milk, which is 87% water, is a whole food. Complete and balanced, it is sometimes called the "perfect food" and "white blood" because its composition is so close to that of blood.

Raw milk is a complete protein. Some of the vitamins and minerals in milk are A, B1 (thiamine), B2 (riboflavin), B3 (niacin), B5 (pantothenic acid), B6, B12, C, D, E, calcium, folic acid, magnesium, phosphorus, potassium, and zinc.

Some people may have a propensity to resist accepting the positive information presented about raw milk, not because the information is faulty but because it is unknown to people and therefore strange and bizarre. It encroaches into concreted paradigms that have never been confronted. As human beings, we tend to fear what we do not consider normal and acceptable by the society that has shaped our thinking. We shy away from foods that are unknown to us. The unusual seems extreme if we are unfamiliar with it.

Yet what people now consider unusual was normal for countless generations. Most modern doctors would never prescribe real milk and mammoth dairy manufacturers declare it unsafe. But this purportedly unhealthy and suddenly dangerous food was commonly consumed as a healthful and healing food by many traditional cultures, including biblical peoples. It is interesting that during its formative years, the Mayo Clinic used raw milk to treat and cure many serious diseases, with excellent results.[13]

Raw milk has been known to normalize blood pressure and stabilize cholesterol levels. Milk can put an end to chronic bronchitis. The prevention and treatment of many gastrointestinal disorders, especially colon cancer, can be aided by the addition of raw milk to the diet.

A natural antibiotic, milk fights bacterial and viral infections, particularly when diarrhea is a symptom.

Raw milk's calcium helps children develop strong bones and teeth and fights osteoporosis, osteoarthritis, arthritis, and rheumatoid arthritis. In addition to excess sugar consumption, commercial milk has been implicated in contributing to arthritis and other bone and joint problems. Ron Schmid explains that this is because "pasteurization changes the way calcium is arranged in milk and disturbs its normal utilization. Often young and early-middle-aged adults with back problems have been large drinkers of commercial milk. Evidence indicates the synthetic vitamin D2, often added to milk also contributes to this type of calcium metabolism problem, which I have never encountered in a raw-milk drinker. Nor have I encountered any older people who developed arthritis while drinking raw milk."[14]

THE MILKY WAY

Almost everyone can benefit from organic raw milk, with the rare exception of people who are severely lactose intolerant. Also, people who have ulcers should not drink milk of any kind because it appears to aggravate the acids in the stomach that contribute to ulcers.

For the majority of the population, though, organic raw milk is safe and healthy. Remember the following basic principle when choosing a food to place into your temple: If God created it for human consumption and placed His stamp of approval on it in the Bible, then it is beneficial, despite what the fluctuating media might say. The key, like all other foods, is to moderately consume it in the state closest to its origin.

Raw milk is not legally available for human consumption in all states. Among states where raw milk may be legally sold, laws vary. Some states allow health food stores to distribute raw milk. Other states allow raw milk to only be purchased from approved farmers. Others have cow share programs, in which you purchase a "share" of a cow and are then able to purchase its milk.

It seems strange that the laws against raw milk, which is so beneficial, are more stringent than laws against alcohol and tobacco, two products that take the lives of thousands of Americans every year. These harmful substances can be found at nearly every corner market and grocery store in America, yet raw milk, which people have been consuming for thousands of years, is subjected to censure and opposition.

If you are one of the growing number of people who want to feed their bodies real milk, take the time to find out the regulations in your state. Discover where you can purchase certified organic raw milk. This milk is routinely inspected and subjected to strict government guidelines. If purchasing organic raw milk is not feasible, at the very least purchase milk that is organic and has been pasteurized as gently as possible.

TWENTY

SURF AND TURF

And Solomon's provision for one day was…
ten fat oxen, and twenty oxen out of the pastures,
and an hundred sheep, beside harts, and roebucks,
and fallowdeer, and fatted fowl.
I Kings 4:22-23

Though he enjoys it for a while, my husband can only tolerate soups, salads, and smoothies for so long. When I start hearing, "When are we going to eat some real food?" I know that it's time to plan some heartier meals – some stick-to-your-ribs, non-rabbit food.

The Bible frequently uses the word "meat." More often than not, however, it is simply another word for "food" and does not necessarily specifically represent "meat" in the sense that we think of it today. For example, Romans 14:17 says, "the kingdom of God is not meat and drink; but righteousness, and peace, and joy in the Holy Ghost." In other words, "the kingdom of God is not food and drink…"

However, meat as we define it today is found in the pages of Scripture, referred to in both the Old and New Testaments. In the chapter entitled "Don't Diet – Do it Right for Life" we established that the Bible does not espouse vegetarianism. In addition to a variety of both wild and domesticated animals, biblical people ate fowl and fish.

There are at least thirty different types of birds mentioned in the Bible. Some of the "clean" birds that Jewish people were permitted to eat were pigeons, partridges, quail, doves, chicken, turkeys, geese, and duck.

Evidently, some people were quite skilled at setting traps for birds (I Samuel 26:20; Proverbs 1:17; Amos 3:5).

The harvesting and eating of fish is mentioned numerous times throughout the Bible. During New Testament times, the Sea of Galilee was the site of a thriving fishing industry.

Net fishing was the most common fishing method. Simon Peter, Andrew, James, and John were fishing entrepreneurs that made a living from net fishing (Matthew 4:18-22). When they responded to Jesus' invitation, they became fishers of men instead of fishers of fish.

Two less common fishing methods were spear fishing and rod and line fishing (Job 41:7). One of the more interesting references to rod and line fishing is found in Matthew 17:27, where Jesus told Peter that if he would "cast an hook," he would find money in the mouth of a fish. This money was to pay taxes. Wouldn't it be wonderful if just dropping a hook into the lake could pay modern Caesars?

The many biblical references to fish verify that it was indeed a familiar food to inhabitants of the Holy Land. One of the gates in Jerusalem was called the Fish Gate (II Chronicles 33:14; Nehemiah 3:3). It must have been okay for children to eat fish, since Jesus used an example of fathers giving fish to their sons to illustrate His loving care (Matthew 7:9-11). Jesus prepared a meal of fish and bread for His disciples (John 21:9). Who knows? Maybe they had fish sandwiches – minus the tartar sauce. After His resurrection, Jesus Himself ate "a piece of broiled fish" (Luke 24:41-43).

Though no particular species of fish are identified in the Bible, there are over thirty kinds just in the waters of the Jordan River Valley. For the most part, fish was fairly inexpensive and plentiful. Commonly dried and salted for preservation purposes, fish was a convenient traveling food. Mosaic law declared only fish with fins and scales fit for consumption (Leviticus 11:9).

Especially during leaner times, most poor people only ate meat during times of special festivities such as weddings and religious feasts or when special guests came to visit. Regular use of such meat seems to have been generally confined to the wealthy.

But another reason why meat was not commonly consumed may have been because it was difficult to preserve. When an animal was slaughtered or taken in hunting, lack of refrigeration required that it be cooked in its entirety right away. Meat was nearly always boiled or roasted.

Both domesticated and wild animals, including goats, oxen, deer, and even gazelle, are specifically listed as being used for food. Along with broth and unleavened bread, Gideon prepared a young goat for the angel of the Lord (Judges 6:19). The faithful father celebrated his wayward son's return with a feast that featured a fatted calf (Luke 15:30). Nehemiah's daily portion for those he hosted was "one ox and six choice sheep" (Nehemiah 5:18). Lambs and sheep, repeatedly mentioned throughout the Bible, were used for food, wool, and sacrifices. Righteous Abel was a keeper of sheep (Genesis 4:2). Abigail prepared "five sheep ready dressed" for David and his men (I Samuel 25:18).

The Bible establishes that consuming meat, fish, and fowl is acceptable. Current nutritional and scientific knowledge reinforces the Bible's approval of animal foods, verifying that they are healthful components of modern diets, when eaten as close as possible to the state in which God intended them to be eaten.

FROM THE SEA

In varying amounts, fish contains minerals copper, iodine, magnesium, potassium, selenium, and zinc. Among others, vitamins A, B6, and D are found in fish. Fish is low in calories and sodium, is an excellent source of protein, and contains healthy polyunsaturated fats.

A significant component of many varieties of coldwater fish is omega-3 essential fatty acids, which are dynamic health advocates. They promote cardiovascular health. These gems are known as inflammation fighters, regulating the immune system and providing relief for sufferers of rheumatoid arthritis. Omega-3 essential fatty acids contribute to proper prenatal and postnatal neurological development and aid brain function and mental alertness in adults. They provide relief for psoriasis, bronchial asthma, glaucoma, migraine headaches, and diabetes. Additionally, they help regulate blood sugar, decrease the risk of lupus, and contribute to kidney health.

One type of fish that is worth special attention is salmon. An excellent source of omega-3 oils, salmon is high in protein and contains vitamins C, E, and beta carotene.

Wild salmon is superior to farm raised salmon. Atlantic salmon is farm raised. Farmed fish usually have higher levels of fat and calories than their wild caught counterparts. Also, their meat and skin usually store higher levels of contaminants, thanks to the feed, water, and occasional antibiotics they are raised with. Pink dyes are generally added to farmed salmon or a supplement is added to their feed to color their skin. This ensures that they look the same as wild salmon, whose skin is naturally pink when they eat their normal diet.

Interestingly, although Atlantic salmon originated in the Atlantic Ocean, it has been introduced to seas around the world. So salmon labeled Atlantic salmon at the supermarket was not necessarily raised in the Atlantic Ocean. Other names for Atlantic salmon are sea salmon, kennebec salmon, Sebago salmon, black salmon, and salmo salmon.

Alaskan salmon is always a safe choice. All Alaskan salmon is wild because there are no salmon farms in Alaska. Taken from uncontaminated waters are five varieties of Alaskan salmon: Chinook, chum, coho, pink, and sockeye.

The benefits of fish are many but contamination of the environment calls for caution when choosing which fish we will eat. Sewage treatment plants, paper mills, chemical plants, and oil industries are usually located near water, which becomes the recipient of industrial waste and a variety of chemicals. Rainwater carries agricultural pesticide residues from the field to nearby streams, rivers, and lakes. Organochlorine pesticides and industrial pollutants, heavy metals, organophospate pesticides, dioxins, carbamates, plastic materials, and solvents all pollute our rivers and streams. Fish absorb these unnatural substances. Study after study finds that fish harbor chemicals that have not been used for years. These unseen toxic materials move up the aquatic food chain into the human body.

Most likely to contain toxic residues are fish that live in polluted waters. Fish that live near the shores where industrial pollution occurs are particularly susceptible to chemical exposure. One rule of thumb to keep in mind is that larger fish tend to contain more contaminants than smaller fish.

Among the many chemicals that infect our environment and thus contaminate the food we eat are three villains that we need to be aware of. They are PCBs (polychlorinated biphenyls), DDT (dichlorodiphenyltrichloroethane), and mercury.

PCBs are a group of organochlorine industrial pollutants that were once widely used. They have been banned. Unfortunately, they are toxic and have a long life. Since they do not break down well, PCBs that were used years ago are still in the environment. They enter the food chain and eventually make their way into human bodies.

PCBs are suspected of interfering with normal neurological and developmental growth in infants and children. Adults whose systems are overloaded with PCBs may experience liver damage, weakened immune systems, impaired nervous systems, and reproductive problems.

DDT is an organochlorine that was developed in 1939, just prior to World War II. It was originally designed to destroy disease-causing insects so that U.S. troops in the South Pacific Islands could fight undeterred by sickness.

From its beginning, DDT was lauded for its cutting edge ability to destroy not just one or two types of insects, but *hundreds* at one time. The strongest pesticide known to man, it seemed to be the answer the farming world had been waiting for.

Unfortunately, DDT did not undergo adequate testing before it began to be indiscriminately and widely used by civilians in 1945. In the late 1940s warning signals began to sound about DDT's toxicity but the United States did not ban its use until 1973.

By that time, extensive use of such a powerful substance had made its mark on our ecosystem. Most insects are actually beneficial to plant life but DDT indiscriminately killed them along with the harmful insects, upsetting soil ecology and natural environmental order. As is the case with many pesticides, insects began to become resistant to it, requiring heavier doses or something different.

This organochlorine single handedly contaminated our soil, water, and bodies, as no other substance was able to do at that time. It is a chemical whose power is still being felt. Soil and water samples routinely reveal the presence of DDE, the breakdown compound of DDT. Traces of it are still frequently detected in fish.

DDT makes itself at home in the body's fatty tissues. It has a long half-life of eight years. This means that it will take eight years for the body to rid itself of *half* of the DDT ingested. DDT is suspected of disrupting normal hormonal function. It is toxic to the body. In addition to regular times of detoxification, it is good to avoid foods that contain DDT residues. It is ironic that the inventor of DDT, a Swiss scientist by the name of Paul Muller, was awarded a Nobel Prize. He was lauded for his contribution to humanity, but today we are reaping the negative consequences of his discovery.

Some industries leach mercury into the environment. This occurs when rain and snow transport mercury from these manufacturing plants into lakes, streams, rivers, and oceans. In the water, mercury is chemically changed to methylmercury, which contaminates fish. When humans eat contaminated fish, the levels of methylmercury are potentially quite toxic.

Mercury has been linked to Alzheimer's disease. It also can negatively affect the brain development of fetuses and young children, impairing cognitive, motor, and sensory functions. Pregnant women should limit their consumption of fish that are known to have a high mercury content.

When purchasing canned tuna, choose "light" tuna, which is usually skipjack, a variety of tuna. It contains much less mercury than "white" albacore tuna. Albacore, bluefin, bigeye, and yellowfin tuna tend to have a high mercury content.

Because of their high PCB, DDT, and mercury content the following fish should never be eaten: American eel, bluefish, spotted seatrout, weakfish, and wild striped bass.

Other fish containing varying amounts of contaminants should be eaten sparingly, if at all. Women of childbearing age, pregnant women, and small children especially should limit their consumption of the following: blue crab, Atlantic croaker, white croaker, summer/fluke flounder, winter/blackback flounder, king mackerel, blue marlin, orange roughy, farmed Atlantic salmon, shark, swordfish, tilefish, Albacore tuna, bluefin tuna, bigeye tuna, and yellowfin tuna.

The following fish are somewhat more acceptable, though they may still have low levels of contaminants: Conger eel, Florida Pompano, grouper, Atlantic halibut, Pacific halibut, lingcod, Spanish mackerel, mahimahi, white marlin, striped marlin, monkfish, opah/moonfish, wild Eastern/American oyster, Atlantic Pollock, Pacific pollock, mutton snapper, red snapper, yellowtail snapper, Pacific rockfish/rock cod, black seabass, Chilean seabass/toothfish, English sole, wild Atlantic sturgeon, wahoo, and winter skate.

While the list of fish to avoid or limit may seem lengthy, there is an equally long list of fish that are uncontaminated by industrial and chemical pollution.

These clean fish include U.S. farmed abalone, anchovies, American shad, Arctic char, black pomfret, calamari, U.S. farmed catfish, farmed caviar, farmed quahog clams, Atlantic cod, Pacific cod, black cod/sablefish (Alaska), Dungeness crab, Florida stone crab, Mid Atlantic blue crab, snow crab, farmed crawfish/crayfish, haddock, Pacific halibut (Alaska), hake, Atlantic herring (US/Canada), Pacific herring, lobster, farmed oysters (Pacific/European), Atlantic/Common/Boston mackerel, farmed and wild blue mussels, perch, wild Alaskan salmon, sardines, Atlantic calico scallops, farmed bay scallops, shrimp, silk snapper, vermilion snapper, sole, farmed striped bass, white sturgeon, squid, tilapia (US/Central American), farmed rainbow trout, and skipjack tuna.

Particularly observant readers noticed that some shellfish and other fish that are considered "unclean" according to Mosaic law were included in the list of acceptable foods. Previous discussion was limited to external pollution of our waters and the extent to which different fish are affected.

Once again we reiterate that New Testament believers are not bound to follow Old Testament dietary laws. However, to pass over this issue in relation to sea creatures will leave questions in readers' minds.

"Unclean" animals such as lobsters and crab seem to be fairly resilient in regards to manmade chemicals and pollutants. But many people consider shellfish and "unclean" fish – such as carp – the scavengers of the sea. Even domestic fish tanks have a clean up crew, usually a large, bottom-feeding fish that keeps the water clean by eating what the other fish will not eat. On a much larger scale, the ocean has a janitorial team. Some of these fish filter the water, cleansing it of bacteria and aquatic toxins. Because a percentage of these toxins settle in the flesh and skin of these fish, some people prefer to abstain from eating them.

I personally do not like shellfish; I find even the smell of it when it is cooking quite repulsive. But those who do enjoy the taste of shellfish have a choice as to whether they will indulge their cravings or not. Choose from the bounty of the sea the fish that will most benefit your health.

The extrinsic (chemical pollution) and intrinsic (natural sea pollution) contamination of fish scares some folks away from consuming any fish at all. But being informed equips us to make educated choices at the fish counter. Research the pros and cons of the fish available in your area. When we choose fish that is clean and unpolluted and harvested in a sustainable manner, we can reap the marvelous health benefits of God's sea creatures.

Fish is very easy to prepare. Branch out beyond the one or two varieties of fish with which you are familiar and try some different types of fish. Don't eat the same kind of fish all the time. The best ways to cook fish are baking and broiling. Many people prefer fried fish but frying can actually conceal the taste of the fish. With just a little seasoning or a light sauce, baked or broiled fish is absolutely delicious.

FROM THE FARM

Beef, chicken, and pork are the three primary meats found in American grocery stores. Though other meats are available, we will limit our discussion of farm-raised meats to these and wrap up our discussion with a brief look at lamb.

Beef

Beef, along with other red meat, has received a bad rap. The powers that be have imbedded in people's minds the certainty that they are going to have a heart attack if they eat a steak or a hamburger. Is there validity to the hype? Is beef really the culprit for America's modern diseases?

We all know the rhetoric: Beef (and other whole foods like whole raw milk and butter) contains saturated fat. Saturated fat raises cholesterol levels. Increased cholesterol clogs arteries and causes heart attacks. It's so simple that it must be true, right? Just for grins, think out of my brain – the brain of an average American that operates out of common sense.

Point #1: Beef was consumed long before heart attacks became so widespread. One hundred years ago when heart disease was rare, the average family lived on a small farm and ate the food they raised, including grass fed beef. Early American wives didn't waste anything and the fat of their animals was used to cook with, including beef fat (lard).

Point #2: If saturated fat and dietary cholesterol are the causes of heart attacks and the solution is to eat a low fat diet – as the parroted mantra goes – and Americans are eating less saturated fat than a century ago, then why is America in a severe cardiovascular crisis?

Point #3: In the twentieth century, when saturated fat and beef consumption fell, rates of heart attacks and cancer were on the rise. Strange, but while this was happening, the consumption of several likely contributors skyrocketed: sugar, boxed, bottled, and canned processed foods, hydrogenated oils, oxidized cholesterol, chemical food preservatives, colorings, and flavorings.

Stress from faster-paced and complicated lifestyles increased.

Labor jobs took a backseat to desk jobs. Many people abandoned life on the family farm, moving into concrete jungles. Thus, less day-to-day exercise and an increasingly mechanized and computerized society promoted an inactive lifestyle. Overweight and obesity began to be serious widespread issues, whereas previously the weight of most people did not reach a dangerous level.

Thus, to blame America's health problems on saturated fat, which *decreased* in the last century, while there are so many other factors that contribute to poor health, is nothing short of absurd.

Point #4: Most of the fat in arterial plaque is unsaturated (74%); 26% is saturated. 41% of the unsaturated fats are polyunsaturated fats. This fact puts a kink in the "saturated fat clogs arteries" line of thought. It is highly possible that it is not saturated fat that is responsible for clogged arteries, but too many refined, overheated, and chemically altered polyunsaturated fats, which have a prominent place in the Standard American Diet.

Point #5: Saturated fat is not the all-powerful villainous health enemy that it is made out to be. Saturated fat gleaned from pure sources such as organic coconut oil, real butter and milk, and naturally raised beef improve immunity, fight infections, and aid digestion. It boosts metabolism and supplies the body with energy. Saturated fat enhances calcium absorption, serves as a vehicle for the distribution of fat-soluble vitamins, and helps build healthy cell walls. When consumed in proper proportions, saturated fat from pure sources can be a beneficial addition to the diet.

Beef from free range, pasture fed, antibiotic-free cows is a healthy food. Naturally raised cattle provide us with meat that is rich in vitamins A, B12, and E, zinc, antioxidants alpha-lipoic acid, beta carotene, lutein, and zeaxanthin, enzymes, CLA, and beneficial stearic acid. Grass fed beef is nutritionally superior to commercial, grain-fed beef. It's vitamin, antioxidant and omega-3 fat content is higher. Grain-fed cattle yields meat that contains too many omega-6 fats, but grass fed meat provides a balanced (about 1 to 1) ratio of omega-3 fats to omega-6 fats.

If you were confined to a dark, tiny space, crowded together with other humans, fed food your body was never intended to eat, and injected with hormones to make you bigger, would you be happy and healthy? Just as humans need exercise, sunlight, and proper nutrition, cows have needs that must be met if they are to thrive and provide quality meat.

Unfortunately, commercial cattle are raised with economics in mind. The less space used to maintain a cow means less money spent on accommodations. So cattle are placed in small stalls that give them little or no room to move around. Since the objective is to bring a cow to market weight as quickly as possible, his lack of exercise means that he will not burn off as much food as he normally would if he was outdoors roaming around a green pasture.

To further help a cow quickly reach his market weight, he is fed a special diet, consisting mostly of pesticide-laden grains. Growth hormones aid the fattening process. Factory beef is almost always fattier than the beef from free range, grass fed cows, which makes it more tender and juicy. People rarely stop to consider that the reason for this flavor is the unnatural methods used to produce the steak they are eating.

Additionally, because crowded conditions and unnatural feed create a hotbed for dangerous bacteria to proliferate, antibiotics are routinely administered to cattle. Just like when pesticides are overly used on crops, pathogenic bacteria become resistant to antibiotics, requiring stronger and more potent antibiotics.

When at all possible, purchase naturally raised, grass-fed, if possible organic, beef.

Chicken

Americans are eating more and more chicken, thanks to the anti-beef, saturated fat, fat-will-make-you-fat campaign. Our overemphasis on chicken might not be so bad if we were eating old fashioned chickens that were allowed to live the way chickens used to live: outdoors with plenty of room to exercise, eating their favorite foods of insects, grubs, worms, and a few greens along the way, enjoying the sunshine and fresh air.

Today's chickens never have the opportunity to stick their beaks into the ground and forage for a tasty lunch because they will never set foot on anything except a manmade floor or the bottom of a metal cage. A typical chicken house hosts from 20,000 to 40,000 chickens in approximately 18,000 square feet. This equates to one-half to one square foot per chicken. These chickens hardly have room to turn around.

These factory chickens are allowed to live only six weeks. During their brief lives they will be given growth hormones and substandard, fattening food designed to make them as big as possible in a short amount of time. It is not uncommon for these chickens to have difficulty walking. A few of them even have heart attacks because they become so large so fast. If these chickens were humans, we would classify them as "morbidly obese."

Once again the public has been deceived. This time marketers use words like "meatier, juicier, bigger" in their attempt to convince us that the large whole chickens and chicken parts at the supermarket are better. My husband and I jokingly refer to these chickens as "bionic."

If you want to avoid these chemical chickens, look for chicken that has been naturally raised and pasture fed. This will ensure that it was raised without the insults of growth hormones, poor quality feed, and antibiotics. Because they are not "mass produced," this chicken costs more but clean, uncontaminated chicken is well worth the extra expense.

Pork
Why is it that the typical all-American breakfast includes some form of pork? You have your choice of bacon, sausage, or breakfast ham. No matter whom you ask, pork just does not have a good reputation. It is suspected of being carcinogenic. And cooking does not destroy any pathogens pork may contain.

Unfortunately, modern pig farming has added fuel to the fire. Factory raised pigs live indoors, confined to crowded pens, unlike small-farm pigs, who happily root through meadows and woods at their leisure.

But all pigs will eat just about anything, including things that are dead, which is one of the primary reasons many people dislike pork. Preservatives are added to pork, which make it additionally undesirable.

For those who can't imagine life without pork, at least carefully limit your intake and buy pork products that are organic, naturally raised and/or locally raised on a small farm. Consider purchasing natural turkey bacon or turkey sausage. Though it does not taste like pork, it is quite tasty and is a nice alternative to pig products.

Lamb

Lamb is one of the few animals that generally escape the commercial methods applied to the raising of other animals. Though a few farmers fatten lamb on antibiotic grain prior to slaughter, most do not. Their lambs are pasture fed and do not receive growth hormones or unnecessary antibiotics.

I wish that I could get over my "little lambs are so cute that I don't want to eat them" hang-up because the nutritional profile of lamb is similar to that of beef. Lamb is sanctioned in the Bible, referred to from Genesis to Revelation. Jesus is called "the Lamb of God" (John 1:29).

FROM THE FIELD

Anyone that knows me may find it hard to believe, but I own a gun. My dad gave me a 20-guage Mossberg when I was a teenager. I've never killed an animal with it though. I have what you might call the "poor deer" syndrome. I'm sure no one would like to take me hunting because if I saw an unsuspecting animal traipsing through the woods, I would warn it away before the hunter could get it in his sights. I have seen all kinds of animals in the wild: deer, moose, loons, eagles, foxes, bears, and even a pheasant. But the only way I could shoot these beauties (obviously, some are illegal to kill anyway) is with a camera. I admit it – I'm an emotional female!

I do enjoy target shooting and my husband tells me that I don't do too badly. But I could never bring myself to kill an animal unless all of the grocery stores ran out of food. But for some guys (and a few gals too) hunting is an enjoyable hobby and provides them with tales to tell their grandchildren. Responsible hunters stock their freezers with meat and share it with neighbors and family.

In spite of my personal aversion to hunting, there is nothing wrong with hunting wild game and using that meat for food. And though – because of my "poor deer" mentality – I will not knowingly eat venison, I readily admit that there are tremendous benefits to eating wild game.

Wild game's crowning characteristic lies in its absence of human tampering – no antibiotics, no growth hormones, no unnatural feed, no crossbreeding. And for the most part, wild game animals are free of pathogens that could harm humans.

Most wild game is leaner and lower in calories than red meat. It tends to contain more EPA (Eico Sapentaenoic Acid), a type of omega-3 fatty acid, than raised meats. EPA lowers artherosclerosis risk, which is a precursor to heart attacks and stroke. Proper proportions of omega-3 and omega-6 fats are present in most wild game.

Wild game requires special preparation to ensure that the meat is tender. But enthusiasts find the extra effort no trouble at all. Some common wild game are antelope, bear, buffalo, caribou, deer, duck, elk, geese, moose, pheasant, quail, and turkey. Most of these animals are classified as "clean" according to Mosaic law.

Researching the nutritional pros and cons of the animals you are considering hunting for food will equip you to direct your interest toward the wild game that will best meet the nutritional needs of you and your family.

MYSTERY MEATS

When I was in high school, I had the same history teacher for three different classes. Sometimes he liked to talk about his own history, which included time spent working at a factory where bologna and hot dogs are made. His nostalgic recollections were so descriptive and thorough that I have eaten no more than five hot dogs and no bologna at all since that time.

Bologna and hot dogs are not what could be classified as "superior quality, top rate" foods. They are the waste products of the meat industry, the bottom of the food chain, so to speak. If you just must feed your kids hot dogs, please *at least* buy hot dogs that are uncured and preservative and nitrite free.

Other mystery meats to avoid are canned ham, canned I'm-not-sure-what-it-is meats, processed and preservative-added deli meats, salami, and pepperoni, and no-refrigeration-required sausages. Some natural food stores stock natural deli meats and uncured salami and pepperoni.

TWENTY-ONE

THE SKINNY ON FATS

For the LORD thy God bringeth thee into a good land,
a land of brooks of water, of fountains and depths that spring
out of valleys and hills; A land of wheat, and barley, and vines,
and fig trees, and pomegranates; a land of oil olive,
and honey; A land wherein thou shalt eat bread without
scarceness, thou shalt not lack any thing in it;
Deuteronomy 8:7-9

Fat-free, low-fat, good fats, bad fats, trans fats –
what does it all mean? In recent years there have
been a lot of conflicting reports about fat and its
effect on our bodies. We have been told "Fat makes you
fat." So we have watched our fat gram intake. The low-
fat, fat-free fad has made us petrified of animal fat and
butter. We equate "fat" with "bad, very bad." In recent
years, we have heard that saturated fat makes you fat,
raises cholesterol, and increases heart attack risk. Yet
Americans are fatter and unhealthier than ever.

In lieu of fat, Americans have filled themselves
with refined sugar, processed foods, margarine, shortening, and refined oils, never realizing that products labeled "fat-free" are usually filled with chemical and synthetic substitutes that are much more harmful to our
bodies than the fat that occurs naturally.

The truth is that the foods we have shunned are
actually foods our bodies need. Consumed in proper
proportions, our bodies require a certain amount of fat.
It is the *type* and *ratio* of fats that we eat that is important. Not all fat is bad. Not all cholesterol is bad. We
need a little of both.

There are three major sources of naturally occurring fatty acids. Most foods contain a combination of all three, in varying proportions.

First, there are monounsaturated fats. You will find these in olive oil, canola oil, walnuts and walnut oil, avocados and avocado oil, almonds and almond oil, hazelnut oil, peanut oil, and other nuts and seeds.

Second, there are polyunsaturated oils. These are found in soybean oil, corn oil, sunflower oil, safflower oil, and fish oil.

Third, there are saturated fats. These are found mostly in tropical oils and animal products such as milk, cheese, butter, beef, and pork.

Let's take a closer look at each of these.

MONOUNSATURATED FATS

These fats safeguard against cardiovascular disease and cancer. The fats of the olive oil-rich Mediterranean diet, purported to be very healthful, are mostly monounsaturated. Our bodies make monounsaturated fatty acids from saturated fatty acids and use them in many ways. Monounsaturated fats are liquid at room temperature and can be used for cooking. These are sometimes referred to as omega-9 fats.

Macadamia nut oil is monounsaturated oil that is rich in antioxidants. (Buy expeller pressed macadamia nut oil; the refining process removes many of the antioxidants.) It has a nutty aroma and buttery flavor and may be used in place of butter. It is great on vegetables, in soups, or drizzled over popcorn.

A word about canola oil is in order. Canola oil (formerly called rape seed oil) has recently received much acclaim as a beneficial oil. It has a high oleic-acid content, which is good. However, canola oil is from a hybrid, not pure, seed. The jury is still out on the possibility of vitamin E deficiency and other drawbacks from canola oil usage. If you do use canola oil, use it sparingly and not exclusively and always use organic canola oil.

Oleic acid is the monounsaturated fatty acid most commonly found in our food, the predominant component of the oil from olives, and is also present in almonds, pecans, cashews, peanuts, and avocados. The word "oleic" comes from the word "olive."

Olive Oil

Olive oil was usually the oil chosen for the anointing of prophets, priests and kings, men that were consecrated to spiritual and governmental leadership (Leviticus 8:12; I Samuel 16:13; I Kings 19:16). The simple act of anointing indicated that they were being set apart for special purposes.

Olive oil was prized for its culinary uses. An important component in bread, it was also common to dip bread into olive oil mixed with spices.

Olive oil was useful as a medicinal ointment and was an ingredient in soap. Shepherds would smear olive oil on the faces of their sheep to keep bugs away from them.

Most people are familiar with the phrase "thou anointest my head with oil" (Psalm 23:5). Traditional customs of hospitality entailed washing and drying the guest's feet upon his entry into the house. The guest's head was also anointed with oil. A slave or the lowest person in the household usually did this.

Addressing the Pharisee at whose house He was a guest, Jesus commended the woman who slipped in and anointed His feet and head. "Seest thou this woman? I entered into thine house, thou gavest me no water for my feet: but she hath washed my feet with tears, and wiped them with the hairs of her head. My head with oil thou didst not anoint: but this woman hath anointed my feet with ointment (Luke 7:44, 46).

The Greek word for Christ is "Christos," which refers to the Messiah, or the Anointed One (Luke 4:18; Acts 4:27; 10:38).

Olive oil has stood the test of time and remains one of the most beneficial, safest, not to mention delicious vegetable oils available. It is excellent in salad dressings and makes a delicious sauté.

Olive oil provides a good balance of fats. It is 70-75% monounsaturated fat, 12% polyunsaturated fat, and 15% saturated fat. It contains natural antioxidants, especially vitamin E.

This age-old oil also positively affects osteoporosis, arthritis, cataracts, constipation, and gallbladder disease. Olive oil contributes to the stability of cell membranes, reinforcing their ability to stifle free radicals, making olive oil a necessity in cancer prevention, especially breast cancer. Olive oil helps lower blood sugar and also serves as a liver cleanser.

Olive oil fights arterial plaque buildup and high blood pressure and improves the health of blood platelets. In Mediterranean countries such as the Greek island of Crete, where olive oil is the predominant oil used, heart disease is very low.

It is possible to purchase olive oil that is extracted in a fashion similar to that of Bible days. Olive oil that was brought to the temple as an offering was from the best olives and was from the first pressing.

"Extra-virgin" olive oil is the result of the first pressing of the olives. This oil is gently extracted. If you purchase "organic, extra-virgin, first pressing, expeller pressed" olive oil, you can be certain that you are using a pure olive oil that will yield the most nutritional benefits. This oil is a golden yellow color with a greenish cast.

"Virgin" olive oil is the result of the end of the first pressing or the second pressing. Subsequent pressings yield a product that is classified as "pure" or "refined," misleading terms since their pristine state is altered by high temperatures and over-processing.

POLYUNSATURATED FATS

Polyunsaturated fats are a major source of energy for our bodies. They help our brains stay sharp, clot our blood, and help prevent the formation of cancer cells. They regulate the function of every cell including our hearts, arteries, and nerves.

Polyunsaturated fats maintain a liquid form whether they are at room temperature or stored in the refrigerator. They are highly reactive and should never be heated or used in cooking.

These fats cannot be manufactured by the human body and so we call them "essential" fatty acids (EFAs). We must obtain them from the food we eat. The two EFAs most commonly found in our food are linolenic acid (omega-3) and linoleic acid (omega-6).

Omega-3 fatty acid is found in flaxseeds, flaxseed oil, walnuts, and leafy green vegetables. The oils of cold-water fish such as herring, mackerel, salmon, sardines, trout, whitefish, striped bass, bluefish, and tuna are great sources of omega-3s.

Omega-6 fatty acid is found in the following oils: corn, safflower, peanut, sunflower, cottonseed, borage, hemp, and evening primrose. When properly balanced with omega-3s and not overly heated or processed, omega-6 fatty acids are beneficial. Some good sources are whole grain cereals, whole grain bread, raw nuts, raw sunflower seeds, peanuts, beans, naturally raised poultry and eggs.

Many people have an imbalance of omega-3 and omega-6 fats, with omega-6s tipping the scale. Modern farmers have tipped the balance way too far in the production of vegetables, eggs, fish and meat. What the animals are fed determines their ratio. For example, organic eggs usually have a 1-1 ratio, which is ideal. Supermarket eggs have a 19-1 ratio.[1]

Omega-6 fatty acids are found in a lot of processed foods and hydrogenated foods. Consuming great amounts of omega-6s without the counterbalance of omega-3s creates an unnatural ratio and encourages disease. "A 1997 study revealed that these diseases [heart disease, allergies, asthma, autoimmune disease, obesity, diabetes, and cancer] began to rise in the Japanese for the first time in history *after* they started eating more omega-6 oils in a westernized diet."[2]

It is in our best interest to curtail our intake of refined omega-6s, sourced from processed foods such as commercial baked goods, refined omega-6 oils, and commercial salad dressing, pork, margarine, and fried foods.

Try using a little flax oil when you make salad dressing. Buy flax seeds and grind them as needed in a coffee grinder. Sprinkle them over salads or yogurt. Eat wild-caught cold-water fish. The list of benefits from omega-3 fatty acids is almost endless.

SATURATED FATS

In recent years many people have shunned saturated fats in favor of polyunsaturated fats, the majority of them being omega-6 EFAs, and the result has been an imbalance of dietary fats. Keep in mind the principle of enjoying in moderation foods that God has created. If He created it and gave it to us for food, then we can eat it, as long as we alter its original state as little as possible.

Saturated fats enhance our immune systems. They are antimicrobial and help protect us against harmful microorganisms in the digestive tract. Our bodies make saturated fatty acids from carbohydrates and we need them to properly assimilate EFAs. Saturated fats are solid or semi-solid at room temperature and can be used for a variety of cooking and baking purposes.

Saturated fatty acids are found in dairy products such as whole milk, cream, and cheese and meats such as beef, veal, and lamb. Coconut oil, palm kernel oil, and natural vegetable shortening are also sources of saturated fats.

Coconut oil especially deserves a commendation. Rather than contributing to heart disease, coconut oil benefits the cardiovascular system. Coconut oil boosts the body's immunity. Coconut oil contains fewer calories than other commonly used oils and is beneficial as a weight loss aid. The body does not hoard the fat in coconut oil, but converts it into energy.

FAT FACTS

- Fats provide building blocks for membranes.
- Eating fat with a meal slows down nutrient absorption so we can go for longer periods of time without feeling hungry.
- Fat is a carrier for vitamins A, D, E, and K.
- Dietary fat converts carotene to vitamin A.
- Fat aids mineral absorption.
- Fats from animal and vegetable sources provide us with energy.

OIL PROCESSING

Conventional oil processing takes perfectly good foods, such as sunflower seeds and olives, and transforms them into nutritionally depleted oils. These oils are subjected to high heat, bleaching agents, deodorizers, the de-gumming process, and additives. The book *Nourishing Traditions* contains a good description of the common procedure used to produce most oils.

"Oils processed in large factories are obtained by crushing the oil-bearing seeds and heating them to 230 degrees Fahrenheit. The oil is then squeezed out at pressures from 10 to 20 tons per inch, thereby generating more heat. During this process the oils are exposed to damaging light and oxygen.

"In order to extract the last 10 percent of the oil from crushed seeds, processors treat the pulp with one of a number of solvents – usually hexane. The solvent is then boiled off, although up to 100 parts per million may remain in the oil. Such solvents, themselves toxic, also retain the toxic pesticides adhering to seeds and grains before processing begins.

"High-temperature processing [creates] dangerous free radicals. In addition, antioxidants, such as fat-soluble vitamin E, which protect the body from the ravages of free radicals, are neutralized or destroyed by high temperatures and pressures.

"BHT and BHA, both suspected of causing cancer and brain damage, are often added to these oils to replace vitamin E and other natural preservatives destroyed by heat."[3]

The Israelites' method of extracting oil from the olive was a much safer, gentler process that preserved the integrity of the oil. Heat was never applied during the extrusion process.

Olive berries were gathered by hand or carefully shaken from the tree with a light reed or stick. They were then ground with a round millstone, bruised in a mortar, or crushed in a press of stone or wood rollers. Some olives were made into oil with the aid of fancy footwork (Micah 6:15). Gethsemane (Hebrew: gath-shemen) at the Mount of Olives referred to the place where an oil mill, or olive press, was located.

When genetically engineered foods are used to make processed oil, insult is added to injury. Corn, soy, and canola are the top three oils that are made from genetically engineered crops.

Choose organic, unrefined, cold pressed, non-GMO oils. This will ensure oils that have been produced without chemical solvents, unnecessary high temperatures, and added preservatives.

TERRIBLE TRANS FATS

Much of the negative implications applied to saturated fats may in fact be due to the overabundant use of trans fats in the typical American's diet. They are found in about 75% of conventional chips and other salty snacks, 50% of all cereals, and 90% of cookies.[4] Trans fats are found in hydrogenated vegetable shortening, margarine, pastries, commercial baked goods, cakes, doughnuts, pies, corn chips, salad dressing, candy – the list goes on and on.

Trans fats have been the junk food manufacturers' windfall. Trans fats stabilize food flavor and make products last longer. By extending the shelf life of packaged foods, they have a longer sell cycle and manufacturers make more money.

Trans fatty acids are created when hydrogen is pumped into liquid oils. The result is a molecular structure that will keep these oils solid at room temperature. This forms a substance completely foreign to our bodies and one we have a difficult time breaking down.

There is a link between trans fats (alias "junk food") and obesity. Some experts believe that trans fats make our cells less resistant to insulin and in this way contribute to obesity. (The answer is not to sue fast food chains for creating junk food junkies. The answer is to stop driving your car there and take personal responsibility for the food you are taking from your hand to your mouth.)

Read labels. Manufacturers are now required to list the amount of trans fat in their products. Look for the words "trans fatty acid," "hydrogenated oil," or "partially hydrogenated oil" and do not buy those products. Also, if a product is labeled "low-fat," it probably has trans fats. Avoid eating at fast food restaurants as much as possible. Most fast food is cooked in hydrogenated oil. Avoid margarine and conventional shortening; choose butter, olive oil, other healthy oils, and organic trans fat free shortening instead.

Since the FDA made trans fat labeling mandatory and consumer awareness has risen, many grocery manufacturers are removing trans fats from their products. They realize that if they want to continue turning a profit, they must quit using that bad stuff that makes their products taste so good. *If they really cared about our health, it wouldn't be there in the first place.*

What's really pathetic is that, instead of seeking natural alternatives to trans fats, manufacturers use extra sugar or other harmful food additives to ensure that their product tastes the same as before. So don't think that just because a product boasts "Trans Fat Free" in big bold letters, that it is safe. Keep reading. Just because something says "trans fat free" doesn't necessarily mean that it's good enough to eat.

GET SKINNY ON THE RIGHT FATS

If fat naturally occurs in a food, it will have some beneficial properties. The key to health is eating a balanced variety. Based on the information presented above, evaluate where you obtain the majority of your dietary fat. If you eat a lot of meat but little olive oil or fresh salads, you may need to eat a little less meat and add more greens to your diet.

Don't allow the ever-shifting media to dictate your food choices. Start reading, studying, and experimenting with new healthy products. You will find there is a whole new way of eating available to you. You have nothing to lose but weight and nothing to gain but energy and better health.

TWENTY-TWO

FRESH PRODUCE

You knew this was coming, right? You first heard it when you were just a child: "Johnny, eat your vegetables. They're good for you." Sometimes the command to eat the "good stuff" was accompanied by a bribe: "Eat three more bites of asparagus and then you can have dessert."

Regardless of the appropriateness of their methods, your parents' desire for you to eat more fresh produce was not a power struggle or a torture experiment, though it may have seemed that way to your young mind.

If the final decision was left to kids, most of them would choose cookies and potato chips rather than nutritious foods that are necessary for the healthy growth and development of their bodies during formative years. Even most of us adults still choose junk food instead of the wholesome, delicious fruits and vegetables that our bodies crave. We have conditioned our taste buds to like what is bad for us, shunning the food that our bodies need to protect us from sickness and disease.

Fresh fruits and vegetables contain vitamins, minerals, amino acids, and natural sugars. Constipation is a dangerous problem for many people; in fact, some nutritionists consider it to be the root cause of numerous diseases. Regular consumption of fresh produce ensures adequate fiber intake, which encourages regular bowel movements, keeping the body clean and toxin free. These delicious foods also protect the body from free radicals and help prevent cancer, heart disease, stroke, and diabetes.

THE BIBLE AND FRESH PRODUCE

Careful study reveals that the Bible has a lot to say about fresh fruits and vegetables, as well as beans, nuts and seeds, the topics of this chapter. Biblical foods are often used in both figurative and literal contexts; fruits and vegetables are no exception.

It is interesting to note that it was God who planted the very first garden. He named it Eden, which meant that it was a beautiful, pleasant, and delightful place (Genesis 2:8). Agriculture and horticulture began in Genesis and are mentioned extensively throughout the Bible.

One archeological dig unearthed a limestone plaque that dates back to 950-918 B.C., about the time of Elijah and the early kings of the divided kingdom of Israel. Called the Gezer Calendar, it was probably a schoolboy's exercise recited in singsong style. It describes the agricultural operations of that time:[1]

> His two months are olive harvest;
> His two months are grain planting;
> His two months are late planting;
> His month is hoeing up flax;
> His month is barley harvest;
> His month is harvest and festivity;
> His two months are vine-tending;
> His month is summer fruit.

God gave very specific laws for the sowing and reaping of crops. He commanded His people to give the land a Sabbath rest to keep the ground fertile and healthy (Leviticus 25:1-5). There are many biblical references to pruning also (Joel 3:10; John 15:2).

Some of the fruits and vegetables that were native to the land of Israel and nearby countries during Bible days were figs, grapes, olives, pomegranates, and dates. Fruit orchards were not uncommon and almonds and lentils were locally grown.

There was a healthful variety of fresh produce available to biblical people. Similarly to the United

States, where some crops flourish best in the South and others in the North, the plains and mountains of Bible lands created diverse agricultural environments. Such varying geographical and climatic conditions enabled the enjoyment of many kinds of fruits and vegetables.

Since Palestine was the crossroads for the African, European, and Asian continents, it became the center for commerce and trade and the Jews benefited from the flavorful and healthful foods of foreign lands. Also, the Jews often brought back foods native to the countries where they spent time in captivity. Some of these foods were apricots, oranges, mulberries, walnuts, and pistachios.

FOCUS ON BIBLICAL PRODUCE

We are going to take an in-depth look at these fruits and vegetables that were common and familiar to biblical people. You may wonder, "Why should we use biblical foods to guide our study of fresh produce? What's so special about these particular foods, when 21st century advancements in transportation enable us to get food from all over the world, from New Zealand's kiwi to Chile's bananas? Why focus on the produce grown in just one small area of the world?"

There are many reasons why studying biblical foods is a worthwhile endeavor. You see, God always provides the very best for His people. He was not only interested in keeping the Israelites spiritually pure and safe from idolatry and evil influences, He wanted them to be physically healthy as well. This is evidenced by the detailed dietary and agricultural laws He gave Moses. Modern Mediterranean foods are the same ones that God's people have been enjoying for thousands of years. They are the very same foods spoken of throughout Scripture. Many of Jesus' parables revolved around the common produce of His time. They are some of the most healthful foods on the planet.

Though many of them may be unfamiliar to us, by learning about the foods that God chose for His people to eat, we will expand our food horizons to the land where Jesus walked. At the same time, we will find that the parables and spiritual teachings that use biblical produce as object lessons will make more sense to us.

Indeed, due to the ethnically diverse selection of fresh produce available to us today and the space limitations of this book, it would be impossible to adequately cover the benefits of every fruit and vegetable known to man. Most of us know that oranges are a great source of vitamin C and bananas contain a lot of potassium, but we don't stop to think that down through the years God's chosen people also enjoyed the nutrition of a variety of fruits and vegetables. As a matter of fact, the nature of these foods is absolutely fascinating and in some cases, surprising.

By no means do you have to limit your produce selections to those mentioned in the Bible. But after realizing that these foods are a powerhouse of nutrition, you will probably start choosing foods that you routinely passed by because of their unfamiliarity and because you did not know how to prepare them. Hopefully you will be motivated to sample these "new" foods, find that you like some of them, and increase the diversity of foods you eat. By using biblical foods as a springboard, we can glean some important selection, preparation, and preservation principles that will apply to all of our fresh produce options.

It is imperative to understand that the Hebrew, Greek, and Aramaic (Chaldean) languages, in which the Bible was written, are much more descriptive and expansive than English. Because of their complexity and because they reflected cultures vastly different from our own, studying the original words used will yield a greater understanding than can be grasped by casual reading.

For example, when we read the word "corn" in the Bible, cornfields of the great American Midwest come to mind. We picture corn on the cob slathered with butter and sprinkled with salt and pepper. However, the corn we are familiar with is not the same as the "corn" mentioned in the Bible. Corn as we know it was not consumed in Israel during Bible days. It was entirely unknown to the inhabitants of that part of the world.

Instead, "corn" usually referred to wheat; the word may have occasionally referred to other grains such as barley, millet, or spelt (fitch) as well. These grains, in addition to being made into bread, could be parched (roasted) or cracked and made into gruel. Understanding the biblical meaning of the word "corn" changes our mental images of familiar passages of Scripture.

For instance, when Jesus' disciples plucked "ears of corn" and rubbed them in their hands to separate the grain from the chaff, the tradition-minded Pharisees classified their action as work, which was forbidden on the Sabbath day (Luke 6:1). John 12:24 makes more sense when we realize that "corn" was really grain: "Verily, verily, I say unto you, Except a corn [grain] of wheat fall into the ground and die, it abideth alone: but if it die, it bringeth forth much fruit."

It is interesting that many times when the word "corn" is used, it is in italicized letters, meaning that the word "corn" was not in original Scripture at all, but was added by the translators for ease of readability. (See Deuteronomy 25:4, Ruth 2:14, and I Samuel 25:18.) So examining the linguistic roots and the biblical, historical and botanical history of certain foods helps us realize that our definitions sometimes dramatically differ from their true meanings that originated in a long ago culture in a faraway place.

So for comprehension purposes, we must explore the meanings indicated by the languages used to write the Scriptures. For each of the biblical foods discussed in this chapter, the original words are referenced. I am not an expert on the Hebrew, Greek, and Aramaic languages but have researched the original words for biblical fruits, vegetables, herbs, and spices to the best of my ability. The interested reader is encouraged to use the original words provided for further study.

Berries
Hebrew (bramble): atad/Greek (bramble bush): batos

Judges 9:8-15 records an interesting analogous dissertation. Jotham contrasts the strength and character of the olive tree, fig tree, and vine to the bramble bush, portraying to the people the futility of putting their trust in Abimelech, an evil and deceitful man. The bramble bush grows low to the ground and offers no protection, safety, or refuge. In the New Testament, Jesus illustrated how our true character is revealed by the fruit we bear. He said that a man cannot gather grapes from a bramble bush (Luke 6:44). The word used in Judges 9 and Luke 6 is also used to refer to the bush that Moses saw burning in the desert (Acts 7:30).

Bramble fruit includes blackberries, dewberries, raspberries, and loganberries.

Though the Bible does not explicitly mention them, botanical historians say that blackberries were a bramble fruit that was native to Bible lands. Blackberries are useful to help cure constipation, anemia, obesity, weak kidneys, rheumatism, arthritis, gout, and skin problems. They are also a good blood cleanser. Other berries are very beneficial also.

Citron
Hebrew: etrog

The citron is a fruit unfamiliar to most Americans but it has been cultivated by Jewish people for many generations. The Jews used the citron tree during Feast of Tabernacles celebrations. Historians, including Josephus, cite that the phrase "goodly trees" in Leviticus 23:40 is a reference to the tree upon whose boughs the citron grew.

The citron was a traditional Jewish symbol, as is evidenced by its use on coins minted in 136 B.C. When the Greeks encountered it during the time of Alexander the Great's conquests, they named it the "Persian apple."

The citron is a rather large, elongated, yellow fruit with a thick, bumpy skin. It has a sour, slight lemony flavor and a pleasant smell. The pulp is used primarily for making jellies and preserves. The skin is candied and used in cakes and puddings. Citron can also be used to flavor meat. The thick peel enables citron fruit to last a long time, whether it remains on the tree or is harvested and stored.

Cucumbers
Hebrew: qishshu

Because the children of Israel forsook the Lord, the prophet Isaiah said that they were left "as a lodge in a garden of cucumbers" (Isaiah 1:8). He was referring to a temporary shelter that was built to house the attendant who guarded the cucumber fields from thieves and wild animals during growing and harvest seasons. After it had served its purpose, the attendant departed and the little cottage was left desolate, at the mercy of the elements which would cause it to decay.

Cucumbers grew extensively in Egypt (Numbers 11:5). The mud along the Nile was very conducive to their growth. Since cucumbers are 99% water, the nomads of Palestine found cucumbers a convenient and refreshing food as they traversed the hot, arid land. Cucumbers became popular with the Greeks and Romans as well.

Said to be the best known diuretic, cucumbers are crisp and cool. They contain an enzyme called erepsin, which helps digest proteins. An alkaline vegetable, the potassium in cucumbers enables them to be useful for treating both high and low blood pressure. The silicon in cucumbers aids calcium absorption. Most of the nutrients of the cucumber are found in its skin.

Add cucumbers to sandwiches and salads or munch on them as a snack. Because of their high water content, an entire cup of cucumbers has only 13 calories.

Dates

Hebrew (palm tree): tamar/Hebrew (desert date): tsori
Greek (palm tree): phoinix

During their wilderness wanderings, the Israelites camped for a time in Elim. Elim was noted for its twelve fountains of water and its seventy palm trees, which made it an appealing attraction for weary travelers (Exodus 15:27; Numbers 33:9). The ancient city of Jericho was called the "city of palm trees" (Deuteronomy 34:3). A female leader of Israel gave guidance and counsel to the people "under the palm tree of Deborah," an open-air office of sorts (Judges 4:5). Bethany, the town where Jesus raised Lazarus from the dead, was called the "house of dates." It was branches of date palm trees that the people placed on the road during Jesus' triumphal entry into Jerusalem (John 12:13).

The many biblical references to date palms show that dates were a common food to the Jews, as well as other nationalities such as the Assyrians and Babylonians. The date palm was a symbol used on Palestinian coins.

Dates were eaten fresh or dried and were sometimes pressed into cakes. The syrup was extracted from dates to make a delicious date honey. Traditional nomadic Arabs still enjoy dates with a form of milk, sometimes living solely on just those two foods for weeks or months at a time. Now as then, dates are valued because they are a great source of easily digestible energy.

Quite long-lived, palm trees begin bearing fruit in their fourth year and produce their greatest crop when they are about eighty. Thousands of dates are harvested from a single tree each year. A new set of branches is produced annually, making the lofty palm tree a majestic sight; fully-grown date palms can be 100 feet tall. A date palm thrives under oppressive circumstances. Given this knowledge, Psalm 92:12-14 takes on new meaning: "The righteous shall flourish like the palm tree...They shall still bring forth fruit in old age."

Dates are a good source of potassium, calcium, and iron. They also have small amounts of minerals and B vitamins. Dates have the ability to serve as a natural aspirin. They can also act as a gentle laxative and have been used medicinally to treat stomach ailments.

Dates are approximately 75% sugar and are an excellent replacement for candy. A few years ago we vacationed in California, which produces nearly all of the dates grown in the United States. Knowing that I like dates, my mother-in-law introduced me to "date shakes," which was easily one of the sweetest things I've ever tasted in my life. It was delicious but only a small amount is needed to satisfy the most voracious sweet tooth. "Dates, raisins, figs, prunes, and other dried fruits are too often relegated to a secondary role in the meals of industrialized societies. These are the sweets (fiber-and nutrient-rich) that we *should* make an important part of our diet."[2]

There are several varieties of dates, though not all are easily obtainable in the United States: Barhi, Blonde, Deglet Noor, Halawi, Medjool, and Zahidi. One of my favorite sweet snacks consists of Medjool dates stuffed with fresh walnuts.

Figs
Hebrew: teen/Greek: sukon

From front to back, Scripture abounds with references to figs. Symbolic of peace and prosperity, figs were one of the most common foods throughout biblical history. Our introduction to figs is given by Adam and Eve, as they sew fig leaves together in an unsuccessful attempt to cover their nakedness after sin stole their innocence (Genesis 3:7). This first mention of figs lets us know that fig trees were one of the trees in the Garden of Eden. In Revelation, the closing book of the Bible, we find figs being analogously used to describe the occurrences of the sixth seal (Revelation 6:13).

Just as Adam and Eve sewed fig leaves together thousands of years ago, people of the Holy Land still sew fig leaves together. Instead of using them for clothing, however, these attached leaves serve as wrappings for fresh fruit.

Figs are eaten fresh or dried. Dried figs were often pressed into cakes or threaded on long strings, making them a convenient food for traveling. Bethphage, a town on the Mount of Olives, was famous for its figs; Bethphage means "house of unripe figs."

The twelve men sent to scout out the Promised Land brought back figs (Numbers 13:23). The children of Israel bemoaned the lack of figs in the wilderness (Numbers 20:5). Along with other provisions, a wise woman by the name of Abigail prepared two hundred cakes of figs for David and his followers (I Samuel 25:18). Cakes of figs were one of the foods eaten during the joyous celebration when David became king of Israel (I Chronicles 12:40). The prophet Isaiah ordered a lump of figs to be placed on Hezekiah's boil, after which treatment Hezekiah recovered from his previously incurable illness (Isaiah 38:21). Jesus cursed the unfruitful fig tree (Matthew 21:19; Mark 11:13-14). Before they met, Jesus "saw" Nathanael under the fig tree (John 1:48). Such supernatural knowledge convinced Nathanael that Jesus was the Messiah.

Figs come in varying shapes, sizes, and colors. The most common types of figs are Adriatic figs, Black Mission figs, Calimyrna figs, and Kadota figs.

Figs are high in natural sugar. (Dried figs are over 55% sugar.) In fact, a white, sugary film on figs is entirely normal. Enjoyed in moderation, figs are a good choice when you want to eat something sweet or need a little energy. Avoid commercially dried figs because they usually contain preservatives such as potassium sorbate and sulfur dioxide as well as added refined sugar.

Figs are a terrific source of fiber, magnesium, potassium, calcium, manganese, copper, iron, vitamins C, B1, and B6. Figs can be used to treat low blood pressure, anemia, gout, liver problems, menopausal symptoms, and skin diseases. Figs have been used in the past to treat gangrene and scurvy.

A natural laxative, figs are a great remedy for intestinal disorders. Hemorrhoids, constipation, and colitis can all benefit from the addition of figs into the diet. The seeds in figs serve as tiny colon cleansers and can help prevent colon cancer. Figs destroy intestinal parasites and bad bacteria and encourage the proliferation of acidophilus, which is beneficial bacteria.

Garlic
Hebrew: shum

Garlic grew abundantly in Egypt and the Israelites reminisced about it during their sojourn in the wilderness (Numbers 11:5). Correlating with the biblical reference to garlic, history also tells us that garlic was given to Egypt's pyramid-building slaves to increase their stamina and protect them from disease, thus making them of greater value to the Egyptians.

For thousands of years, garlic has crossed national, ethnic, and social boundaries to become the seasoning of choice for cultures around the world. In addition to flavoring a variety of foods, garlic has a long history of being a healthful and healing agent. It is sometimes referred to as "Chinese penicillin" and the former Soviet Union called it "Russian penicillin." It seems that most everyone recognizes the healing nature of garlic. "One raw crushed clove contains the antibiotic equivalent of one hundred thousand units of penicillin and has proven more effective than either penicillin or tetracycline in suppressing certain types of disease-carrying agents."[3]

"The ingredient that gives garlic its strong smell – allicin – is what gives garlic its potent antibiotic properties. In hundreds of scientific experiments, allicin extract from raw garlic has been shown to destroy the germs that spread diseases such as botulism, diarrhea, dysentery, staph, tuberculosis, and typhoid. Garlic has the broadest spectrum of antimicrobial substance known in the natural world. It is an antibacterial, antifungal, antiparasitic, antiprotozoan, and antiviral."[4]

This medicinal food contains vitamin A, vitamin C, selenium, calcium, and magnesium. Used during World War I to prevent gangrene, garlic is a great infection fighter and superbly combats the viruses that cause colds and the flu. Garlic boosts the body's immunity and is good for the digestive system. It helps eliminate lead and other toxic heavy metals from the body. Also, garlic fights inflammation and improves circulation, making it useful in the treatment of arthritis and rheumatism.

Garlic is beneficial for the prevention of certain cancers, providing protection against oxidation and free radicals, especially benefiting the stomach, colon, and esophagus. Studies have found that garlic may help prevent breast, endometrial, prostate, and testicular cancer as well.

Garlic is good news for our hearts too. It can help prevent heart disease because it cleanses impurities from the blood, slows blood coagulation, reduces both systolic and diastolic blood pressure, and lowers blood cholesterol levels. (Note: Garlic can act as a natural blood thinner, so before you integrate garlic into your diet, consult a physician if you are taking pharmaceutical blood thinners.)

Elephant garlic is a variety of garlic that, like its name implies, dwarfs regular garlic in size, though it is not quite as pungent.

The somewhat socially offensive odor of garlic keeps some people from eating it. To combat garlic's odor, chew a sprig of parsley. The chlorophyll in parsley reduces garlic's strong aroma. If your hands contact garlic, wash them in lemon juice and salt, then rinse.

If you desire the benefits of garlic but want to eliminate "garlic breath" altogether, an odorless supplement form of garlic developed by the Japanese called Kyolic aged garlic extract is available.

Grapes

Numerous Hebrew, Aramaic, and Greek words translate to the English word "grapes" and their byproducts. Grapes were a food so intertwined in the lives of both Old and New Testament people that they are referred to from Genesis to Revelation.

When Moses sent twelve men to spy out the Promised Land, they returned carrying "a branch with one cluster of grapes" from a place called Eshcol, which was so named because of the abundance of grapes that grew in that area (Numbers 13:23-24). According to the Law, strangers were allowed to eat of another's vineyard, as long as they did not carry any grapes away with them in their own container (Deuteronomy 23:24). In fact, vineyard owners were commanded to leave some grapes on the vine for foreigners and poor people (Leviticus 19:10). Vine-tenders knew to guard against foxes, which would destroy the harvest while it was still young and tender (Song of Solomon 2:15).

If finances allowed, families built towers to live in during grape harvest time. This temporary home also served as a watchtower. Isaiah 5:2 describes the process of building a productive vineyard, including the construction of such a tower: "And he fenced it, and gathered out the stones thereof, and planted it with the choicest vine, and built a tower in the midst of it, and also made a winepress therein: and he looked that it should bring forth grapes." Jesus referred to this type of watchtower in His parable about the man that built a vineyard and then traveled to a far country (Matthew 21:33-41).

In Bible days, grapes were eaten fresh or pressed into fresh grape juice and vinegar. Some of the references to honey in the Old Testament probably refer to grape juice that was boiled down into thick jelly-type syrup called "dibs." This grape honey was spread on bread or diluted with water and drunk. This may be the "honey" referred to in Genesis 43:11, when Israel commanded it to be sent to Joseph. Some grapes were fermented to produce "strong drink."

Other grapes were dried into raisins. These were a convenient and highly nourishing food, especially useful for travelers. When David and his household left Jerusalem because of Absalom's traitorous actions, Mephibosheth sent David food, including "an hundred bunches of raisins" (II Samuel 16:1). To revive him, an Egyptian man that had not eaten or drunk for three days was given bread, water, figs, and raisins (I Samuel 30:12).

Grape leaves were stuffed with rice, lamb, and spices and then cooked in the leaves. Still today, the French wrap some of their cheeses in grape leaves. Grape seed oil is an exotic product of grapes, yielding a delicate and pleasant flavor.

The Jews were not the only people who cultivated and harvested grapes. The Hittites and the Egyptians, as well as other nations, capitalized on the benefits and many uses of grapes. The Philistine city of Gath actually means "wine press."

The grape vine is a climbing shrub. Carefully tended grape arbors are beautiful. There are approximately 1500 varieties of grapes. The most common variety in the United States is the Thompson Seedless.

Grapes are a beneficial quick-energy food and are great virus fighters. They contain calcium, potassium, zinc, vitamins A, B, and C, soluble and insoluble fiber, and phenolics, which are powerful antioxidants. Boron is a mineral present in grapes that helps prevent osteoporosis. Grapes contain caffeic acid (a cancer fighting agent) and ellagic acid, which has anti-mutagenic and anti-carcinogenic properties, helping protect the body's DNA. A phytonutrient in grapes called resveratrol protects the heart, helps prevent cancer, and combats inflammation and arthritis. Resveratrol is found in the skins, leaves, and seeds of red and green grapes, with red grapes yielding more than green.

Grapes with seeds are one of the best sources of tartaric acid (cream of tartar). The combination of tartaric acid and fiber in grapes creates a healthy environment in the colon. Because of their cleansing and laxative traits, grapes expel poisons from the body, providing relief for constipation, gastritis, and chronic acidosis.

They support the health of the digestive tract, liver, kidneys, and blood.

Sun drying grapes preserves the nutrition of grapes so they can be enjoyed year around. Raisins are a great source of iron, potassium, boron, B vitamins, dietary fiber, carbohydrates, and phenolics. Actually, all of the benefits of grapes are magnified in raisins. Because of their concentrated sugar content, they should be enjoyed in moderation.

Conventionally grown and produced raisins, because they are concentrated grapes, contain more pesticide residue than any other fruit. Try to always buy organic raisins. They are grown without the use of chemical fertilizers and fumigants such as methyl bromide.

Mandrakes
Hebrew: duwday

Mandrakes are a bright red fruit belonging to the potato family. The insides of mandrakes are soft and pulpy. They have a sweet taste and unusual smell. Probably the best known reference to mandrakes is found in Genesis 30:14-17, which illustrates why mandrakes are known as the "love fruit." In addition to the folk belief that mandrakes improved fertility, some have found mandrakes to be useful for treating vertigo. Ironically however, eating too much mandrake fruit can cause dizziness. (See Song of Solomon 7:13.)

Melons
Hebrew: abattiyach

Melons were one of the things the children of Israel pined away for while in the wilderness (Numbers 11:5). There are essentially two types of melons: muskmelons and watermelons. Muskmelons include cantaloupes, honeydew, Casaba, Persian, and Crenshaw melons.

Historians are uncertain whether the melons the Israelites longed for referred to the muskmelon or the watermelon. One thing that is certain is that watermelons were grown in Egypt and ancient Israel. They were cultivated along the fertile banks of the Nile River. To-day, watermelons from Jaffa (Joppa) are especially prized in Israel; they can be purchased just outside Jerusalem's Damascus Gate.

All melons are cooling, re-hydrating, and cleansing. They contain over 90% water; thus, they require little work of the digestive system.

Melons have a rapid transit time. If eaten with or directly after heavier foods that take longer to digest, melons sit in the small intestines and ferment. If you experience digestive discomfort when eating melons with other foods, you may want to eat them a good while before you eat anything else.

Mulberries
Hebrew: baka

Mulberries are the fruit of the tree called "the weeping tree." Its thin branches drape nearly to the ground, giving it an appearance similar to the weeping willow tree that we are more familiar with in the U.S.

The biblical incident that comes to mind in relation to mulberries is David's victorious, God-led battle against the Philistines (II Samuel 5:23-24). Bible students know that the valley of Baca is indicative of tears and weeping (Psalm 84:6). Baca can also be translated to mean "valley of mulberry trees," a thought that helps us further develop our understanding of mulberry trees.

Trade made mulberries available to biblical people, who cultivated them for their fruit. Resembling large blackberries in appearance, mulberries are usually eaten fresh. They are also used to make juice, jam, or pies.

Mulberries have traditionally been used to treat stomach ulcers, aid digestion, calm the nervous system, and strengthen the blood.

Olives
Hebrew: zayith/Greek: elaia

The olive tree is one of the oldest trees known to

mankind. It is first mentioned in the Bible when the dove Noah sent from the ark brought back an olive leaf, which signified "that the waters were abated from off the earth" (Genesis 8:11). Sin and destruction were being replaced by renewal and peace. Still today, the leaves and branches of the olive tree are symbols of peace. (Incidentally, an herbal supplement called olive leaf extract is highly effective at fighting all types of viruses, harmful bacteria, parasites, and fungi, thus bringing balance and peace to the body's immune system.)

Because his trust in God produced stability in his life, David likened himself to a "green olive tree in the house of God" (Psalm 52:8). God used the following picturesque analogy to describe how He would bless the man that feared Him: "Thy wife shall be as a fruitful vine by the sides of thine house: thy children like olive plants round about thy table" (Psalm 128:3).

A good source of essential fatty acids, vitamin E, vitamin A, many of the B vitamins, zinc, copper, iron, calcium, magnesium, and phosphorus, olives were an important part of the daily lives of the Israelites. Olives were used for food, light, religious ceremonies, body cleansing, and skin ointments. Olive oil was especially valued. The virtues of olive oil were extensively discussed in "The Skinny on Fats," a chapter dedicated to the study of oils.

Although olive trees are native to Bible lands, they require care and cultivation. "Olive trees were grown by inserting a graft from a cultivated tree into a wild stock. The wild stock was then cut down to the ground. The tree takes about fifteen years to grow to maturity, and then it bears fruit for centuries. Some olive trees are more than 1,000 years old. Paul says that when Christianity followed the Judaism of the Old Testament, it was as if, contrary to normal practice, a wild olive were being grafted into a cultivated stock (Romans 11:24)."[5]

Though some olive trees are cultivated in the United States – mainly in California – Spain and Italy produce more than 50% of the world's olives. Spain produces mostly green olives while Italy produces mostly black olives. (Black olives are just very ripe green olives.)

In order to preserve olives, they are packed in salt water. There are several varieties of olives, all of which have their merits and specific uses. Kalamata olives, a Grecian specialty, are a favorite of my husband's. Some supermarkets have olive bars. These make it convenient to purchase small quantities of different types of olives so you may sample them and see what might suit your taste buds.

Onions
Hebrew: betsel

Numbers 11:5 is often used to illustrate how some people disdain God's blessings and protection on their lives and desire to return to "Egypt," a type of the sinful world of bondage from which God delivered them. People often mention the foolishness of the Israelites for wishing that they were in Egypt where they ate leeks, onions, and garlic. While it is positively true that it is very foolish to want to abandon God's protection in favor of willingly subjecting ourselves to the worldly system's harsh taskmaster, there is more to this story than initially meets the eye.

Numbers 11:5 mentions leeks, onions, and garlic, three things given a bad rap because of their pungent odor. However, this passage also mentions fish, cucumbers, and watermelons, foods that most people find pleasing to their palates. So it seems that the food itself may not have been the primary reason the Hebrews wanted to go back to Egypt.

Intermingled amongst the children of Israel was a "mixed multitude" (Exodus 12:38; Numbers 11:4). This "mixed multitude" probably consisted of Egyptians who had accompanied the children of Israel into the wilderness. These people were not of the seed of Abraham and it is highly doubtful that they revered and worshipped Jehovah as the one true God. They did not have a covenant relationship with God as the Hebrews did. Scripture seems to indicate that they incited widespread discontent among the Israelites. They began to complain about the manna that God provided. Their unthankful spirit infected the people of God.

When people begin to take for granted God's provision and protection, they longingly look back at the world, remembering how gratifying the world was to their fleshly nature. Seldom do they stop to consider that such seasonal fun is only a façade that will quickly lure them back into cruel bondage.

In this instance, the Israelites recalled the fish, watermelons, cucumbers, leeks, onions, and garlic, forgetting the pain and suffering they endured. Whatever manna was, it must have been a very nourishing and complete food, because God himself created it for the Israelites to live on. However, nowhere does Scripture tell us that the foods eaten in Egypt were forbidden, bad or sinful.

The point of Numbers 11 is not that leeks and garlic are inferior foods, but that the Israelites quickly lost sight of the power of their God. Their relationship with Him was in need of serious repair. They very easily allowed themselves to be influenced by things that they should have left behind in Egypt.

Actually, onions, as well as garlic, are among some of the most healthful foods on the planet. Although Numbers 11:5 is the only biblical mention of onions, they were widely used throughout Bible times. Thirty to forty species are currently grown in Palestine.

There are several hundred species of onions. Some of the varieties are Bermuda (Spanish) onions, chives, Maui onions, pearl onions, and shallots. Cipolline onions are great to have on hand when making kabobs. Yellow and white onions are by far the most common onions to the American kitchen. Vidalia onions of Vidalia, Georgia and Walla Walla onions of Walla Walla, Washington both have distinctive flavors.

Scallions are also called green onions. Interestingly, the word "scallion" is derived from Ashkelon, a Philistine city. Leeks are similar in taste to onions, but they are sweeter and milder. Leeks (Hebrew: chatzir) were a component in medicinal remedies. They are useful when treating obesity, kidney problems, coughs, and intestinal disorders.

All onions contain positive health-supporting properties. Onions can serve as a pain reliever, expectorant, and diuretic. They are a remedy for kidney and bladder problems and ease intestinal gas pains by cleansing the gastrointestinal tract. They help regulate blood sugar and may also help prevent cancer.

Onions are infection fighters and serve as antibiotics which combat bacteria, fungi, and parasites. They serve as external antiseptics. Just five minutes of chewing raw onions will kill all the germs in your mouth, including the ones that cause tooth decay, making it sterile and clean.

Our hearts benefit from onion consumption as well. They help to raise HDL cholesterol while lowering LDL cholesterol. They improve blood coagulation, helping to prevent abnormal blood clots. The alarming symptom of high blood pressure (hypertension) can be eliminated by the inclusion of onions in a healthy diet.

These many benefits of onions should motivate us to find ways to eat more of them. Onions can be eaten raw or cooked. Eaten raw, onions cleanse the body's pores. Onions contain a bioflavonoid called quercetin, which is a cancer fighter that is not destroyed by cooking.

Pomegranates
Hebrew: rimmown

Pomegranates are one of the most interesting fruits that God created. The outside of pomegranates gives little clue of what is inside. The hard, reddish-brown rind provides a covering for edible seeds that are crunchy, juicy, and delicious. Due to its many ruby-red seeds, the word pomegranate literally translates to "apple with seeds or grains."

Pomegranates can be enjoyed by eating the seeds or drinking juice extracted from the fruit.

Grenadine is red syrup made from pomegranates. I first heard of grenadine when my high school French teacher brought some to class for us to taste.

Military minded individuals might find it interesting that the root meaning of the word "grenade" is "something that contains grains or seeds." The French were familiar with the pomegranate's ability to, when opened, scatter its many seeds in all directions. So when a weapon was invented which, when detonated, scattered pieces of metal all around, the French naturally applied the word "grenade" to it.

Pomegranate trees can live a long time, upwards of 200 years. They have grown wild and been cultivated in Bible lands for many years. In addition to grapes and figs, the twelve men chosen to scout out the Promised Land brought back pomegranates (Numbers 13:23). The priests of the Lord wore garments that had hems decorated to look like pomegranates (Exodus 39:24-26). While Jonathan and his armor bearer were undertaking a daring offensive against the Philistines, "Saul tarried...under a pomegranate tree" (I Samuel 14:2). Hundreds of brass pomegranates were skillfully crafted to adorn Solomon's Temple (I Kings 7:42).

Pomegranates provide fiber, potassium, vitamins C and B, copper, and magnesium. They cleanse the body and are useful for treating bladder disorders.

THE GREAT APPLE DEBATE

Avid Bible readers are quite familiar with Scriptural references to apples. It is intriguing that research of the use of apples during Bible days reveals a wide array of conflicting strains of thought, making it difficult to conclusively determine what "apples" referred to. Most scholars agree that "apples" as we define them in modern times were not indigenous to the Mediterranean during Bible days. The only apples similar to what we know were of very inferior quality, equated with the crab apple.

What was native and accessible were citron fruits, pomegranates, and apricots; some people believe that the biblical "apple" was one of these three. As a result of my studies, I personally believe that "apple" especially does not refer to the citron fruit, and it was probably not a pomegranate either. In Joel 1:12, we find the pomegranate tree and the apple tree both mentioned. Two distinctly different Hebrew words differentiate between the two: rimmown (pomegranate) and tappuwach (apple).

Apricots seem to be the most likely definition for the biblical "apples." Familiar to the Assyrians and Babylonians, apricots were introduced to Palestine from Armenia. Solomon's phrase "comfort me with apples" may be a reference to the revitalizing aroma of apricots (Song of Solomon 2:5; 7:8). Proverbs 25:11 says that "a word fitly spoken is like apples of gold in pictures of silver." Still today, apricots are known in Cypress as "golden apples."

However, the improbability of apples being eaten in Bible times does not negate their wonderful health-building properties. Apple cider vinegar, the product of aged apple cider, is deserving of special note. For centuries, it has been praised for its ability to cure many diverse ailments and diminish the effects of others. A rich source of essential amino acids, enzymes, and minerals – notably potassium – apple cider vinegar helps control weight, serves as a natural antibiotic, cleanses the colon, mends urinary tract infections, provides PMS relief, promotes healthy skin, flushes toxins from the body, and eases the pain caused by stiff joints and arthritis.

Commercial vinegars have been refined, distilled, and pasteurized. They are void of health promoting properties. Be sure to buy apple cider vinegar that is organic, raw, and unfiltered. This naturally fermented apple cider vinegar is usually aged in wood and transferred to glass bottles and is just as healthy and vibrant as the apple cider vinegar that Hippocrates administered to sick folks in 400 B.C.

HOW DOES YOUR GARDEN GROW?

Horticulture was a familiar art to the inhabitants of the Holy Land. The first gardener mentioned in the Bible is God. "And the Lord God planted a garden eastward in Eden" (Genesis 2:8). God promised Zion, a figurative reference to His bride, the Church, that He would "make her wilderness like Eden, and her desert like the garden of the Lord" (Isaiah 51:3).

King Solomon was a botanical genius, an expert in cultivating herbs and vegetables. His gardens were not flower gardens, but orchards and vineyards, trees and shrubs of great variety. He said, "I made me gardens and orchards, and I planted trees in them of all kind of fruit" (Ecclesiastes 2:5). From front to back, the Song of Solomon is filled with references to Solomon's gardens. In great detail, he discusses the variety of plants, spices, fruits, and nuts that grew there. His gardens must have been beautiful, since everything Solomon did he did to excess and he spared no expense.

King Ahab wanted Naboth's vineyard so that he could make it into "a garden of herbs" (I Kings 21:2). Scholars say that this "garden of herbs" was probably a royal kitchen garden that yielded both herbs and vegetables.

Gardens are used figuratively to refer to peace and prosperity. The Lord said that He would make His people like "a watered garden" (Isaiah 58:11). Because of the abundant blessings of God in our lives, we can be called "the planting of the Lord, that he might be glorified" (Isaiah 61:3). Isaiah predicted that the Messiah would "grow up before him as a tender plant, and as a root out of a dry ground" (Isaiah 53:2).

Personally, the extent of our gardening has been confined to the cultivation of tomatoes and a few herbs such as parsley and basil. If your location and lifestyle allow you the opportunity to grow a garden, take advantage of the benefits of homegrown foods. Not only will you reap nutritional benefits if you reduce your dependency on store-bought produce, but you will save a bundle of money as well.

In place of synthetic and potentially harmful pesticides, insecticides, and fungicides, investigate the potential of herbs (such as neem) to prevent bugs from overtaking your garden. These herbs are safe for your garden, the environment, and your health. Use organic compost and practice crop rotation to mix nitrogen into the soil and keep it healthy.

LEGUMES

Legumes are the family name for a variety of beans and peas. Some of the members of this family are adzuki beans, black-eyed peas, lima beans, peas, peanuts, black beans, canellini beans, great northern beans, navy beans, and pinto beans.

Legumes satisfy hunger and supply long-lasting energy. They are easy to store and inexpensive, making them a convenient and healthy food. Many crops deplete the soil of nutrients, but not beans. While beans are growing, they add nitrogen back into the soil.

Common legumes known to modern Mediterranean people are garbanzo beans (chickpeas), lentils, fava beans (broad beans), and the common green pea. Garbanzo beans are used to make hummus and falafel.

Lentils (Hebrew: adash) and beans (Hebrew: powl), which means "thick" or "plump," are specifically mentioned in the Bible (Genesis 25:34; II Samuel 17:28; II Samuel 23:11; Ezekiel 4:9). Though sometimes beans and lentils were eaten alone, it seems that they were usually a key ingredient in stews and pottages, with garlic and meat sometimes added. The bread and lentils that Esau traded his birthright for is probably the most famous reference to legumes in the Bible.

Lentils are one of the easiest legumes to implement into one's diet. They are one of the few beans that do not require soaking. They cook quickly and can be used in soups, stews, salads, side dishes, and casseroles. Choose from red, brown, green, yellow, orange, or French (dark green-blue) lentils or use a combination for a splash of various colors. (Note: Yellow and orange lentils lose their shape faster than the other varieties.) Lentils are a good source of folic acid and pureed lentils can help those with stomach ulcers and colitis.

Though it is a bit off of the beaten bean path, carob (Greek: keration) is definitely worth mentioning. Famished and penniless, the Prodigal Son longed to partake of "the husks that the swine did eat" (Luke 15:16). These husks were not the remains of corn-on-the-cob.

They were instead the pods of the carob tree, which is native to the eastern Mediterranean region. Most carob pods were used to feed livestock. However, very poor people also ate carob pods. They were also eaten during times of famine, which is what the Prodigal Son was experiencing when he "came to himself."

At one time carob seeds were used by goldsmiths to measure gold by "carat" weight. Because they were shaped similarly, carob beans were commonly called "locusts." A food additive in common use today is "locust bean gum," also called "carob bean gum." "In Palestine, a molasses named dibs is prepared from ripe carob fruits."[6]

Carob products abound in health food stores. It is often used as a substitute for chocolate. Although it does not taste like chocolate, when it is ground into a powder, carob looks like chocolate and has similar cooking and baking properties. Its obvious advantage over chocolate is that it does not contain caffeine. Rich in vitamins A and B complex, carob is naturally sweet, is low in fat and high in protein.

The pectin in carob makes it beneficial for the treatment of stomach disorders and diarrhea. Carob also has a reputation for helping asthmatics. Years ago, carob seeds were in demand by singers because of carob's ability to soothe the throat and bring healing to the respiratory tract.

One of the star characteristics of legumes is that they are a good source of soluble fiber, which aids in lowering LDL cholesterol, reduces blood pressure, and helps stabilize blood sugar. This fiber prevents and cures constipation and reduces risk of some cancers.

Legumes are high in potassium, iron, thiamine, and vitamin C. They are a good source of complex carbohydrates.

Because they lack some of the essential amino acids, legumes' protein is incomplete. But when legumes and grains are combined, they form a protein similar to that in meat. In Bible days beans were ground into flour, mixed with wheat or barley and baked into breads. This is seen in Ezekiel 4:9 where beans and lentils (legumes) were combined with wheat, barley, millet, and spelt (grains) to make bread which contained a complete mix of proteins.

If you want to obtain the benefits of legumes yet you are concerned about the gastrointestinal distress their consumption sometimes causes, rinse and soak them overnight. Never cook legumes in their soaking water; always rinse them in fresh water when they are done soaking. Also, adding a little ginger, epazote, bay leaf, cumin, anise, fennel, or summer savory during cooking will aid digestion.

While dry beans are naturally low in sodium, most canned beans have had a lot of salt added to them. Be sure to rinse them before you use them.

NUTS AND SEEDS

The next time you want a snack, instead of reaching for potato or corn chips, M&Ms, or packaged cookies, eat a handful of raw nuts. A snack of nuts is much more satisfying than a candy bar or a bag of chips because nuts will actually supply nutrition to your body whereas a candy bar and potato chips only satisfy temporarily and supply no nutrition to your body. The Jews use nuts in desserts. Kibbet, a Hebrew word that means "treat," is a combination of dates, figs, raisins, and nuts.

Nuts are a good fat and are a great source of protein and energy. They are packed with necessary vitamins, minerals, fiber, and antioxidants such as B complex vitamins, folic acid, potassium, magnesium, manganese, iron, phosphorus, calcium, boron, vitamin E, zinc, copper, and selenium, among others. Many nuts are slightly sweet and, once you have weaned yourself away from refined sugar, they will pleasantly satisfy your sweet tooth. Various studies have concluded that eating a moderate amount of nuts can reduce your risk of heart attack and adult-onset (Type II) diabetes.[7]

There is such a wide variety of raw nuts to choose from that you are certain to find some you really like that suit your specific health needs. Try almonds, walnuts, pistachios, cashews, chestnuts, hazelnuts (filberts), pecans, Brazil nuts, macadamias, and pine nuts. There are three nuts in particular that were well known to biblical people: almonds, pistachios, and walnuts.

A good source of healthy fats, carbohydrates, and protein, almonds (Hebrew: shaqad) contain vitamin B2 and calcium, making them good for the teeth and bones. A poultice of ground almonds can remove sunburn spots and are a good addition to the diet for weight maintenance. The oil extracted from almonds is used in some quality face creams, perfumes, medicines, and even baked goods.

Almonds were very familiar to Biblical people. Along with other foods, Jacob told his sons to take almonds to Joseph in Egypt (Genesis 43:11). The Lord reestablished His approval of Aaron's position by causing his rod to bring forth buds, blossom, and yield almonds overnight (Numbers 17:1-8). When the almond tree is in full bloom, its blossoms are white. The statement "the almond tree shall flourish" is a reference to the white hair of the aged (Ecclesiastes 12:5).

Pistachios (Hebrew: boten) originated in Syria and Persia but became popular throughout Palestine. Pistachios were the "nuts" that accompanied the almonds that Jacob sent to Joseph (Genesis 43:11). Considered a luxury, pistachios were eaten raw and were also used in the preparation of various sweet treats such as ice cream and Turkish delight.

Many Bible scholars believe that the "garden of nuts" referred to in the Song of Solomon was a walnut orchard. Walnuts were always planted in the lowest parts of the valleys, which would explain why Solomon "went *down* into the garden of nuts" (Song of Solomon 6:11 – italicized emphasis added). Walnuts (Hebrew: egowz) were highly regarded in Bible lands. They came to Israel from Persia and the Greeks called the walnut the "Royal Persian." The Hebrew phrase "egowz melech" meant "the king's nut." During Jesus' time, walnut trees grew along the Sea of Galilee, providing refreshing shade.

Walnuts help build muscles and healthy teeth and gums. They contain antioxidants gamma tocopherol and delta tocopherol. The serotonin in walnuts helps control hunger and improve metabolism. Walnuts help correct liver ailments and aid in lowering cholesterol levels. During the Middle Ages, "walnuts were considered so powerful that they were included in a prescription to ward off the dreaded Black Plague that swept Europe."[8]

Nuts contain enzyme inhibitors that can cause digestive discomfort. Some nutritionists suggest soaking raw nuts in salt water overnight then drying them out in a warm oven for easier digestion. (Cashews, unlike other nuts, should only be soaked for six hours.)

Purchase nuts that are raw and unsalted. This means that they have not been heated or altered in any way. Start using nut butters that are nothing but freshly ground nuts. You will still get the fantastic benefits of the nuts yet avoid hydrogenated oil and the adverse effects of processing that accompanies commercial nut butters. All raw nuts and seeds may be stored in the refrigerator or freezer for greater freshness but walnuts and pecans particularly should be. They become rancid quickly. Cashews contain a little less fat than other nuts.

And while you are beginning to enjoy the taste and health benefits of raw nuts, try some raw seeds too. Sunflower, pumpkin (pepitas), and sesame seeds are some commonly used seeds. Tahini is made from roasted, ground sesame seeds. Tahini combined with honey makes halvah, a Middle Eastern candy. Keep flax seeds handy and grind them as needed. Sprinkle a tablespoon into baked goods, cereal, and granola, salads, and shakes.

Sprinkle nuts and seeds on your salads, add them to your granola, and use them in cooking and baking. Look for recipes that call for the use of nuts and seeds. Enjoy a variety of nuts and seeds regularly.

A FRESH LOOK

In addition to those used in Bible lands, God has provided us with a wonderful variety of fresh produce. The multiculturalism of North America has introduced us to formerly obscure foods that are delicious and nutritious. Due to the plethora of information readily available about ethnic fruits and vegetables as well as common produce such as oranges, grapes, bananas, and apples, this book does not address those foods in particular.

Cruciferous vegetables, sometimes called the cabbage family vegetables, include broccoli, cauliflower, Brussels sprouts, bok choy, collard greens, mustard greens, watercress, turnip greens, radishes, rutabaga, horseradish, and cabbage. The active ingredient in cruciferous vegetables is indoles, which protects against cancer, especially breast and ovarian cancer. Cruciferous vegetables are good sources of folic acid, vitamin C, and beta carotene. (The body converts beta carotene into vitamin A, which aids the immune system and prevents cancer.)

Carotenoid vegetables include tomatoes, watermelons, pink grapefruit, apricots, carrots, spinach, collard greens, romaine lettuce, leeks, squash, and sweet potatoes. These dark green and bright, colorful fruits and vegetables also contain beta carotene, as well as alpha carotene, gamma carotene, lycopene, and lutein.

Chlorophyll is the element that makes plants green. The darker the vegetable, the more chlorophyll it contains. Chlorophyll purifies the blood and is an antioxidant. It protects us from toxins, particularly those that result from smoking, fried foods, and charcoal grilled foods. Some examples of chlorophyll vegetables are spinach, kale, collard greens, beet tops, and parsley.

Bioflavonoids are necessary for vitamin C to be properly absorbed into the body. They are found in peppers, plums, honey, citrus foods such as lemons and grapefruit, and some whole grains.

Fruits and vegetables are important sources of antioxidants. I once heard an analogy that simply explained the important job of antioxidants in their fight against free radicals. In this analogy, free radicals are like destructive fire in our bodies which, if unchecked, will cause our bodies to be consumed by cancer. Antioxidants are like the fire department that is present the second the fire starts and works diligently until the fire is extinguished.

Fresh fruits and vegetables supply soluble and insoluble fiber. Fiber keeps the body clean, preventing buildup of toxins. This greatly decreases the risk of hemorrhoids, constipation, and colon cancer.

In addition to fruits and vegetables, sources of soluble fiber include garbanzo beans, lentils, navy beans, barley, oats, and rice.

Insoluble fiber is found in whole grains, dried beans, and the skins of fruits and vegetables.

Some fiber supplements available today are psyllium seed, flax seed, rice bran, and oat bran. Be sure to drink plenty of water when using fiber supplements. Keep in mind that fiber supplements should not be consumed at the same time as mineral and vitamin supplements.

Variety is still the spice of life. The potato is one of the most popular vegetables in America, eaten mostly in the form of French fries or potato chips, distortions which minimize or destroy the benefits of the potato. With such a great variety of vegetables available to us, it is unfortunate that we do not take advantage of them.

The conclusion of a study conducted by researchers at Colorado State University found that "smaller amounts of a large variety of fruits and vegetables may be more beneficial than larger amounts of the same old, same old. It might not be more kinds of antioxidants, but rather the interaction of all those antioxidants that's important."[9]

Be adventurous. Try some new foods at ethnic markets, health food stores, and farmers markets. Just beyond your comfort zone of iceberg lettuce, tomatoes, apples, oranges, and bananas is a whole world inviting you to experience healthy, fun foods brimming with flavor and nutrition.

Sometimes my husband and I have "Vegetable Days." These are days when we eat only vegetables. In the summer, when the farmers markets are brimming with delicious, fresh produce, we take advantage of their bounty to feast on God's creative delights.

AT THE MARKET

Whenever possible, choose organically grown produce over conventionally grown produce. Organic produce contains more polyphenols, antioxidants, minerals, vitamin C, beta-carotene, and flavonoids than foods that have been grown in mineral-depleted soil and sprayed with manmade chemicals. Remember that bigger, shinier, perfect looking produce sometimes has cosmetic help along the way. Some of the best tasting produce is not necessarily the prettiest.

Conventional produce notorious for having a lot of pesticide residue are peaches, strawberries, apples, celery, imported grapes, spinach, bell peppers, nectarines, cherries, pears, lettuce, and potatoes. When purchasing these foods, choose organic versions if at all possible. Produce with the least amount of pesticide residues are onions, avocados, sweet corn, pineapples, mango, asparagus, sweet peas, kiwi, bananas, cabbage, broccoli, and papaya.

Fresh fruits and vegetables are the most beneficial. Frozen is the next option. When fruits and vegetables are flash frozen, have not been heated to high temperatures, and have not had sugar or preservatives added, they retain most of their vitamin content. They are a good choice if fresh produce is unavailable. Only use canned vegetables in a pinch. Much of their vitamin content is lost during processing. They are subjected to high cooking temperatures and usually have any number of additives in the can with them.

IN THE KITCHEN

A few of the agents used to preserve and wash fresh fruits and vegetables are potassium bromide, polyacrylamide, and sodium 2-ethyl-1-hexylsulfate. Some chemicals have been found to be toxic, skin irritating, and harmful to the central nervous system. By the time these foods reach your table, these chemicals have not all been rinsed off. Even if it looks clean, wash your produce just before eating or cooking it. Don't overlook produce with skins and rinds that are inedible, such as bananas and watermelons; they have been handled by a lot of people during their journey from the field to your kitchen. Use a solution of pure water, baking soda, and lemon juice and scrub your produce with a vegetable brush that will penetrate into crevices where dirt and microbes can hide. Be sure to keep your vegetable brush clean.

When you purchase fresh organic fruit and vegetables with edible skins, be sure to eat the skins. The skins are alive with flavor and healthful properties.

Preparation of vegetables is key to preserving their nutritive content. Steaming is the preferred method for cooking vegetables. High pressure and low pressure boiling are not as good as steaming but better than microwaving.

In the name of convenience, some people cook almost all of their food in a microwave oven but microwaving is probably the least healthy cooking method. Do you like broccoli? If you microwave it, almost all of the flavonoids are removed. There is a reason why we say we are going to "nuke" our food when we use the microwave: the microwave zaps the nutrition right out of it. Microwaving alters the molecular structure of food, damaging its vitamins, minerals, fats, and proteins. Mothers especially should avoid heating Baby's milk in the microwave. Doing so affects the amino acids in the milk and can be detrimental to a little liver and central nervous system.

Many people use a microwave oven to defrost meat. Defrosting without a microwave takes only a few minutes of forethought. Another common use of microwaves is reheating leftovers. It really does not take all that much time to reheat food on the stove. The little extra mess is a fair exchange for nutrient retention.

Just in case you can't imagine life without a microwave oven, I am living proof that you don't really need it. I can count on one hand the times I have used a microwave oven in the last eight years. I don't miss it one bit.

So eliminate or at least greatly limit your use of a microwave oven. Trade in limp, microwaved broccoli smothered in synthetic cheese for broccoli with its nutrition intact that has been simply and healthily prepared.

Regardless of whether you choose to steam, boil, or bake your vegetables, don't overcook them. They should still be slightly firm, not wilted or shapeless.

Educate yourself about the benefits of fermented vegetables and experiment with making your own. My husband makes pickles using the process of lactic acid fermentation. They have an excellent flavor that is far superior to pasteurized store-bought pickles. Many other vegetables such as cabbage (which produces sauerkraut and kimchi), beans, beets, pumpkins, and squash can be used to make lactic-fermented foods. Lacto-fermentation proliferates healthy bacteria and increases vitamin content, while inhibiting unfriendly bacteria. This process benefits digestion, boosts metabolism, supports systems that are lactose intolerant, and fights cancer.

AT THE TABLE

Express your thanks for the food you are about to eat. Jesus exampled this for us before He fed the multitude and before He ate the Last Supper with His disciples (Matthew 15:36; John 6:11). As we thank the Lord for the food He has provided for us, we can also ask Him to help us eat wisely and temperately.

Any endeavor that is undertaken without the help and blessing of God will simply be a work of our own willpower. When it comes to changing long ingrained dysfunctional eating habits, willpower usually fails because it requires that we rely on our own fluctuating strength. From start to finish, our lives should be inseparably intertwined with His will as we fulfill His purpose for our lives. It should be our desire that He receives glory out of the positive changes we make in our lives in regard to health and nutrition.

During meals, moderation should always be our goal. Even if our meal is very healthy and entirely organic, we can overextend ourselves (our tummies!) if we eat too much.

We tend to put more on our plates if our plates are large. No rocket science required here; it's just the American way. Large plate = large amounts of food. The solution? Eat on smaller plates – and don't keep refilling them.

If you are in the habit of adding a lot of salt to your food at the table, experiment with different spices and use freshly ground pepper, cayenne pepper, and sea salt-herb blends instead of refined salt. Many people don't really enjoy the true flavors of food because they add too much salt to their food.

Branch out from your taste buds' comfort zone. Learn to enjoy celery with raw almond butter instead of hydrogenated, processed peanut butter. Savor the flavor of a crisp apple *without* caramel sauce. Snack on carrot sticks that are not smothered in ranch or blue cheese dressing.

Slow down and enjoy life. Though you may be busy all day, learn to look forward to and enjoy mealtime. Eating on the run should be the exception, not the rule. Though we may not be able to spend two or three hours lingering at the table as is customary in some European countries, mealtime should not be conducted in Indy 500 style. If your life is fast paced, learn to view mealtime as a time to relax. Especially if you or someone in your family has taken extra time to prepare a healthy meal, show your appreciation by slowing down and enjoying it.

Goal oriented people might be tempted to rush through meals in an attempt to finish the meal so that they can go on to do something else. Don't spend your entire mealtime thinking about all the things you need to do. Don't consider mealtime wasted time. If you are a task-oriented person, keep a small notepad handy. During a meal, if you think of something you need to do, jot it down on your notepad and forget about that task until mealtime is over.

Enjoy your family and converse with them while you are eating. Keep the conversation positive and uplifting. Ask questions to get to know one another better. If you live alone, occasionally ask a friend over for a meal. Mealtime is a time to share our thoughts and connect with each other.

Keep all media turned off during mealtime. If the phone rings and the call does not require immediate attention, inform the caller that you are eating with your family and arrange to call him or her back later. This is not rude; it is setting a boundary around the relationships you are trying to build with the most important people in your life – your family and friends.

Chew your food slowly and thoroughly. Many of us gulp or inhale our food rather than chew it. The more you chew your food means less work for your digestive system.

Take smaller bites and take the time to savor every bite of food. The goal is not to see how much food you can put into your mouth at one time. Also, finish the first bite before inserting the second bite.

When we eat this way, we may find ourselves not eating as much as we used to though we are not consciously trying to limit our food intake. Our slower eating habits will signal our bodies that they are getting full. Also, when mealtime becomes important, we will find it less necessary to snack between meals, grazing and nibbling our way through the day.

EATING HEALTHY ON A BUDGET

When I talk to people about the benefits of eating healthy foods, invariably the first thing I hear is, "It is so expensive to eat healthy. Fresh fruits and vegetables and organic food cost so much more than regular food." Most organically grown fruits and vegetables contain at least 20% more vitamins and minerals than conventional produce that processing has corrupted. Though you might pay a bit more for organic produce you are actually getting more bang for your buck.

You can purchase fruit, vegetables, meat, honey, maple syrup, cheese, and even homemade soap from farm stands or farmers markets. Oftentimes produce is cheaper and definitely fresher when it is bought directly from the source than from the supermarket. The less distance food has to travel to reach your table, the fresher it will be. And supporting local farms and gardens in your community will help you establish relationships with people who have the same health goals as you do. Many of them will be thrilled to encourage, help, and inform you as you learn how to eat better.

If food cooperatives are available in your area, you may want to join one. These provide you with local, seasonal produce at a fraction of the cost you would pay at the supermarket. Pick-your-own farms and orchards are not just ways to improve your diet but time spent with a friend or family member picking strawberries, apples, or peaches will make a lot of good memories as well.

Not only does purchasing locally grown food benefit your health and your pocketbook, it is also better for the local farmer's pocketbook. Much more money is spent on marketing than the actual growing and harvesting of food. According to the USDA Agriculture Fact

Book, for every $1.00 spent on farm-raised food, the farmer's share is only 19¢. The rest is used for packaging, transportation, advertising, wholesalers, retailers, manufacturers, assemblers, etc. When you support small local farmers they get to keep more of the profit, which will empower them to continue growing fresh, healthy food for you.[10]

Clip coupons. Many health food stores offer free magazines that contain coupons. Some stores even have coupon books available. You can download free coupons from your favorite health food manufacturers' websites. Use your coupons in conjunction with sales and stock up on staple items. I've saved as much as 80% of my shopping bill just by using coupons and taking advantage of sales. This takes a little time but it is time well spent. "A penny saved is a penny earned."

Consider any extra money spent on good produce or staple items an *investment* in your health and the health of your family. Pay now (on delicious, healthy foods) or pay later (on expensive, painful surgeries and medications).

When beginning to eat healthy, the first few months may inflate your budget as you stock your kitchen. The transition can be easier financially if, as you use up your unhealthy foods, you replace them with healthy ones. When you replace soda with water, pre-packaged deli meats with home cooked whole chickens, and cookies, donuts, and potato chips with fresh produce, you will actually save money.

Become familiar with the bulk section of your health food store. There you can purchase quality herbs, spices, nuts, seeds, grains, legumes, and even sea salt, usually at a fraction of the cost of packaged products. As finances permit, gradually purchase "tools" such as a juicer, grain mill, and steamer that will equip you to achieve homemade health.

As you prepare meals made from whole foods and decrease your fast food meals and purchases of junk food, in time you will see great returns on the investments of your finances, time, energy, and effort.

TWENTY-THREE

HERBS AND SPICES

D uring Bible days, herbs and spices were an integral part of daily life and they are still too important for us to overlook. Many of them were multi-purpose. In addition to seasoning food, they were aromatic and medicinal.

Ezekiel 47:12 says that the fruit of the trees could be used for food and their leaves for medicine. Revelation 22:2 states that "the leaves of the tree were for the healing of the nations." God used the healing properties of nature to show how completely and lovingly He would restore and heal His people.

God instituted that the fruit, leaves and bark of trees and plants could be used for food and medicine, providing health and healing. Some millennia-old remedies are still in use today and have the ability to marvelously improve our health. Knowing that some of the same herbs used in the Patriarchs' day are still available to us speaks of the wonder of God's care and forethought for His people. Long before scientists analyzed them and pharmaceutical companies capitalized on some of them, healing herbs and spices were in common use by "primitive" nomadic people that lived in tents. Herbs and spices truly are God's medicine cabinet.

If you choose to take advantage of the benefits of herbs for healing, it is recommended that you consult a certified herbalist to determine the correct dosage and proper combination of herbs you need to use. Individuals who specialize in homeopathic, herbal, and nutritional therapy can create a personal profile for you to aid your application of God's bounty.

When using herbs and spices for cooking, choose fresh rather than dried whenever possible. The bottled spices at most mainstream grocery stores are far from fresh and oftentimes contain additives to extend their shelf life. Of course, the optimal scenario is to grow your own herbs. Keep in mind that you can purchase or create herb blends to be a flavorful replacement for salt when seasoning is needed. Experiment with different herbs and spices. Get out of your comfort zone of using just the few spices with which you are familiar and you will discover a whole new world of delightful flavors.

The word "herbs" in the Bible is often an umbrella term that covers not just herbs such as rue and mint, but also encompasses vegetables. Herbs, especially the "bitter herbs" that accompanied the Passover meal, were probably a combination of herbs and vegetables (Exodus 12:8). Gathered fresh, these plant crops consisted of chicory, dandelion, endive, lettuce, sheep sorrel, mint, and watercress. The Egyptians mixed green herbs with mustard and dunked their bread into the mixture or mixed the herbs together and ate them like a salad. The Hebrews probably learned about bitter herbs from them.

It is interesting that the "herbs" used for the Passover meal were sweet at the beginning of the growing season but by the time of the Exodus, they were bitter. This was symbolic of the 430 years the Israelites spent in Egypt. At first, when Joseph brought his family into Egypt, they were blessed with food and protection. Life was good and all was well. But after Joseph died and a new king sat on the throne, life for the children of Israel began to become harsh and bitter (Exodus 1:6-14).

Due to the great availability of herbs and spices from around the world, we will focus on just herbs and spices referred to in the Bible. We will further narrow our discussion by choosing specific herbs and spices that may be particularly interesting and intriguing to the curious Bible student.

Though some of these herbs and spices are familiar and readily available, we will explore others simply for the sake of reinforcing our understanding of the importance biblical people placed upon these culinary and medicinal jewels. While this very brief sampling will be sufficient to demonstrate how vital these nutrient-packed foods were to the lives of our spiritual ancestors, hopefully we will be motivated to experiment with uncommon and unusual herbs and spices.

Additionally, rather than looking through 21st century, westernized eyes, enlightening our comprehension with knowledge of Bible lands and customs will make our times of Bible reading and study more enriching.

Aloes
Hebrew: ahaliym/Greek: aloe

Aloes of biblical times were different from the aloe vera plants that some of us grow and keep handy in case of burns, cuts, or open sores. However, they were just as renowned for their wide range of healing and beneficial properties. Aloes were even used for embalming, since they keep their fragrance for many years. Aloe has a long, illustrious history that has traversed cultures and continents. Christopher Columbus made this entry in his diary: "All is well, Aloe is on board."

"The USDA gets more letters about aloes as a folk remedy for skin cancer than any other species, except possibly eggplant."[1] People have discovered aloe to be a tried and proven healing agent.

Aloe can be used topically to treat burns, including sunburn. Even skin that is inflamed or burned due to radiation exposure can benefit from the application of aloe. Used to soothe and beautify skin, aloe also helps heal acne and treat jaundice. Aloe serves as an emollient in a variety of skin and hair products. Heated aloe leaves can be applied to abscesses, bruises, wounds, skin inflammations, and sprains. One folk remedy purports that a plaster of aloe leaves or juice can cure some tumors. The water used to rinse aloes can serve as eyewash for inflammation of the inner eyelid.

Aloe juice or gel can be used to treat a variety of internal ailments. Fevers, coughs, sore throats, colds, pneumonia, edema, whooping cough, and gallbladder ailments can all benefit from aloe's anesthetic and anti-bacterial properties. Aloe can also be used to purge the stomach and lower intestines.

(See Numbers 24:6, Psalm 45:8, and Song of Solomon 4:14 for more Scriptures about aloes.)

Balm
Hebrew: tsori

Balm is the shortened form of balsam. Probably the most commonly known biblical reference to balm is heard in Jeremiah's cry as he laments Israel's spiritual condition in Jeremiah 8:22: "Is there no balm in Gilead; is there no physician there? why then is not the health of the daughter of my people recovered?"

The balsam tree grows east of the Jordan River in the land of Gilead; hence, the term "Balm of Gilead." When the oil was extracted from the fruit, the balm was used medicinally. It was highly regarded as a pain reliever and was a valuable aromatic spice.

(See Genesis 37:25; 43:11; Jeremiah 46:11; 51:8; Ezekiel 27:17.)

Capers
Hebrew: abiyownah

Included in Solomon's list of the ailments that sometimes accompany old age is the cessation of something called "desire" (Ecclesiastes 12:5). "Desire shall fail," he declared.

In ancient times, capers were served as an appetizer; the flower buds of the caper were named "desire shall fail" because caper berries abated hunger until the main course was served. Solomon had observed how the taste buds and appetite of aged people tend to lessen. In our vernacular, instead of saying "desire shall fail" we might say "appetite will decrease."

It is interesting that capers are still used today during some appetizer courses. The capers commonly available to us are harvested from the wild or cultivated and preserved in brine.

Cinnamon
Hebrew: qinnamown/Greek: kinamomon

One of the components of the holy anointing oil was sweet cinnamon (Exodus 30:23). More than a wonderful aromatic, cinnamon can be used to cleanse and detoxify the body. A digestive aid, cinnamon soothes the stomach, relieves pain, and eases the discomfort of coughs and congestion. Cinnamon oil is a tremendous virus fighter. The potential of cinnamon to help type 2 diabetes patients is encouraging. Studies show that cinnamon may help regulate blood sugar by increasing insulin efficiency.

For thousands of years, cinnamon has been highly valued for its varied uses. In addition to being an important ingredient in incense and holy anointing oil, cinnamon has served as a spice, medicine, perfume, and food preservative. Typical culinary uses today include the addition of cinnamon to hot apple cider, fruit salads, cakes, breads, and tea.

Note: Cassia, also mentioned in the Bible, is very similar but slightly inferior in taste to cinnamon. For example, to obtain the same flavor of first-rate cinnamon, twice that amount of cassia is needed.

(See Song of Solomon 4:14 and Revelation 18:13.)

Coriander
Hebrew: gad

Since the Israelites had never before seen manna, they compared it to coriander seeds, with which they were familiar (Exodus 16:31). Coriander is a plant of the carrot family. It grows wild in Palestine and Egypt. It is still a very popular spice among the Egyptians and Indians, who add it to meat and some breads. It is also used to flavor pastries, candies, salads, curries, and soups.

Coriander can be used medicinally to treat minor stomach discomfort. It can also be used topically to soothe joint and muscle pain.

Frankincense
Hebrew: lebonah/Greek: libanos

The literal translation of "frankincense" is "free (frank) lighting (incense)." Frankincense is the gum resin obtained from the bark of a tree. It burns freely and is glittering and white. The pure nature of frankincense made it appropriate for use in worship unto the Lord. Some of the offerings the Israelites brought before the Lord were presented with frankincense and oil on them (Leviticus 2:1).

Probably what comes to most people's minds when they hear the word "frankincense" is its presentation to Jesus by wise men from the east. It is no coincidence that the three gifts offered to Jesus when he was just a child – gold, frankincense, and myrrh – symbolized His identity and mission. Gold was given to kings, thus affirming the divine nobility of this child born in obscurity and humility. Frankincense represented His perfect purity and holiness. Myrrh was used during embalming procedures. Giving myrrh to the young child Jesus provided insight into His future that would consist of hardship, suffering, and cruel death. Joseph of Arimathaea and Nicodemus used "a mixture of myrrh and aloes" when they prepared Jesus' body for burial (John 19:39-40).

Hyssop
Hebrew: ezowb/Greek: hussopos

Hyssop, a member of the mint family and a type of marjoram, was an aromatic shrub that boasted clusters of yellow flowers. At maturity it achieved only three feet in height. It grew abundantly in dry, rocky crevices and was cultivated on terraced walls.

In the dialogue of Solomon's great wisdom, I Kings 4:33 states that he expounded on "trees, from the cedar tree that is in Lebanon even unto the hyssop that springeth out of the wall." The tall, majestic cedar was contrasted to the humble hyssop. The identification of these two particular trees served to define Solomon's vast wisdom.

Hyssop may be used as a cooking spice and in therapeutic teas. Hyssop can help prevent blood coagulation. It is also effective at concealing unpleasant odors.

However, the most outstanding quality of hyssop is found in its cleansing ability. It is a natural decongestant that relieves respiratory problems and cold and flu symptoms. Because of its infection fighting power and purification properties, it serves as a beautiful biblical symbol of spiritual cleansing. In fact, hyssop plays a part in some of the most significant biblical events.

The tenth and final divinely delivered message that God sent to Egypt's Pharaoh, the one which helped Pharaoh decide that it was in his best interest to liberate the Hebrew slaves, was the death of every firstborn in the land of Egypt. Only the obedient Hebrews who placed the blood of the Passover Lamb on their doorposts were spared this terror. The blood was applied with the use of "a bunch of hyssop" (Exodus 12:22). "A bunch of hyssop" was a natural "brush" which made it the ideal tool for applying the blood to the doorposts. Symbolically, this blood separated the Hebrews from Egypt. Egypt is a type of the worldly, anti-God system, a realm in which sin and iniquity dominate those that abide there.

The next mention of hyssop is in relation to the cleansing of lepers. Leprosy, a type of sin, is a disease that slowly eats away at a person's skin. Lepers were required to separate themselves from non-leprous people because any contact they had with healthy people would contaminate them with leprosy too. It was the responsibility of the priest to determine if an individual was leprous or not.

If the priest determined that a person was healed of leprosy, he would conduct a purification ceremony in which a living bird and hyssop were bound with scarlet string to a cedar board. The bound bird was dipped into the blood of a sacrificial bird. The blood was then sprinkled seven times onto the leper. The living bird was set free and the leprous-free person was free to re-enter society (Leviticus 14:1-7). A similar procedure was followed for the cleansing of a house that was once leprous (Leviticus 14:48-53).

The combination of cedar wood, hyssop, and scarlet is used elsewhere: in the burning of a red heifer, which provided "water of separation" and "a purification for sin" (Numbers 19:1-9).

When someone touched a dead body, he was considered unclean. He became clean by allowing an undefiled person to use hyssop to sprinkle a combination of water and the ashes of the red heifer onto him (Numbers 19:14-18).

David, who discovered that a love-trust relationship with God was far superior to strict adherence to Mosiac law alone, drew upon hyssop's important cleansing abilities. No doubt he had many times observed hyssop being used during sacrifices that were made to atone for sins. After the prophet Nathan confronted him about his sin of adultery, David cried out to God, "Wash me thoroughly from mine iniquity, and cleanse me from my sin. Purge me with hyssop, and I shall be clean: wash me, and I shall be whiter than snow" (Psalm 51:2,7).

David was dissatisfied with ritualistic sin atonement. He wanted his *heart* to be cleansed. He desired a restoration of his relationship with God. He used hyssop to describe how he wanted God to cleanse his heart. He didn't want just ceremonial cleansing; he wanted inner cleansing. He wanted to be clean "in the inward parts" and "in the hidden part" (Psalm 51:6).

(See John 19:29 and Hebrews 9:19.)

Mint
Greek: heduosmon
Mint is a sweet smelling herb that grows wild

throughout Palestine. Mint is mentioned in Matthew 23:23 and Luke 11:42, where Jesus exposes the Pharisees' ritualistic tithing of the smallest herbs while they avoid judgment, mercy, and faith – the real "meat" of the law.

As well as its medicinal uses, mint was used to flavor salads, fish, fowl, and meat, especially the Passover lamb. The Romans and the Greeks used mint to prevent milk from spoiling. They also ate mint after meals to aid digestion.

The floors of Jewish synagogues were strewn with mint, which filled the air with its sweet scent.

Today mint is used to ease menstrual cramps and morning sickness. Mint is an antispasmodic; it soothes uterus muscles. Colds, flu, motion sickness, heartburn, fever, headache, insomnia, and nausea may all profit from mint's healthful properties.

Note: Some authorities believe that women with a history of miscarriages should avoid peppermint as a treatment for morning sickness. To be safe, consult a physician or trained nutritionist before using peppermint remedies.

Mustard
Greek: sinapi

Jesus compared the kingdom of God to a grain of mustard seed, which was the tiniest seed known in Jesus' day. Just as the grain of mustard seed, once it was sown, became very great, so would the kingdom of God expand into great proportions if a man would simply sow the seed (Matthew 13:31; Mark 4:31; Luke 13:19).

Jesus also used a grain of mustard seed to give a lesson about faith. He said that if a believer has faith the size of a grain of mustard seed, he can move a mountain or transplant a tree into the sea. Jesus was demonstrating the power of faith. The tiniest amount has tremendous spiritual potential (Matthew 17:20; Luke 17:6).

Mustard is a plant that grows wild in Palestine along roads and in fields, especially along the Sea of Galilee. It can reach a height of about 15 feet and has very large branches, which would certainly be inviting to birds, which like to eat the seeds. The mustard's flowers are yellow.

What comes to most of our minds when we think of mustard is the condiment. Table mustard comes from the seeds of the mustard plant. Some people also enjoy mustard's leaves as a vegetable.

As for mustard's healthful properties, people have used it as a decongestant and antiseptic and it is said to significantly increase metabolism. It has been used to treat hardness of the liver and spleen. The seeds are reported to help heal carcinoma and throat tumors.

Some of the most interesting reported remedies of mustard: Tea made from mustard has been said to cure hiccups. Mustard oil is said to stimulate hair growth. And the application of mustard is purported to heal scorpion bites. That's certainly good news for any Texan who might find an unwanted surprise in his boot!

Parsley

Though parsley is not expressly mentioned in the Bible, it is nonetheless an important ingredient in the preparation of Middle Eastern dishes. It grows abundantly in Israel and is traditionally used in Passover meals. Use it in salads and as a flavoring for meat, fish, and poultry.

Parsley is a vibrant source of vitamins A and C. It is a mild laxative and strong diuretic; it may help regulate blood pressure. Need to freshen your breath? Chew on a few sprigs of parsley. Do allergies plague you? Incorporate parsley into your diet. Parsley prevents histamines from forming. (Histamines are the chemical that triggers allergy attacks.) Hay fever, hives, and upset stomachs all can be relieved by parsley.

Saffron
Hebrew: karkom

Saffron is the world's most expensive spice and understandably so, when one considers that it takes

4300 flowers to make just one ounce of saffron. Solomon referred to this distinctive spice (Song of Solomon 4:14). Saffron was imported to Palestine but many other cultures also enjoy its distinct flavor and unique yellow color. From Indian curries to Spanish paella to French bouillabaisse, it is a key ingredient in a wide variety of dishes. Experiment with saffron the next time you prepare rice or soup.

In the past, some people used saffron as a perfume. They even strew it onto the floors of public buildings and at places where weddings occurred. Due to its pricey nature, though, a naturally scented candle might be a better option when you want a pleasant aroma to fill the place where you host your next social event!

Spikenard
Hebrew: nerd/Greek: nardos

Spikenard plays a central role in some of the most beautiful love stories in the Bible, stories that excellently illustrate the relationship God longs to have with His Bride. The Song of Solomon 1:12 says that "while the king sitteth at his table, my spikenard sendeth forth the smell thereof." Solomon's bride desired to be found fair and pleasing to her love, the king. One of the ways she expressed her attraction to him and sought his favor was through the use of the precious perfume called spikenard.

Jesus was the recipient of worshipful adoration that found its expression through the sweet perfume of spikenard. (Note: It seems that myrrh was also used to anoint Jesus. For more in-depth study, compare the accounts of Jesus' anointing in Matthew 26:6-13, Mark 14:3-9, Luke 7:36-50, and John 12:1-8.)

Contained in an alabaster box, a lovely and valuable stone vase that was specially designed to contain precious oil, ointment, or perfume, spikenard was a gift quite suitable for kings. When the seal of the alabaster box was broken and the ointment was poured out, the aroma that filled the atmosphere was a fitting symbol of the worshipper's pure love and unadulterated devotion.

Since, for the average laborer, its value was equivalent to about a year's wages, a pound of spikenard was a very precious possession. Imported from India in alabaster boxes, spikenard was set aside to be used only on the most special occasions. A highly honored guest would be the recipient of spikenard poured from alabaster boxes onto his feet and head.

The New Testament compares the relationship of Christ and the Church to a man and his bride. As such, it is significant that, in the biblical accounts of spikenard, it was women that used this spice to express their feelings of gratefulness to the One they loved above all others.

One source declares spikenard to be a "lowly herb, the emblem of humility."[2] When we consider just how much Jesus has done for us, deep gratitude and a sense of indebtedness wells up within us. We are motivated to express to Him how much we love Him. His devotion to us prompts us to humble ourselves before Him and serve Him.

A broken alabaster box of precious ointment was once an expression of honor and love – a gift of the highest classification. Today, all Jesus wants is us – our wills, our complete devotion, and our undivided commitment. He just wants to know that we love Him more than anybody or anything, that He means more to us than all of the money and possessions in the world.

As beautiful as it was, a broken alabaster box of precious ointment is not what got God's attention; it was only a means of expression, an outward representation of the heart. It is just as true today as it was then: a heart that is broken and humble is what captures God's attention (Psalm 51:17). Jesus said, "They that are whole have no need of the physician, but they that are sick: I came not to call the righteous, but sinners to repentance (Mark 2:17). Jesus specializes in things that are broken. When we acknowledge that we need Him and that He is our only hope, He is then able to step in and fix that which is broken in our lives.

As our relationship with Jesus develops, our trust and adoration grow. Giving to Him does not stem from a sense of obligation or duty alone, but is the expression of a heart filled with a longing to respond to His goodness and love.

The value of spikenard is a beautiful illustration of worship. The picture of a woman humbling herself before the Master in a posture of servitude can help us refocus and remember the awesome opportunity we have for close, intimate communion with the Lord, the lover of our souls.

Wormwood
Hebrew: la`anah/Greek: apsinthos

The word "wormwood" means "bitterness, calamity, poisonous, accursed." In the Bible, wormwood typifies bitter sorrow and distressing calamity. Similar in nature to gall and hemlock, wormwood is a potentially toxic plant/herb. Ironically, however, wormwood was used early on medicinally to promote healthy digestion and in a culinary setting to season foods such as pork and lamb.

It is interesting and perhaps fitting that down through history wormwood has also been used to spice alcoholic beverages. One drink called absinthe used wormwood leaves. This beverage "caused mental and physical illness until it was forbidden – by the Swiss in 1907, and later in many other countries."[3]

(See Deuteronomy 29:18; Proverbs 5:4; Jeremiah 9:15; 23:15; Lamentations 3:15, 19; Amos 5:7; 6:12; Revelation 8:11.)

SALT AND SEA VEGETABLES

Jesus said, "Salt is good" (Luke 14:34). Salt was a very important commodity to biblical people. It was a purifier and a preservative as well as a commonly used food seasoning (Job 6:6).

Salt was used not only during food preparation, but also as an antiseptic. Newborn babies were bathed and salted (Ezekiel 16:4). At times in history, salt has played an integral role in trade and commerce. Roman soldiers were given "salt money," which was part of their pay that was used to purchase salt; this is the origin of the word "salary."

In the Bible, places such as the Valley of Salt and the City of Salt were named for their association with salt (Joshua 15:62; II Samuel 8:13). The most common geographical association with salt, though, is the Salt Sea; today it is called the Dead Sea. Located at the southern end of the Jordan Valley, the Dead Sea contains no marine life because of its heavy mineral content. The Dead Sea is about nine times saltier than the oceans, which contain 2-3% salt. It is the chief source of salt for inhabitants of that part of the world.

Historians believe that Sodom and Gomorrah were located near the southern tip of the Dead Sea. After seeing photographs of tall pillars of salt which form on the salt beds of the Dead Sea, it is easy to picture Lot's wife being turned into a pillar of salt (Genesis 19:26). It is interesting that Arabs call the Dead Sea "Bahr Lut" (Sea of Lot).

The Lord told the children of Israel, "With all thine offerings thou shalt offer salt" (Leviticus 2:13). All animal sacrifices were sprinkled with salt when they were offered unto the Lord (Mark 9:49). This was called "a covenant of salt." The Salt Covenant originated as a covenant between God and man. It signified an everlasting agreement. It was a pledge of faithfulness and perpetual devotion.

When two men initiated a Salt Covenant between them, it was a binding agreement of mutual fidelity, loyalty, friendship, hospitality, dependability, and guaranteed protection. Salt's preservative ability symbolized the enduring nature of the covenant. The Arabic word for "salt" is the same word as "compact" and "treaty."

Understanding the Salt Covenant is integral to our relationship to God and His body – our brothers and sisters in the Lord – and our obligation to be "the salt of the earth." Matthew 5:13 tells us: "Ye are the salt of the earth: but if the salt have lost his savour, wherewith shall it be salted? it is thenceforth good for nothing, but to be cast out, and to be trodden under foot of men."

When Jesus told us that we are "the salt of the earth," He was saying in essence, "Just as salt provides necessary nutrition to the human body, you are to provide others with the opportunity to have salvation. As salt creates thirst, you are to season others' lives so that they will thirst for Me. Just as salt is an enduring element, you are to endure. As salt purifies, you are to remain pure and help others become pure as well. Be loyal and faithful in your commitment to me, as I am to you, and others will see Me in you and receive salvation."

But how does salt lose its savor? How do we lose our ability to be a seasoning lifeline to the world around us?

From casual appearance, the salt harvested around the Dead Sea all looked the same. Only when the salt was closely examined could its saltiness and useful qualities be determined. Though on the surface it may have looked like savory salt, when it was collected some salt was determined to be completely flavorless and worthless, good for nothing but "to be trodden under foot of men."

Salt's lack of savor was due to its exposure to the elements; the wind, rain, sun, and air all take their toll on the salt. It is only the salt that was somewhat hidden from the elements, *connected to the rock*, that maintained its saltiness.

When we stay connected to the Rock, Christ Jesus, who is the Source of life, we have access to Him. As we partake of His nature, we take on His "salty" characteristics.

When Jesus told His disciples "Have salt in yourselves, and have peace one with another," He was instilling a New Testament Salt Covenant (Mark 9:50). Our Salt Covenant with the Lord, which signifies our dedication and sold-out commitment, will naturally overlap into a covenant with our brothers and sisters.

Salt was used to heal wounds. While there will be times when, like David, we will feel betrayed and hurt by familiar friends that we trusted, we must forgive, pray for them, and seek restoration and peace (Psalm 41:9). Peace with one another is the best and most savory salt we can offer the world because Jesus said, "By this shall all men know that ye are my disciples, if ye have love one to another" (John 13:35).

When people see our unbreakable connection to the Rock and our unbreakable connection with one another, the foundation for their salvation has been laid. Now they too can partake of the Salt Covenant.

Salt is mentioned so frequently and favorably in the Bible that it is to our advantage to examine this subject closely. There is a lot of talk today about the overuse of salt. Too much dietary salt is blamed for many serious health conditions. Yet the Bible never once condemns its use. Salt has been used throughout history to preserve and season many foods. People the world over used salt to dry and smoke the animals they hunted and the fish they caught. Butter and cheese were two other foods that were commonly salted.

Salt (sodium chloride) is essential for life and our bodies contain about 3-1/2 ounces of it. It is present in our tears, perspiration, muscles, and bodily fluids. Sodium is the vehicle that carries water throughout our bodies. Together, water and sodium are necessary for the maintenance of healthy blood pressure. Sodium aids digestion, balances blood sugar, and helps build strong bones.

In and of itself, salt – as Jesus said – is good. Unfortunately, however, due to diets high in processed foods which contain exorbitant amounts of salt, most of us get way too much of a good thing. One source figured that the average American consumes ten pounds of salt annually. This seems preposterous until we consider that almost all processed foods contain sodium. Some processed foods with high salt content: canned and instant soups and broths, bouillon cubes, potato chips, salted peanuts, pretzels, catsup, salad dressings, canned, bottled, and packaged gravies and sauces, soy sauce, processed cheeses, smoked fish, bacon, hot dogs, lunch meat, bologna, and corned beef. (Note: MSG is a hidden source of sodium.) Factor in the salt we add during cooking and baking, the salt we add to our cooked food, the salt we consume from restaurant food, the salt we drink supplied by our municipal water supply, and ten pounds of salt per person is quite plausible.

Too much salt disturbs the body's water balance. This means that the kidneys are not able to function properly, which in turn can create cardiovascular problems. Excess salt can cause water weight gain; this too has subsequent negative consequences.

While many people understand that they need to decrease their sodium intake, most are not aware of the importance of maintaining a proper balance between sodium and potassium. Sodium and potassium work together outside and inside the cells of the body. When there is an imbalance between the two, it takes a toll on the kidneys and blood pressure abnormalities may result.

Very few people are actually sodium deficient. People that sweat a great deal may need to replenish their salt supply, due to the loss of sodium through perspiration. (One sign of sodium deficiency is frequent leg cramps.) If you are one of those rare sodium deficient people, don't use refined table salt for your sodium needs. Enjoy whole foods; almost all of them contain some sodium. Healthy foods with high sodium content are naturally raised beef and poultry, celery, beets, carrots, artichokes, turnips, chard, spinach, and parsley.

The bright white free-flowing table salt that can be found in most American households is extremely refined. Salt naturally harvested from lakes and oceans contains as many as 80 important trace minerals in the proper proportions required by our bodies. The high temperature and chemicals used to process salt destroy all of those minerals. Some of the chemicals that are used to refine salt are magnesium carbonate, calcium silicate, sodium silicoaluminate, tricalcium phosphate, destrose, and sodium ferrocyanide. Remember the little girl holding an umbrella as snow-white salt pours freely from the salt container? Aah...advertising at its finest. One of the signs of really good salt is that it clumps together and it is not pure white; it hasn't had anti-caking chemicals and bleach added to it.

During the salt refining process, naturally occurring iodine is removed. In 1924, potassium iodide was added to salt to prevent goiter (enlargement of the thyroid gland). Goiter is the result of iodine deficiency. While the human body needs iodine, most iodized salt has been stripped of its optimal nutrition. Unrefined salt contains iodine that has not been altered. It just makes common sense that unrefined, unaltered salt with its iodine intact and the consumption of sea and land vegetables that contain iodine is the best way to meet iodine requirements.

Rock salt is mined from underground salt deposits. Salt is also harvested from lakes, seas, and oceans. Salty seawater is collected and evaporated by the sun or vacuum dried. When choosing salt, make sure that it is unrefined and unaltered.

Sea vegetables are mineral rich salt alternatives. They satisfy the taste buds' desire for something salty and can be used instead of salt to season foods during cooking. Some of the more common sea vegetables are dulse, hijiki, Irish moss (carrageen), kelp, nori (laver), kombu, and wakame.

PART IV

PRACTICAL PRINCIPLES

Finishing Touches

TWENTY-FOUR

MORNING MANNA

But when the morning was now come, Jesus stood on the
shore: but the disciples knew not that it was Jesus.
As soon then as they were come to land, they saw a fire of
coals there, and fish laid thereon, and bread.
John 21:4,9

There are a lot of good reasons to eat breakfast – a healthy breakfast. You give your metabolism an early boost, decrease your sugar cravings, and reduce your susceptibility to obesity, which in itself creates a host of problems. Skipping breakfast makes you 4.5 times more likely to be overweight.

Breakfast is the most important meal of the day. By the time you wake up and sit down at the table, your body has been without food for quite a while. It is time to refuel. Would you expect your car to transport you to work if you did not put gas in it? Of course not. Yet, we do that to our bodies all the time. You don't have to eat a big breakfast every day, but at least get in the habit of eating something nutritious to jump-start your metabolism.

QUALITY COUNTS

It's not good enough to just eat breakfast. Consider that the *type* of fuel you give your car counts too. Some cars require specific types of fuel, and all cars benefit from *clean* fuel. The same is true with our bodies. If we put junk in our bodies, they will not perform optimally and will eventually break down.

Sugary breakfast cereals, commercial granola bars, high calorie bakery pastries, doughnuts, preservative laden sausage and bacon, pulp-free orange juice, coffee, white toast slathered with margarine, and fake eggs are just some of the breakfast foods America loves and *sub*sists on. No wonder they're headed for the coffee pot or the candy bar vending machine by mid-morning. Their blood sugar has taken a nosedive because their breakfast did not consist of a fiber-rich meal that would sustain them throughout the morning.

There are many healthy and delicious breakfast options. Oatmeal is the healthy breakfast standby. If you don't like plain oatmeal, add a little cinnamon and pure maple syrup. Make a quick omelet and throw in some healthy additions – the choices are limited only by your creativity – bell peppers, onions, even chicken. Don't be afraid of eggs, despite what the media says. They are the perfect protein. God made them; they were eaten in Bible times. They will give you long lasting energy. Make breakfast burritos with whole-grain tortillas. Try turkey bacon in place of pig bacon. Grapefruit is an excellent breakfast choice, as well as berries, apples, and many other fruits. They provide a wonderful variety of vitamins that are absent from the typical American breakfast that consists of white bread and more white bread. Try yogurt, but not just any yogurt. Many commercial yogurts are filled with added sugars, artificial coloring and synthetic preservatives. Choose a plain yogurt, preferably a locally made yogurt, and sweeten with pure maple syrup if necessary. Add fresh blueberries, strawberries, blackberries, or peaches. Yogurt contains A, D, and B-complex vitamins. It's a great source of probiotics (good, friendly bacteria).

Experiment with different breakfast foods as you veer away from the standard American breakfast. Buy breakfast foods that will give your body optimum energy and performance. If you deliberately and carefully choose to eat something healthy first thing in the morning, you will be more likely to choose healthy foods throughout the day. You will have started out on the right foot and the course of the day will naturally follow.

BREAKFAST WITH THE KING

Not only is it important to start the day out right with healthy food for our bodies, but we need spiritual food as well. David wrote, "My voice shalt thou hear in the morning, O LORD; in the morning will I direct my prayer unto thee, and will look up" (Psalm 5:3). Time spent in prayer and Bible reading early in the morning, before the hustle and bustle of the day presses in upon us, establishes the course of the day. By spending time in prayer and the Word, we make Jesus the number one priority each day. When our focus is right, we are peaceful and satisfied all day long, regardless of what may come our way.

When we don't pray first thing, it seems like something is missing, something is awry. We don't feel quite as contented and assured. When we don't pray, we say by our actions, *I don't need God today. I can make it on my own.* We wouldn't get in a car with a nearly empty gas tank or a weak battery and expect it to transport us to our destination. When we don't take time to recharge our spiritual batteries at the beginning of the day, we keep ourselves from operating at peak performance. Our flesh is alive and well every morning and, like the apostle Paul, we have to crucify it on a daily basis (I Corinthians 15:31).

By submitting our fleshly will to the will of God at the onset of the day, God empowers us to resist the devil (and our flesh) throughout the day. We are less likely to sin when we crucify our flesh as the day dawns because we have a greater awareness of the presence of God.

Praying first thing in the morning establishes a clear channel of communication with God. We get tuned in to His voice. Throughout the day, we will not be walking according to our own reasoning, but we will be walking in the Spirit. Beginning our day with prayer and reading the Word equips us to be used of God in a greater dimension because we open our minds and spirits to Him, making it easier for Him to speak to us when He wants and needs to.

In prayer we put on spiritual armor, so that we

can be victorious in battle. When we get up in the morning, we clothe our physical bodies with garments to cover and protect us. Likewise, we need to go to the closet
of prayer to clothe ourselves with protective armor and
equip ourselves with spiritual weapons. We can then
realize our maximum potential for the day and be ready
to meet its challenges.

Praying in the morning is only one time of day
that the Bible advocates, but it is special because it provides focus. This time should not be viewed as a dutiful
appointment or a fulfillment of an obligation, nor should
it be motivated by a sense of guilt. Rather, it should be
the result of a desire to develop a consistent walk with
God that is defined by a 24-7 God consciousness. Walking with God is achieved when we follow Him and align
our will with His. One of the primary ways to achieve
this is through humbling ourselves in prayer first thing
in the morning.

BREAKFAST OF CHAMPIONS

When we partake of the Bread of Life first thing in
the morning, we are supplied with power, faith, direction, peace, and mercy. God designed our spirits to
crave a sumptuous early morning feast.

Even if we aren't very spiritually or physically
hungry first thing in the morning, we are wise if we eat a
healthy breakfast anyway. If we don't, chances are good
that we will eat something later in the day that is not
good for us, because we get spiritually and physically
weak and reach out for anything to give us quick energy.

Along with feeding our bodies healthful, God
created foods first thing in the morning, getting charged
spiritually gives us long lasting energy. A New Testament believer, supercharged both spiritually and physically, is savory salt, a radiant light, and a powerhouse of
faith. He is equipped to live a godly life, fulfill God's purpose for the day, and win the battle against the powers
of Hell, all because he took the time to enjoy the best
meal of the day, spiritually and physically.

TWENTY-FIVE

PLAN OF ACTION

*"I decided to take an aerobics class.
I bent, twisted, and jumped up and down for an hour.
But, by the time I got my leotards on, the class was over."*[1]

You won't find the following commandment in the Bible: "Thou shalt exercise thirty minutes every day." Physical fitness is not expressly addressed in the Bible. One reason for this is because daily physical labor was an intrinsic part of most people's lives. Remember, they were not exactly on the cutting edge, technologically speaking. There were no drive-thru restaurants, personal digital assistants, remote car starters, and high-speed jets. Everything our biblical forefathers did involved physical activity. Eating, traveling, working, even worship all required more than quick, mechanized movements such as the click of a mouse or a phone call to the pizza joint. They walked almost everywhere they went so they didn't need treadmills. Physical inactivity and ensuing health complications were simply not common issues for people of Bible times.

Just as you will not find a verse commanding you to implement an exercise regimen into your daily schedule, neither will you find a verse that states: "Thou shalt *not* exercise thirty minutes a day."

Some people love to refer to I Timothy 4:8 in an attempt to prove the futility of physical fitness. "For bodily exercise profiteth little: but godliness is profitable unto all things, having promise of the life that now is, and of that which is to come." From my studies, I have found two lines of thought regarding this verse. Neither of them prove that physical exercise is a complete waste of time and of no benefit to the born again believer.

The first view of this verse is found by exploring the world of Ephesus, the city where Timothy lived. Grecian influence was great in this magnificent city. A massive stadium was built explicitly for athletic purposes. The Greeks greatly prized physical strength and ability and exercised for entertainment purposes. The Greek word for "exercise" in I Timothy 4:8 is "gumnasia." Some people draw the conclusion that Paul was telling Timothy to avoid overemphasizing physical fitness at the expense of things of eternal importance.

Though Paul may have been using Grecian influence to illustrate a point, most Bible scholars believe that Paul was admonishing Timothy to avoid the asceticism falsely associated with godliness in Timothy's day. The Essenes were a group of people who believed that strict self-denial made them more pure.

Paul was warning against trying to achieve true righteousness through fleshly means. In this context, actual physical exercise is not in view whatsoever, rather, attempting to accomplish spiritual things through carnal means. This seems a plausible explanation, especially considering that the preceding verse tells Timothy to "refuse profane and old wives' fables" and to "exercise" himself "rather unto godliness" (I Timothy 4:7). Actually, Paul addresses false ideas of godliness throughout this entire letter. Essentially, Paul did not want Timothy to get distracted by the unbalanced and false teachings of his day.

Either way, Paul was *not* saying, "Don't exercise your body." Elsewhere, Paul taught spiritual lessons using a topic familiar to him and other apostolic believers – physical fitness. Consider Hebrews 12:1 ("Let us run with patience the race that is set before us") and II Timothy 4:7 ("I have fought a good fight, I have finished my course"). Paul had God given authority to direct the New Testament Church. If God did not want the Church to be physically fit, the apostle Paul would undoubtedly have warned against it in his teachings.

WHY EXERCISE?

As an adolescent, I much preferred reading a book to playing basketball or running down the street. I lacked coordination and balance and found sedentary activities more to my liking. In my early twenties I began to realize that an unbalanced, inactive lifestyle was not beneficial for me. So I began to try new athletic activities and to my surprise, found out that I enjoyed them. My coordination improved too.

In such a sedentary culture as ours, it is necessary to consciously exercise in order to achieve and maintain good health. If you struggle with developing an exercise routine, maybe what you need is to be educated about the long-term benefits of doing what is good for your body. There are many great motivating reasons to exercise. While you are exercising to take care of your temple, you might discover that you actually enjoy it.

"Experts find that the risk of developing at least half of all illnesses associated with aging – even heart attacks, diabetes, and broken bones – can be eliminated with regular workouts. One five-year study of 10,000 men found that the mortality rate of those who were most active and fit was one-third the rate of those who were out of shape. The better physical shape you're in, the longer you'll probably live. Regular physical activity not only staves off the physical effects of aging but also keeps your brain and mental functioning sharp as you grow older."[2]

"The closest thing to a 'magic bullet' for maintaining youth and optimal health is a well-balanced combination of exercise and proper nutrition. The entire body benefits from this formula. Regular exercise improves digestion and elimination, increases endurance and energy levels, promotes lean body mass while burning fat, and lowers overall blood cholesterol while increasing the proportion of 'good' cholesterol (HDL) to 'bad' cholesterol (LDL). Exercise also reduces stress and anxiety, which are contributing factors to many illnesses and conditions."[3]

FITNESS FOCUS

"Exercising" and "dutiful torture" are terms that go hand in hand for many people. Fortunately, exercise does not have to be an unpleasant chore. There are many ways to get your quota of daily exercise. All of these listed here will, to varying degrees, burn calories, improve heart rate, increase oxygen intake, and strengthen muscles.

Lifestyle Fitness

This is by far the easiest form of exercise to incorporate into your life. I define lifestyle fitness as multitask daily activities such as gardening, vacuuming the house, walking the kids to school, and shoveling snow. These are productive activities that we enjoy or do out of necessity anyway.

My dad provided me with a good example of a person committed to lifestyle fitness. He never joined a gym but he was constantly busy and active. For many years he worked four miles from our home. In addition to working 8, 12, or 16-hour shifts at a physical labor job, he bicycled to work when weather permitted. He jogged from his car to the store. He took us on long canoe rides when we were too young to be much help paddling. When climbing stairs, he took two at a time. Vacations nearly always consisted of visits to parks where he was moving, moving, moving – setting up a tent, hiking up a mountain, wading in a stream. No doubt my dad's devotion to lifestyle fitness is one reason why he has never struggled with weight problems.

Incorporate lifestyle fitness into your everyday routine. Consciously examine your days and determine where you could insert extra effort to get your blood pumping. When you go to the mall or go grocery shopping, park at the end of the parking lot. You can walk to the store within the time it would take you to find a parking spot close to the entrance. If you work in a multi-storied office building, get to work a few minutes early and take the stairs instead of the elevator. During your lunch break, do a few minutes of stretches.

If you are an inactive person, think about an active hobby that you would enjoy learning. Deliberately concentrate on putting as much effort into that activity as possible.

Lifestyle fitness is what fitness experts refer to as anaerobic exercise. It gently and deliberately transforms natural real life movements into a means of becoming fit.

Cardiovascular Exercise

Bicycling, running, fast walking, and swimming are examples of this type of traditional aerobic exercise. It promotes cardiovascular health. As your heart rate increases, circulation improves and blood pressure is lowered.

Care should be taken to not overstress joints and ligaments. If you experience actual pain from aerobic exercise, you may be overworking your body.

Weight Training

Also called strength training, this type of exercise makes use of machine or free weights. Weight training contributes to muscle, bone, tendon, and ligament health. It builds muscle mass, which increases your resting metabolic rate, meaning that you burn calories while sitting still, if you regularly train with weights.

Find someone that can teach you about using weights. Learning the correct way to lift and how to properly align your body will help you avoid injury and get the maximum benefit from your workout. Be sure to do each repetition slowly and deliberately. Hold in your abdominal muscles and exhale upon exertion.

TIPS OF THE TRADE

Here are a few tips to make your workout time more enjoyable and effective.

- Before working out, it is very important to warm up by walking or slowly jogging in place, then doing stretches. The older we get the more crucial this becomes. Stretching helps avoid injuries.

Slow down and stretch again at the end of your workout. This is not time wasted.

- Don't do the same thing every day. Diversity will not only prevent working out from becoming boring, but it will work different parts of your body. If you join a gym, the staff can help you develop a routine specifically for you. Strive for a balanced blend of lifestyle fitness, cardiovascular exercise, and weight training, as well as other types of exercise.

- Don't work out seven days a week. Exercising three to five days a week is probably sufficient for some people to stay in shape. Personally, I rarely exercise on Sundays. That is the day I allow my body to rest and repair itself.

- At some point, you will reach a plateau. Don't stop exercising! It is normal to have times when there are no visible or obvious results.

- Drink water before, during, and after your workout, even if you are not noticeably thirsty. If you feel like you need something to eat during or after your workout, don't eat sugary snacks. Instead, choose high protein and complex carbohydrate foods, such as lean meat, raw nuts, or raw vegetables.

- Don't hold your breath while exercising. Rather, take long, deep breaths.

- Don't exercise for three or four hours at a time on a regular basis. 15-45 minutes a day is a great workout for beginners. Frequent, vigorous exercise for too long at one time might actually damage your muscles and joints.

- If you have children, you may want to include them in your exercise time, achieving three goals at the same time: 1) You can spend quality time with them, 2) by your involvement, you can teach them the importance and value of physical fitness and 3) you can get in shape yourself while enjoying the company of your children.

- Try doing something you've never tried before, such as jumping rope, playing ping-pong, or rebounding on a small trampoline. You might discover a few things you really enjoy that can give you a great workout. Remember, we are not all the same. I personally cannot jump rope for long periods of time because it hurts my back. But I love to walk and hike and I kayak whenever I get the opportunity. Working out should be fun, not a chore.

- It's easy to talk ourselves out of exercising when we are tired and lack energy. Ironically, our energy increases when we exercise. So the next time you feel groggy in the middle of the afternoon, take a brisk walk or do some sit-ups to stimulate and invigorate your body and mind.

- Consult a physician before beginning any physical training program. He may be able to assist you in your choice of activity, having knowledge of your health issues and physical limitations.

- Some people don't exercise because it hurts and they are afraid that they are harming their bodies. Always stop exercising if you experience actual pain and consult a physician if necessary. However, when beginning to exercise after many months or years of inactivity, it is normal to experience aching and burning sensations in your muscles. Learn to distinguish the difference between true pain and the feeling of your body being shaped and improved by new exercises.

- Ladies: Don't avoid exercise because you think it is unladylike. Aside from a few sports like cliff rappelling, most activities can be modestly enjoyed. And don't be afraid to work up a sweat – that doesn't mean you aren't a lady; it means you are a human being having fun getting fit.

THE METABOLISM MYTH

It seems that most of us have this strange concept in our minds that we have a slow metabolism. If you think this about yourself, have you ever stopped to question *how* you got a slow metabolism? Were you born with it? Did it come upon you one night while you were sleeping? As odd as it may seem, most of us are not predestined with a slow metabolism.

Metabolism is a multi-faceted and somewhat complicated subject. Different factors such as genetics, body shape, early childhood diet, and ethnicity influence metabolism, but that does not mean that a slow metabolism cannot be at least somewhat altered.

Take a minute to digest this thought: By and large, we have the ability to determine our own metabolism. How? By exercising or not exercising. Metabolism is the rate at which we burn calories. As we exercise, our body's metabolic rate speeds up and begins to consistently operate at a quicker pace. Working out early in the day may be especially beneficial, giving our metabolism a jump-start. The afterburn effects of vigorous exercise increase basal metabolic rate for four to 24 hours. So exercise actually *increases* our metabolism.

When we commit to regular, moderate exercise and give our bodies proper nutrition in reasonable proportions, we lose weight and keep it away. It is very exciting to realize that we are not doomed to an overweight existence because we mysteriously acquired a slow metabolism. For most of us, we have the power to increase our own metabolism.

HELPFUL HINTS

Start small. Be realistic. If you are not very fit, deciding to bicycle two hours every day is setting yourself up for failure. Try bicycling five minutes a day. Set attainable goals and gradually increase them.

Be patient. If you are unfit, it took some time to get that way. And it will take some time to get back in shape. Our weight is going to come off the same way it went on – ounce by ounce.

We live in an "instant" society. Unrealistic lose-weight-quick schemes (pills, shakes, mainstream magazine diet plans) eliminate personal responsibility by not addressing the root cause of our unfit condition: We neglected to take care of our temples. They offer temporary fixes but not lasting changes. Only good nutrition and consistent exercise will bring the results we desire.

So don't be disheartened if you aren't competing in a triathlon within a week. Be content knowing that you are doing what is good for your temple and delight in the small changes you experience.

More important than the amount of time you spend exercising is that you are consistent. If you are extra-busy three days in a row and can only stretch for five minutes a day, that is better than not doing anything at all for three days. Staying in a routine will help you stay focused and maintain momentum. Also, choosing a specific time of day to exercise will promote consistency. Getting fit will not just happen. You must plan for it to happen. (If you fail to plan, then you plan to fail.) Then, you must consistently work your plan.

Don't get discouraged if you fail. Just start again, with renewed purpose. In spite of my best efforts, an overtaxed schedule has prevented me from working out much for weeks at a time. If this happens to you, don't give up just because your routine is derailed. Get back on track and get moving again. You'll be glad you did.

PARTNER PACT

For some people, having an exercise partner is essential in order to stay on target. If you need encouragement to exercise consistently, find a workout partner. It is important that you help each other achieve your goals. Agree to not accept excuses from each other. Having a workout partner will only benefit you if you are accountable to him or her. Illnesses, emergencies, or a call to prayer or Kingdom service should be the only acceptable reasons to not work out. If you don't hold one another accountable, your exercise regimen can become inconsistent and ineffective.

Many people find that having a work out partner makes the time go faster, provides motivation, makes the workout more fun, and supplies a social outlet.

Personally, I like to work out alone most of the time. The reasons are varied. First, my life is very people oriented. My workout time gives me the opportunity to relax my mind and have some "alone time." Second, much of my workout entails walking. I walk rather fast and most people can't keep up with me. While I don't mind slowing my pace sometimes, if I do that too frequently, I won't get the optimum benefit from my walk. Third, when walking alone outside, I use this time to talk to the Lord. It is hard to communicate with God and someone else at the same time. I have had some wonderful conversations with the Lord during my walks. Sometimes I write verses of Scripture on small index cards and memorize them as I walk. As I repeat the verses over and over, I am edifying myself both spiritually and physically.

With all that said, individuals must choose for themselves whether or not they need a workout partner. God did not create us all with a cookie cutter. Do what will benefit and bring you the most satisfaction from your workout efforts.

LOCATION, LOCATION, LOCATION

Some people find it very motivating to belong to a gym. Gyms have staff that will guide and assist as needed and "spot" you when you use free weights. They offer programs to help you achieve your goals. However, carefully scrutinize the gym before buying a membership. Take into consideration the following traits of most gyms that can be detractions to your spiritual life: Immodestly dressed members of the opposite sex who are also there to exercise, television and video projectors with unwholesome content, and loud, obnoxious music. Before signing up, ask Jesus if He would be comfortable going there with you and then listen for His answer.

YMCAs are generally more family oriented than mainstream gyms. Also, many city and town parks have tracks, basketball courts, tennis courts, and fields that are open to the public. Some high schools make their tracks available for use to the public after school hours.

If you are an outdoors person, hiking, canoeing, and kayaking are great forms of exercise. Check your local tourist bureau for information about hiking trails and state parks.

If you choose to work out in the privacy of your own home, the sky is the limit, depending on what form of exercise you choose and how much money you want to invest. You will need to schedule a time when you can exercise uninterrupted. This may be while your children are at school or before you leave for work. Communicate with your family about the importance of uninterrupted workout time. Ask someone else to answer the phone and take messages for you while you are exercising.

If you live in a climate that is extremely cold or hot for a good portion of the year, you will definitely want to invest in home workout equipment. This does not have to be exorbitantly expensive. Educate yourself and decide what brand is best for you. Then read the classifieds in the newspapers, ask around, and you're sure to find some great used equipment for a sliver of the price you'd pay at the fitness store. Many people have perfectly fine, albeit dusty, exercise equipment in their basements.

When you get your great deal home, don't put it in the garage or the basement, unless you positively have no other place for it. For the sake of familial harmony, I don't recommend putting it in the middle of the kitchen, but do make a special fitness corner in your house that is accessible and "user friendly." You will be more likely to work out if your equipment is not hidden between boxes and "stuff" in a dark, cobweb filled basement. Also, the little saying "out of sight, out of mind" is applicable here.

Whether you work out at a gym, a park, or at home, it is important to choose a place where you are comfortable, a place that is a positive and safe environment.

TO SCALE OR NOT TO SCALE

How to best gauge fitness progress is a controversial subject. Some people use a scale, enjoying watching the numbers drop before their eyes. For others, body measurements may be a better gauge. For ladies especially, the latter may be more accurate, as variables such as water weight, time of day, and certain times of the month all seem to dictate, sometimes drastically, our weight. Some of us can fluctuate five pounds a day due to hormonal changes. If this is the case with you, periodically take your body measurements and keep them on a chart to gauge your progress. For most of us, simply how our clothes fit lets us know how we are doing.

Whatever you do, don't obsess over what your scale or chart says. That is a recipe for a roller coaster ride of exhilaration and discouragement. Just keep exercising, knowing that you are doing what is best for your body. Don't focus on the scale; rather, focus on becoming healthy and fit and enjoy the process.

As you exercise, you will start building up your muscles and losing fat, if you have fat to lose. Because muscle weighs more than fat, you may actually gain pounds at some point. Save yourself the discouragement and just keep exercising, despite what the scale or chart says. In time, you will see the digital or written results you desire.

WILL WORK FOR FOOD

There is a principle in the Bible that is foreign to some who are content to let others provide for them when they are fully capable of working. This principle is found in II Thessalonians 3:10-12: "For even when we were with you, this we commanded you, that if any would not work, neither should he eat. For we hear that there are some which walk among you disorderly, working not at all, but are busybodies. Now them that are such we command and exhort by our Lord Jesus Christ, that with quietness they work, and eat their own bread."

This is a great weight loss plan! If you can work but you *won't* work, then quit eating. How much more simple can you get? God told Adam, "In the sweat of thy face shalt thou eat bread" (Genesis 3:19). An able bodied person that refuses to work behaves as though he is entitled to bypass God's universal law.

When a person is inactive and consumes more calories than he can utilize, he tends to gain weight. But a person who works burns for fuel the calories he consumes. He doesn't have time to sit around, eat unnecessarily and compromise his health.

In 21st century America, where most of the population is not employed in strenuous labor, it is possible to be a hard worker yet not use all calories consumed. Physically inactive jobs demand extracurricular times of exercise if one wants to stay fit. Also, monitoring food intake in proportion to the physical activity required by jobs will help keep those spare pounds at bay.

KEEP YOUR BALANCE

When I was in grade school, I learned how to walk on a balance beam. I never was able to do cartwheels or other fancy gymnastic tricks. I was fortunate to go from end to end without falling off! One thing I learned though is that balance is achieved through complete concentration and undistracted focus.

It has been said, "There's a ditch on either side of the road." In relation to exercise, there is danger in both neglect and excessiveness. The dangers of neglecting exercise altogether have already been discussed.

For a select few, overemphasis on exercise presents a danger to their spiritual lives because they consider physical fitness of greater importance than fundamental spiritual disciplines such as prayer and Bible reading.

In polytheistic Greek culture, strength of body and keenness of mind were valued to such a degree that they were revered and exalted above all else. Essentially, Greeks engaged in worship of the human body. We must be cautious that we do not scramble our priorities. While exercise is very beneficial, communication with Jesus is much more beneficial! If our physical being gets fit while our spiritual man deteriorates through neglect, we are unbalanced and in danger of falling.

Remember – first things first! I have found that when I put prayer and reading the Word first in my day, Jesus usually makes sure that I have time to give my body the exercise it needs.

STAY ON TRACK

As with any new discipline that requires consistency, exercising may be hard at first and the desire to give up may be great. It will be tempting to let daily duties distract you. Deviations from regular exercise, even if we intend them to be temporary, can make it hard to get back on track.

Physical fitness must be a priority. (Remember, your body is the temple of God and you only get one.) Even when you are on vacation, take time to exercise and keep in sync with your regimen as much as possible. Also, after noticing a little progress, you may be tempted to let down and give yourself a break. Don't treat yourself too much or you might be right back at Square One.

Once you are in the habit of exercising, you will be motivated to continue by how great you feel. Instead of viewing it as a dreaded chore, in time you will look forward to exercise.

Make exercise a lifelong habit. As we get older, our fitness goals and interests may change. Our bodies may need different types of exercise to stay in shape. Don't get stuck in a box, doing the same thing year after year. When you meet your body's needs through good nutrition and varying types of exercise, it will pay you back with the energy, vitality, and endurance you need to fulfill God's purpose for your life.

TWENTY-SIX

CLEANING THE TEMPLE

And Jesus went into the temple of God,
and cast out all them that sold and bought in the temple,
and overthrew the tables of the moneychangers.
Matthew 21:12

It was an unusual day. It began calmly but developed an exciting twist. Jesus went to the temple in Jerusalem, a beautiful edifice dedicated to prayer and worship. His righteous indignation at what he saw catapulted Him to action. This place that was built to be a "house of prayer" had been transformed into a "den of thieves," a descriptive phrase that aptly described the greed that operated there. Jesus made a whip and forcibly drove out people and animals, upturned tables, and poured the profiteers' money on the temple floor.

The temple was a place where common people came to make sacrifices for sin. They came to the house of God to be reconciled to God. They wanted to get rid of the sin in their lives that strained their relationships with God. They wanted God to be pleased with them.

According to the Mosaic law, the means by which this reconciliation took place was an animal sacrifice – an ox, a dove, a sheep – the sacrifice varied according to the offense and sometimes the monetary abilities of the worshipper.

Underneath the guise of innocent goodwill to offer a convenient service to worshippers, men brought animals to the temple and advertised them for sale. Such profitable business ventures turned the place of prayer into a place of commerce. In addition, moneychangers were on hand to exchange foreign currency for the Jewish half-shekel, which was the required acceptable money for temple maintenance offerings. These moneychangers included hefty commissions in their currency exchanges.

Jesus was angry because people were using His house as a place of unholy gain. They had stolen prayer and replaced it with the love of money. Jesus violently cast out the buyers and sellers and moneychangers. He cleaned out the evil to make room for righteousness.

It is interesting that the Bible records Jesus cleansing the temple on two separate occasions, first at the beginning of His ministry and again at the close of His ministry (Matthew 21:12-13; Mark 11:15-17; Luke 19:45-46; John 2:14-16). It was very important to Jesus that the temple – His house – be clean, pure, and holy.

This very vivid example of spiritual cleansing provides us with a terrific model for physical cleansing.

CLEANING CRISIS

Imagine that you have a neighbor who cares very little about keeping his house and yard clean and tidy. He much prefers golfing, hunting, or relaxing to mowing his lawn and painting his house. One day you come home and are shocked to find him ambitiously pruning shrubs, cleaning gutters, pressure washing his house, and cleaning the debris out of his yard. By the time he is finished, you are amazed. His lawn and the outside of his house are immaculate enough to be featured on the cover of *Better Homes and Gardens.*

So the next day you stroll over and knock on your neighbor's door. You want to commend him for all of his hard work. You hear a muffled "Come in" and you slowly open the door. What meets your eye takes you aback. Your neighbor is lethargically slouching in an old, lopsided armchair. He is surrounded by junk: piles of books and magazines, old pizza boxes, dirty coffee mugs. There are papers and clutter everywhere. It looks like the place hasn't seen a dust cloth or vacuum cleaner in a decade. In your shock you quickly blurt out,

"What's going on? The outside of your house looks wonderful but the inside looks like a pigsty." Fortunately, your neighbor is not too offended by your rudeness and explains to you that he received a notice from the city officials informing him that if he did not clean up his yard and the outside of his house he would receive a hefty fine. That motivated him to clean his house...but only what the city officials could see.

INSIDE OUT

Most of us have a cleansing routine. The order in which we bathe, brush our teeth, and comb our hair varies from person to person but we all spend a certain amount of time each day cleaning our bodies. This is a good thing. Cleansing is such a necessary and common habit that we seldom stop to think about it; we just do it. We're pretty good at cleaning what obviously needs to be cleaned. Since we are ambassadors of Jesus Christ, we should appear as clean and neat as possible. After all, we are representing the King.

However, we seldom stop to think that what is on the other side of our skin might need cleaning too. Who would spend hours every week cleaning and polishing their car but disregard the need for tune-ups, tire maintenance, oil changes, and occasional major repairs? Yet that is what we often do with our bodies. We spend a lot of time maintaining our appearance and are shocked when our body's complex "under-the-hood" systems malfunction. It doesn't matter how pretty a car may be; if it is broken down on the side of the road, just how useful is it? So the inside of our bodies need attention just as houses and cars need maintenance and care in order to be useful.

Many times we become aware of an inner problem because of an outward sign. For example, we realize that something is wrong with our car when we hear an unusual noise or the "Check Engine" light appears on our dashboard. It is a warning sign notifying us that a hidden malfunction has occurred. Many people consider pain their enemy but pain is actually like the "Check

Engine" light on our car. It is telling us to stop and give our bodies some rest and make needed repairs. If we don't listen to our bodies and barrel ahead, thinking that the problem will just disappear on its own, we might find ourselves like a disabled vehicle stranded on the side of the road.

Some people think that they have so many places to go and people to see that they don't have time to listen to the warning signs. They don't want to waste time resting and repairing. Our bodies are not designed to operate ninety-to-nothing without taking time to stop and rest. God rested on the seventh day after six days of creating and working. As God, He surely does not need "rest" as we define rest and He certainly needs no repairs but His seventh day sabbatical set an example for us.

Nobody is superhuman. We are not infallible machines. We must learn to "listen" to our bodies and take care of them when they need attention. They will serve us better if we take simple precautions and routinely clean them from the inside out.

TOXIC TIMES

I grew up in a residential area of north St. Louis. Anyone that has ever been to St. Louis, Missouri in the summer knows that it is miserably hot, very humid, hazy, and sticky. People don't like it but the mosquitoes absolutely love that type of weather. It seems that they travel from all over the world to vacation there each summer. Swatting at them doesn't seem to help because when you kill one mosquito, ten come to its funeral.

Coming to the rescue of hapless citizens, the public works department obtained a big truck which they drove through the neighborhood. This truck belched out a stinky fog that was designed to kill the mosquitoes. I'm not sure how effective it actually was – there always seemed to be a surplus of mosquitoes around – but what I vividly recall is that we were supposed to stay in our houses when the mosquito fog truck went by.

I do not know the extent of the toxicity of the fog that was emitted into our neighborhood. But it is just one example of an environmental toxin.

The word "toxin" comes from the Greek word "toxikon" which means "poison." Toxins are substances that are foreign to the body which will eventually cause harm if they are not properly eliminated.

There are more than 80,000 chemicals, many of them toxic, in use today. Toxic chemicals are used to dry-clean clothes. They can be found in common household products such as cleaning supplies, personal care products, furniture polish, paint thinner, nail polish remover, perfume, and lawn care products.

Toxins are in food and food additives. Farmers are well aware of the toxicity of the insecticides, fumigants, fungicides, rodenticides, antibacterials, and herbicides that they spray on their crops. They understand the danger they present not just to consumers, but also to their own families. Yet they are compelled to use them because these substances seem to offer an easy remedy to control pests, weeds, and fungi.

Other environmental toxins come from secondhand smoke, pharmaceutical drugs, air pollution, and even tap water. Industrial chemicals are sometimes highly toxic and can contaminate the air, water, and earth.

Studies have found toxic amounts of heavy metals such as mercury, lead, cadmium, aluminum, and arsenic in many people. Even many newborn babies have trace amounts of lead, DDT, and mercury in their bodies. "Studies conducted by the Environmental Protection Agency (EPA) show that 100 percent of the people studied had fat stores containing chemicals such as styrene from Styrofoam, dioxin from pesticides, and xylene, a solvent."[1]

These environmental toxins enter our bodies through the air we breathe, the water we drink, the food we eat, and the products we use every day. Some environmental toxins can cause cancer and birth defects. Others are proven neurotoxins.

In addition to external toxins, some of which we cannot control, our own bodies produce digestive toxins. After all of our food has been broken down, waste and small amounts of toxins are what remain, which a healthy digestive system is able to properly expel.

Toxicity from these internal digestive toxins occurs when the body's digestive system becomes sluggish. When waste and toxins sit in your large and small intestines, toxicity levels rise. When the digestive system becomes overloaded, excess toxins will be stored in tissues and the blood.

Too many external and internal toxins, combined with a poor diet and inadequate exercise, can prove too much for our bodies. When our bodies become overloaded with toxins, they can lose their ability to naturally detoxify themselves.

The infirmities that many people think are just signs that they are getting older are many times actually signals that they need to detoxify their bodies. Some very serious sicknesses and diseases are entirely preventable. If you struggle with chronic fatigue, headaches, backaches, allergies, mood swings, depression, gas, bloating, constipation, weight gain, joint and muscle pain, eczema, psoriasis, dermatitis, varicose veins, inflammation, decreased immunity, skin problems, IBS, colon cancer, bladder cancer, gallstones, diverticulitis, or leaky gut syndrome, it is possible that your body is begging for relief from its toxic overload.

There are several things we can do to aid the systems of our body as they work to eliminate toxins. Decreasing mental, emotional, and physical stress, chewing our food more thoroughly, exercising regularly, and reducing the amount of processed food we eat will all assist our bodies in the elimination of toxins.

Since the skin is the body's largest organ, choosing plant-based, non-toxic, biodegradable personal hygiene products will help as well. As for household products, there are a number of plant and citrus based products that work as well or better than those filled with dyes, perfumes, and potentially harmful chemicals.

Additionally, special times of cleansing will improve digestion and prevent toxins from being stored in our bodies.

TEMPLE CLEANING TIME

There are three kinds of housecleaning: 1) daily maintenance, 2) general weekly cleaning and 3) periodic deep cleaning. If we maintain our temples day-by-day, the weekly and periodic times of cleaning will not be as challenging.

I personally do not believe that times of cleansing should be torture. While self-denial is certainly involved and most of us are very unfamiliar with hunger pangs, we should conduct cleanses in such a way that we are invigorated and energized by our cleaning efforts.

There are several cleansing methods. Our bodies are all unique. Your personal health goals will determine the kind and length of cleanse you choose.

The most obvious cleanse is the water only cleanse. Not much explanation is needed here. This is the most stringent cleanse and is not necessarily the best for everyone, especially for those who are new to cleansing.

A less painful introduction to cleansing is dedicating a week or month to decreasing or excluding the consumption of foods that are particularly harmful. Some suggestions are coffee, sugar, potato chips, and soft drinks. When you are finished, you might just love the way you feel so much that you never incorporate those foods back into their normal place in your life.

If your diet consists mainly of sugary, refined foods, anticipate withdrawal symptoms when you begin refusing them. If your body is used to caffeine and sugar, you will realize how controlling they are when you go without them. The most common withdrawal symptom is headaches. Some people develop rashes, feel lightheaded, experience joint pain, or feel like their brains are in a fog. These are indications that the body is cleansing itself of toxins. The adage, "Things sometimes get worse before they get better" applies to cleansing. If you will persevere, your headaches and other symptoms will eventually dissipate and you will feel much better than you did before your cleanse.

A liquid cleanse is not too difficult for beginners. Drink pure water and add freshly squeezed lemon juice, cayenne pepper and a little pure maple syrup. Cayenne pepper clears mucus and maple syrup supplies minerals. Unsweetened cranberry juice added to pure water is excellent, especially for those whose kidneys need to be flushed. A cleanse of fresh vegetable juice is excellent for healing and repairing the body. My husband has drunk nothing except organic raw milk for several days. He reports that the milk is very filling so he does not get hungry and it makes him feel great.

A terrific one-week cleanse would consist of plenty of pure water, raw and lightly cooked vegetables, raw fruit, fresh vegetable and/or fruit juice, light soups, light vegetable, bean and/or grain salads, raw almonds, almond butter, raw pumpkin seeds, and raw sunflower seeds. Some beneficial fruits and vegetables to include are artichokes, asparagus, beets, blueberries, broccoli, cabbage, cauliflower, cherries, collards, daikon, garlic, kale, onions, peaches, and radishes. These foods will cleanse your body while they supply you with energy. During the course of the week, if possible, abstain from all food for a day.

Keep in mind that the foods, beverages, and herbs you use when you cleanse should be organic and toxin-free. After all, your purpose is to cleanse your body of toxins. If you cleaned the outside of your body with dirty water, just how clean would you get? Likewise, it doesn't make much sense to try to detoxify the inside of your body using tainted cleaning agents.

Cleansing is actually a natural process. Remember the last time you or a loved one had the flu? You may not have had much of an appetite. The lack of appetite was your body's way of communicating its need for rest and cleansing.

When people are acutely ill, they sometimes lose their appetite. Obviously, loss of appetite can sometimes be an indicator of something else, but often it is the body's cue that it needs time to rest and repair. Cleansing is very effective for those who have acute gastrointestinal problems and those that are recovering from surgery.

Losing weight should never be the main reason we cleanse. Cleansing on a regular basis may aid weight loss and help maintain a healthy weight, but losing weight should not be our main focus. We should focus on cleaning our temples and recharging our batteries. The purpose of cleansing should be to bring glory to God, not ourselves.

When weight loss becomes the main reason to cleanse, we tend to forget that times of cleaning are designed to aid our entire being; overweight and obesity are just outward symptoms of inside problems. Yes, obesity is a problem in its own right but it is the result of inside issues. As the inside gets cleaned up and our bodies begin operating optimally, we can see excess weight start to dissipate.

Cleansing gives our bodies rest from their work. It rids our bodies of impurities and purifies our blood. It re-empowers the colon, liver, kidneys, lungs, and skin to resume their natural detoxification tasks. Our nervous, cardiovascular, endocrine, reproductive, lymphatic, and immune systems are cleansed of toxins. Organs and tissues are renewed.

Cleaning house is not something most of us really *like* to do, but something we all *need* to do. Many nutritionists tout cleansing as the missing link to vibrant health.

HELPFUL HERBS

Herbs purify the blood, aid digestion, treat inflammation, cleanse the skin, and serve as diuretics. Some herbs are natural laxatives and are useful during cleansing, though they should not be relied on long-term.

Some herbal cleansers are stinging nettle, dandelion, burdock, cleavers, echinacea, red clover, milk thistle, rose hips, golden seal, Oregon grape root, yellow dock, sarsaparilla, chicory root, plantain leaf, poke root, kelp, watercress, olive leaf, grapefruit seed extract, and lemon. Most of these can be used in teas.

Additionally, digestive enzymes such as pepsin, papain, and betaine and the probiotics lactobacillus acidophilus and bifidobacterium bifidus may aid the cleansing process. Antioxidants vitamin C, natural mixed tocopherol (vitamin E), selenium, mixed carotenoids, alpha lipoic acid, and coenzyme Q10, which assist detoxification and neutralize free radicals, should be considered.

If you want to supplement your cleanses with herbs, consult an herbalist or naturopath. He or she can help you determine the proper proportions and combinations that will be safe and effective.

A CLEAN HOUSE FOR OUR MAKER

Until we start cleaning, we don't usually realize just how dirty our house is. We get used to feeling lousy and forget that life can be lived any other way. We grow accustomed to feeling tired, bloated, achy, and foggy-minded.

It's interesting that cleaning one portion of a dirty house will make the unclean area more conspicuous than it was before. Cleansing exposes to us just how much we need it. As we begin to clean our temples and experience such wonderful results, we will be motivated to do all we can do to be as clean and toxin-free as possible.

Some people only clean their houses when they are expecting company. They don't keep their houses clean for themselves and the other people that live there.

The bottom line reason to cleanse is that our bodies house the Almighty God. He deserves a clean house!

TWENTY-SEVEN

RESIDENT THIEF

No time to exercise and prepare healthy, home-made meals, you say? Cutting back, or better yet, *eliminating* the time you *waste* staring at your TV will give you more time for physical activity and meal preparation, not to mention quality interaction with your family and friends. It will free your time to study nutrition and prepare healthy meals rather than depending on nutrient deficient fast food and TV dinners to give your body the fuel and energy it needs.

Consider the following quotes from *Powerful Effects, Powerful Choices*, an outstanding book written by Michelle Dangiuro, filled with compelling, undeniable facts, statistics, and research about the adverse effects of television.

- "In the average American home, the television is on for nearly half of all waking hours."[1] (That's a lot of unnecessary chatter.)
- "If Americans watch the average amount of television – four hours a day, 28 hours a week – they will have spent 13 years of their lives watching TV by the time they are 75."[2] (*13 years*!!! That's about *1/6* of our lives!)
- "Television is now so entrenched in society that 25 percent of respondents to a *TV Guide* poll said they wouldn't give up their TV's for $1 million."[3]
- "66 percent of Americans watch television while eating dinner."[4] (This excludes meaningful communication. Memories made from family meals shared around the table are few when families prefer to eat in front of a TV. Memories are in-

stead relegated to the shallow entertainment the family shares.)

THE NUTRITION LINK

So what does television have to do with health and nutrition?

Dangiuro points out that the term "couch potato" came into use in 1979 to describe the lifestyle and body shape of those spending a lot of time in front of the tube. As we know, overweight and obesity is many times a precursor to serious health issues.[5]

"An extensive 10-year study conducted by the Harvard School of Public Health shows that watching television and Type-2 adult onset diabetes are linked. An estimated 38,000 males, aged 40-75, who watched more than three hours of TV a day were found to have double the risk compared to men who watched an hour or less. Those watching more than six hours of TV daily had three times the risk for Type-2 diabetes."[6]

CAPTIVE KIDS

Is there a connection between juvenile obesity, preventable childhood diseases, and TV viewing? Absolutely. Read on.

"For your kids' health, think seriously about limiting time your children spend watching television. Obesity among 8 to 16-year-olds is lowest among those who watch an hour or less a day. Kids who tune in four or more hours a day have the highest incidence of obesity. 'TV reduction appears the most effective measure in reducing weight gain among children,' says William Dietz, MD, director of the Division of Nutrition and Physical Activity, Centers for Disease Control. And don't forget to set limits for time on the computer and video games as well."[7]

And more from *Powerful Effects, Powerful Choices* about TV and kids: "Twelve medical studies have been conducted since 1985 linking excessive television viewing to obesity. Only four to five percent of American children ages 6 to 11 were seriously overweight in 1983. In 1993, that number jumped to 14 percent. And just guess the number of "junk food" ads aired during four hours of Saturday morning cartoons – more that 200."[8]

MODEL ME

"Even though girls and guys are concerned about the weight and shape of their bodies, television commercials emphasize snack foods with high fat and salt content that can lead to obesity. Television sends mixed messages to children and teens, juxtaposing the thin ideal of beautiful people with commercials for soft drinks, fast food, and other items high in sugar and/or fat."[9] (They're lying to us! How long will we continue to believe and endorse their lies?)

"Commercial images, just like images portrayed in television programs, distort children's self-images. Teenagers report having similar experiences. In a 1997 Body Image Survey, adolescents said that viewing thin and muscular models made them feel insecure about themselves. For adolescent girls, body dissatisfaction has been shown to be positively related to watching movies, serials, and soap operas, and their drive for thinness significantly correlated to watching music videos."[10]

Boys and girls, men and women, form from television their ideas about how they and the opposite sex should look. We *pay* Hollywood to make us feel lousy about our body shape. We make them millionaires so that they can create dissatisfaction in us because our boyfriend/girlfriend or spouse does not look like they just stepped out of the television. TV creates in us a sense that what is unreal [TV] is real and makes us disillusioned and dissatisfied with actual reality.

"The people you see become role models for you (implicitly) and your children (explicitly). They set the subconscious standards for the way we talk, the level of violence we accept, and the size and shape we want our bodies to be. An interesting note appeared in *Focus*, a news magazine from Harvard Medical School, about this

TV effect. This article pointed out that sociologists recently had a rare opportunity to observe a culture before and after the introduction of American TV. The images we've become used to were seen for the first time on the island of Fiji in 1995. This report stated that, by 1998, an incredible 74 percent of girls suddenly thought themselves too fat. Many rushed to diets. Others (15% of girls, average age 17) vomited to control weight."[11]

SIT STILL
Television has bred a nation of sedentary entertainment addicts. "Not only do you have to be sedentary to watch TV (so it encourages inactivity and weight gain), but the shows also trumpet the Barbie form as an ideal, when this is not normal, natural, or healthy. It's...common...for people to sit around watching shows to see the people they want to be. But that very act of watching creates the opposite person on the other side of the screen! It's ironic and sad."[12]

People weren't designed to sit in front of TVs and computers for long periods of time. "Watching TV is a passive, receptive event for the watcher. You are not acting or *interacting* with anything, just receiving like a lump. Set a limit, get off the couch, play a game with your kids. Garden, paint, live your life."[13]

BAD BUGS
It is symbolically fitting that in hospital rooms, it is the television remote control that has the highest level of bacteria. Chuck Gerba – "The Germ Doctor" – is a microbiology professor at the University of Arizona. The tests he conducted found bacteria levels on the television remote to be over three times higher than the bacteria found on the call button, the bathroom door, the toilet bowl handle, the hand rail, the tray table, and bathroom sink faucet handle. Even the dreaded Methicillin-Resistant Staphylococcus Aureus (MRSA) was detected on the remote control.

THE GRAND DECEPTION

The Fat Fallacy, a non-religious book by Dr. Will Clower that promotes food consumption principles similar to those in this book, has some thought provoking observations regarding America's obsession with television:

"Pretend you're from Mars. You can be green, or not. You can have those beetle-black teardrop eyes, or not. But think like someone who is not from this planet when you look around in your house or other people's houses. You, the brilliant Martian anthropologist on sabbatical, repeatedly see an altar in the living room. Many people have them in their bedrooms, too. The sofa, chairs, and coffee table are all arranged facing this shrine out of reverence. It's elevated, often encased in a lovely cabinet. It comes with a remote."[14]

If you use your television to unwind, relax, and provide accessible entertainment, you are not alone. Most people are quick to justify, defend, and try to qualify their enjoyment of television viewing, saying that they can control what they watch.

Another quote from Dangiuro: "People believe that it's not television's technology that's bad, it's how you use TV. Content – that's what counts now. Cut back on the violence, skimp on the sex, and add heaping spoonfuls of educational and inspirational programming to round out a balanced TV/video diet. But if this were true, if the TV itself had nothing to do with the messages being broadcast, then why are so many people addicted to it?"[15]

Television *is* addicting and mesmerizing, in a way that books, newspapers, and magazines are not. It has a pull that is, for the vast majority of viewers, completely irresistible. Most people are drawn to it and powerless to actually control it, in spite of what they say. Thus, they willingly, even eagerly, open up their minds and allow the content of the news reports, programs, movies, and commercials to freely shape the way they think, shop, eat, interact with others, and live.

Few things have as much control and influence over Americans as television. The most pathetic part of it is that it's all a big façade. It's time to blow the cover on TV's grand deception. It's time to get real.

THE BOTTOM LINE

Television is about one thing: Money. The financial masterminds behind television do not have your physical or moral health in mind. Television producers, actors, and advertisers don't care about you. They care about one thing – money. They want it to flow from your bank account to theirs.

Annette, a mother of two children, describes the tantalizing power of television advertising to influence food choices and purchases, most of which are extremely unhealthy: "When you watch television, tell me, how many of the commercials are not related to food, whether it's beer, pretzels, or Burger King? If you don't eat while you're watching television, what are you going to do? I heard that in an hour-long program, 15 minutes of it are commercials. And they're all about relationship – escape to the Bahamas; escape to Applebee's; escape to Budweiser. And they're entertaining, too! My family could sit through a 30-minute sit-com and chuckle a few times, but when the commercials came on, we were hysterical. Advertisers know what they're doing."[16]

"During the course of a year, the typical American child watches more than 40,000 TV commercials. About 20,000 of those ads are for junk food: soda, candy, breakfast cereals, and fast food. That means children now see a junk-food ad every five minutes while watching TV – and see about three hours of junk-food ads every week. American kids aren't learning about food in the classroom. They're being told what to eat by the same junk-food ads repeating again and again."[17]

If you're sick in the hospital because you bought a drug advertised on a TV commercial, believing that it would help you with one thing only to have it create more physical problems because of its adverse side effects, do you think the pharmaceutical company will send you flowers and pay your medical bills? No, they'll beef up their commercials to get more people to use their drug. They don't care about your health. They care about selling their products and promoting their values. They don't care that your child's teeth have 20 cavities in them by the time he or she is ten years old. They just want your child to see that sugary cereal or soda commercial and beg you to buy it when you go grocery shopping.

Use your money on something more productive than padding the pockets of the network providers and entertainment industry.

In your pursuit of better health, consider ditching your TV and investing in something worthwhile – workout equipment, a new pair of walking shoes, membership to the gym. In place of the money you spend every month sitting sedentarily in front of a talking box, you could fill your pantry with healthy staples and buy fresh vegetables that you thought you couldn't afford before.

Remember, you need to be healthy to serve God in the best way possible; you don't *need* a TV, in spite of what most Americans think. You'd be amazed at the time and money available to you when you break the bondage of TV's pretense in your life. Evaluate your priorities. Where we spend our time and money is an accurate gauge of where our priorities lie and what is really important to us.

CONNECTED

We live in a technological age. The Internet can be accessed via cell phones and movies can be watched in the comfort of your own vehicle. Large commercial airplanes have movie screens so passengers can be entertained during their flight. It is not unusual to see kids sitting for hours playing video games. Today, everyone wants to be "connected."

I am certainly not opposed to technology. I own a cell phone, PDA, and laptop computer. I am interested in learning about the latest gadgets on the market. I remember when the Internet first came into existence. I was working for a company that taught me how to navigate it from its beginning. For years there have always been people who have recognized television's blatant flaws. Yet when the Internet appeared, it was freely welcomed and accepted from the onset. While the Internet is an amazing tool that changed the dynamics of the way we communicate and placed literally a world of information at our fingertips, it has also proven to be a channel for great evil. Marriages, ministries, and families have been destroyed because the Internet has easy loopholes that cause good men to fall and kids to learn things they should never know.

The Internet has created an entirely new discussion about television. Inseparable connection between television and the Internet is right around the corner. People that have previously refused to have televisions in their homes will find it there because they brought the Internet into their homes without considering all of the possible ramifications.

It is true that righteousness cannot be legislated. Yet if we hunger for truth, we will naturally desire to be pleasing to God and to carefully monitor what we allow ourselves to see and hear. Owning media devices is a personal choice. But if at any time the devices that connect us to the world and provide us with a plethora of information threaten to break our connection with God, they have then become idols to us. We need to be wise enough to eliminate their influence from our lives.

HIDDEN AGENDAS

Digital communications will soon be the only medium of transfer used for television programming. This shift to digitalization is the bridge to complete television/computer/Internet integration.

Decades ago, when a single computer filled entire rooms, an old time preacher forecasted that the computer would be the avenue by which the Anti-Christ gains the allegiance of the world.

While some people would think this farfetched, consider that television (which will soon be entirely viewed via computerized technology) is the platform for all kinds of agendas. In this regard, television is a much more powerful method of influence than radio, newspapers, or news magazines. This is possible because while people are relaxed and being entertained, their minds are open to the insertion of whatever agendas programmers want to fill them with.

Consider the openness of homosexuality in the media today. Contrast that openness to just 25 years ago. Then, proponents of homosexuality stated that they would use TV as the way to get their message across. Obviously, their plan is working.

Television is such an important part of most families that the attitudes, trends, and behavior portrayed on the screen sets the standards for our society.

MIXED SIGNALS

A man went to Hollywood interviewing camera-toting visitors. One of the questions he asked them was, "Do you watch movies that take God's name in vain?"

Most of them responded, "Yes."

He then asked, "Does it bother you?"

Most of them again said, "Yes."

"But you watch those movies anyway?"

"Yes."

The interviewer then asked the same people, "Would you be offended by a movie that took your mother's name in vain?" All of them quickly responded that they would be offended if their mother's name was used as a byword.

This contrast stunned most people. Obviously they had never considered these questions before. They began to rethink their acceptance of God's name being used so freely as a curse word.

Yet this is just one of television's contradictions, just one of the mixed signals that distort people's sense of logic and reason.

What sane wife would allow a woman to enter her home and try to seduce her husband? Yet each month millions of American wives pay bills for revealing women's magazines, television, and Internet service that are stumbling blocks to her naturally visually stimulated husband.

Most parents would be horrified if their five-year-old witnessed a brutal murder that stole his innocence and gave him horrific nightmares. Yet unmonitored television is a convenient babysitter to keep little Johnny from being underfoot. By the time Johnny graduates high school, he will have seen thousands of brutal murders, thanks to such a caring, protective babysitter.

When a man or woman has an affair, painful turmoil ensues. Feelings of rejection, betrayal, and anger sometimes lead to divorce, which confuses and wounds children and other family members. Yet Americans are enthralled by yet another messy television affair, which, if that happened to them, would devastate them.

Television blurs the formerly clear lines of demarcation. The more of it we ingest, the more desensitized we become. Our consciences become dull. Right and wrong absolutes blend into gray. The transformation happens so gradually that we can't perceive the deception as it occurs.

Why can't we see television for what it really is? Our country is delightfully entertained by behavior and events that would anger most red-blooded Americans if those things happened to them. It's time we think for ourselves and protect our minds and our families.

THE INSIDE SCOOP

Amazingly, some television producers and movie stars recognize that the entertainment world from which they derive their livelihood is nothing more than a cesspool of filth. We would be wise to learn a lesson from those speaking from within the walls of the silver screen.

A popular Asian movie star recently denounced

Hollywood as detrimental to families and society.

Even Madonna does not allow her children to watch TV, which she calls "trash."[18] "Of reports that she doesn't allow Lourdes and Rocco to watch TV, Madonna first says, 'I was raised without television. They watch films, and my daughter always has her nose in a book. I don't get the sense that they feel deprived. I don't know why that's shocking.' But Madonna also admits she is concerned about the impact too much contemporary pop culture should have on her offspring in particular. 'TV is horrifying,' she says. 'Everything is so celebrity-obsessed, and I'm a celebrity. Why confuse my children with that?'"[19]

Philo Farnsworth was the inventor of television. Evidently he did not envision how his invention would someday be used. When, by today's standards, the worst things on TV were mild and harmless, Farnsworth was angry and regretful about television's content. In his book *When Television was Young*, Ed McMahon says that Farnsworth "wasn't particularly proud of his invention. He didn't let his own kids watch TV, telling them, 'There's nothing on it worthwhile. We're not going to watch it in this household, and I don't want it in your intellectual diet.'"[20]

Jesus said that "the children of this world are in their generation wiser than the children of light" (Luke 16:8).

TELEVISION AND YOUR HEALTH

Television is unhealthy spiritually and it endangers familial bonds. Unhealthy relationships with God and others can contribute to a negative mental state that is detrimental to health and physical healing processes.

Television encourages a sedentary lifestyle and the consumption of unhealthy foods. Television programming can create anxiety and it has the potential to raise blood pressure. Rather than being a refreshing escape for people, it adds stress to already stress-filled lives.

The strife, confusion, and violence which are par for the course any day of television's week creates a snowball effect. What affects our minds also affects our bodies.

THE POWER OF PURITY

From the vantage point of someone who has never owned a television, it is absolutely amazing to observe how important people think television is. The attachment to television is such that I'm sure there are many people who would do without a bed or a car but they must own at least one television.

When I was a teenager, I could have had a television in my room if I would have wanted one. Thank God that even in my youth I saw through it's facades; my decision prevented visual images being cemented into my mind that I would have had to fight in my pursuit of purity.

Lest I be misunderstood, I do not think that I am the least bit superior to people who watch television. I pray that I will never have a self-righteous attitude toward others. I just know that my life is more peaceful because of the absence of television. I sincerely want others to know how it feels to have a mind that is clean and a spirit that is void of images and emotions that are transmitted via television.

One of the reasons I don't own a television is because it is so captivating and I, like most people, am not strong enough to resist its draw. On the rare occasions that I do find myself in the vicinity of a television, I find myself watching things I'm not even interested in.

Some people say, "I like to watch the news and keep up with what's going on in the world." It's always the same, just different names and different wars. Others say, "I want to listen to the weather forecast." Step outside and look around. You'll have about as much of a clue as the overpaid weatherman. Some folks favor religious programming, the majority of which uses sensational and flamboyant methods to retain viewers.

Maybe you have been known to say, "I like the history channel." Or the science channel. Or the political channel. Unfortunately you will have to muddle through liberal ideas, opinions, slanted views, evolution, and postmodern nonsense to learn what you could learn at the library.

Is everything on TV bad? Of course not. There are a few wholesome programs.

But let's get honest. Unless you are already so desensitized that you aren't fazed, it is hard to listen to the radio without hearing words that make you want to blush. How much more does TV, which uses audio *and* visual media to flaunt sin, present a challenge for those who desire pure minds?

I am not anti-current events, anti-education, or anti-information. But when people take the approach, "I'll eat the meat and throw away the bones," they encounter a problem: there is very little meat on television. If I have to wrestle through the trash to get to something worthwhile, I will certainly get contaminated during the process.

Our minds retain what we see and hear. What we absorb through our five senses gets down into our spirits, and before we know it, the attitudes that we expose ourselves to become a part of us.

Hollywood opposes everything that God is and everything that He advocates. Holiness. Clean living. Words of faith and love. Living peacefully with others. Not stirring up strife. Not taking pleasure in wickedness. It is a fact that the "works of the flesh" outlined in Galatians 5:19-21 are what make television so alluring and sensational. Television utilizes them all in their efforts to appeal to the minds of men, women, and children.

The Psalmist prayed, "Turn away mine eyes from beholding vanity" and he determined that he would not set any wicked thing before his eyes (Psalm 119:37; 101:3).

Ephesians 5:11-12 admonishes us to "have no fellowship with the unfruitful works of darkness, but rather reprove them. For it is a shame even to speak of those things which are done of them in secret." If we are not to even talk about the wicked things that people do, then surely seeing visual enactments of such perverseness is not acceptable to God.

Philippians 4:8 tells us to fill our minds with things that are true (real, factual, accurate), honest (honorable), just (fair, impartial), pure (clean, chaste, innocent, modest), lovely (acceptable, pleasing), and of a good report (well spoken of, reputable).

I've spent my entire life striving for purity. I've gone against the flow, defied America's twisted passion with ungodly entertainment. I'm not about to throw away all that I have attained. It doesn't bother me that I can't name the most popular anchorwoman on CBS. I don't care that I'm not "in the know" about the most popular shows.

I don't feel the least bit behind the times. Some people might think I live with my head in the sand and that I'm not progressing with the modern world. I could care less if I'm in step with the times; I'd rather be in step with Jesus. And with so little time, I'd rather be reading His Word or enjoying wholesome fellowship and conversation than watching TV. Rather than being tuned in to the world's stage, I'd rather be progressing in my walk with the King of all kings.

A popular radio talk show host recently stated that he wanted to get rid of the televisions in his home because he thought that their content was worthless. But his producer convinced him that, because of his line of work, he needed to stay informed of current events.

This story is often repeated by people who are not necessarily Bible-believing individuals. If they can recognize the entertainment industry for what it is, how much more should those of us who are born again believers renew our commitment to purity?

Our speech reflects our heart. Are we talking more about funny television episodes, outrageous statements made by radio news analysts, or the latest Internet development than we are about an old verse of

Scripture that just came "alive" to us? Do spiritual things still exhilarate us or do other things fill our thoughts? We must ask God to renew our minds and help us desire things that are holy and good. Technology and entertainment will only momentarily satisfy us; being in the presence of God will provide true contentment and lasting satisfaction.

HELLO FAMILY

Some schools have instituted TV Turnoff Week, when students and their parents are encouraged to keep their TVs turned off for one week. Many students like the experiment because they get to actually communicate with Mom and Dad. They get to make memories interacting with their families.

It's sad but true that some people know the fictional lives of soap opera stars better than they know the thoughts, feelings, dreams, and ambitions of their own loved ones. TV characters seem real to them. Television makes some people dissatisfied with their lives, which seem boring when contrasted with the exciting lives of make believe people on television.

I've talked to adults who can recall spending very little quality time with their parents. Their parents' idea of family time was sitting in front of a TV. As a result, families hardly know one another.

When the entertainment fades into darkness, the relationships have usually not grown stronger. A make-believe world is allowed to prevent meaningful communication and personal growth.

ADIOS THIEF

Television viewing is an enemy of our physical and spiritual health, and *we* are the ones responsible for allowing it to influence us. We sit in front of it mindlessly, letting it tell us what to do, what to eat, how to live. We accept what it presents to us almost without question.

Our laissez faire attitude toward television's evils can be likened to a homeowner who invites a thief into his home. Not only does he allow the thief a permanent place of residence, he *pays* him to pillage and destroy what the homeowner has worked so hard to gain and really wants to retain: peace, harmony in the home, a healthy body, a clean mind.

It's time to say goodbye to the thief that is stealing from us. It's time to let him know that his presence is no longer welcome.

THE CLOCK IS TICKING

Replace the time you waste sitting in front of your TV. Take a walk with a friend. Play an outdoor game. Explore a new park or museum. Volunteer to work at your church. Participate in your children's homework and school projects. Experiment with a new healthy recipe.

Quit wasting your time; you probably only have 7 or 8 decades worth. That's too little to waste 1/6 of it doing nothing but filling your mind with spiritual, mental, and physical junk food. *Invest* your time instead. Invest it in the things that really matter and the activities that will keep you healthy, happy, and vibrant.

TWENTY-EIGHT

SWEET DREAMS

He giveth his beloved sleep.
Psalm 127:2

Restful sleep is essential to good health. It allows our bodies to rest, repair, and rejuvenate. Jesus, God manifested in human flesh, had to sleep (Mark 4:38; Colossians 2:9).

If you have trouble getting to sleep at night or if you do not sleep well, there are several things you can do to ensure a good night's rest.

MIDNIGHT SNACKS

Avoid sugary, spicy, salty, and heavy foods. Also, avoid caffeine, found in regular coffee, regular tea, and chocolate, before going to bed. Caffeine is a stimulant. Remember, you're trying to wind down, not wind up!

When we praise and worship God in apostolic services, we exert a lot of physical, emotional, and spiritual energy. After times of exuberant praise and worship we are spiritually and emotionally rejuvenated but our bodies are sometimes a little tired. We tend to want a pick-me-up after such services and head to the table for food and fellowship.

Unfortunately, our late night choices are usually poor ones – quick and sugary or heavy restaurant food. We want to relax and unwind before going to sleep yet we fill our bodies with food that it will have to work hard all night to process. Have you ever wondered why you wake up feeling tired after a full night's sleep? The reason just might be the type of food you eat before bed. Be good to your body: eat light at night. When we eat heavy meals shortly before bedtime, our bodies do not have the opportunity to actively burn the calories we have just consumed. Routinely eating heavy late night meals guarantees us an expanded waistline and is the enemy to successful weight loss. Let your body rest instead of having to work all night processing and digesting food.

Eating with believers is definitely an apostolic thing to do. Acts 2:42 says of the First Church of Jerusalem that "they continued stedfastly in the apostles' doctrine and fellowship, and in breaking of bread, and in prayers." In addition to praying and teaching, the believers fellowshipped and broke bread (ate) together. This is an important part of our spiritual growth. Because it helps to break down barriers, sharing a meal can pave the way to share the gospel and help new believers bond to the body of Christ.

Yet, because the times we meet together for worship, the Word, and prayer are often in the evening, breaking too much bread late at night can actually be detrimental to our bodies. As we know, the condition of each part of us (body, soul, and spirit) affects our entire being.

PRE-SLEEP PLANS

Sometimes our time would be better spent by going home and quietly unwinding instead of staying up late at a restaurant. Not only would this benefit us spiritually, it would allow us time to absorb and bask in the spiritual blessings we received and meditate on the Word we heard.

If you want to fellowship after services, plan ahead and prepare a light snack. You can fellowship in a more relaxed environment, eat lighter, and save money too.

If you do need a little something to eat, choose foods that contain tryptophan. Tryptophan is an essential amino acid that promotes a healthy nervous system. It has a calming effect. Eating foods with tryptophan increases the amount of serotonin made by the brain. Low levels of serotonin can lead to anxiety and sleep disorders. Tryptophan eases tension and stress, encourages a quiet mood, and aids restful sleep by combating insomnia. It helps hyperactive children and adults. Tryptophan aids in weight control by reducing appetite. It is good for heart health and migraine headaches. Tryptophan is necessary for the production of B3 (niacin).

Some sleep-friendly foods that contain tryptophan are brown rice, bananas, dates, fish, peanuts, freshly ground peanut butter, and dairy products. Eggs and cottage cheese are good choices of dairy products. Also, try hummus with whole-grain pita bread, toasted whole-wheat tortillas, or toasted sprouted grain tortillas. Hummus is ground chickpeas (garbanzo beans) and has tahini (ground sesame seeds) in it. Tahini is a good source of tryptophan. Also, don't forget turkey. It also contains tryptophan and is a good choice when you want a little something substantial before bedtime.

SLEEP LIKE A BABY

David said, "I will both lay me down in peace, and sleep: for thou, LORD, only makest me dwell in safety" (Psalm 4:8). Before going to bed, choose to read a portion of Scripture instead of filling your mind with the evening news. The latter has been proven to create feelings of confusion, stress, and anxiety, which inhibit a relaxing bedtime routine. When at all possible, do not engage in stressful conversation. Clear your mind of the problems and stress of the day by meditating on the Word and the goodness of the Lord. One man's advice was this: "Before you go to bed at night, give all your burdens to the Lord. He'll be up all night anyway." Think and speak positively. Use words of faith instead of fear.

If you have trouble with nightmares or troubling dreams, pray and ask the Lord to control your dreams that night. Sometimes dreams are a result of the things we think about throughout the day. Keep your mind pure and clean by thinking uplifting thoughts. God has promised to give us a good night's rest: "When thou liest down, thou shalt not be afraid: yea, thou shalt lie down, and thy sleep shall be sweet" (Proverbs 3:24).

"My mind just won't shut down. I keep thinking about all of my problems and the stress of life. I have to take sleeping pills to get to sleep." Worry is not just the enemy of restful sleep, it is the opposite of trust in God. As paradoxical as it may seem, when we worry we are placing our faith and trust in what we are worrying about. LaJoyce Martin said, "I know worrying works because 90% of the things I worry about never happen." Worry is a waste of time. Take your burdens to the Lord in prayer and leave them there. Get godly counsel from your pastor about stressful family and job situations and implement his advice. When we stew on problems we rob ourselves of peace. Also, unrepented sin will keep us awake at night (Psalm 38:3).

In place of the negative and worrisome thoughts that fill your mind, meditate on God, His goodness, His laws, and His Word (Psalm 1:2, 63:6; 119:148). If you can't get to sleep, pray, meditate on the things of the Lord, and read the Word. Take some time to praise and worship God, refreshing your spirit with His presence. The Bible speaks of night songs (Job 35:10; Psalm 42:8). David, the sweet psalmist of Israel, who had plenty of stressful situations that could have robbed him of his peace and relationship with God, wrote, "Let the saints be joyful in glory: let them sing aloud upon their beds" (Psalm 149:5).

God designed us to live peaceful, stress-free lives. Begin applying the Word to your life. Clear your mind of negative and critical thinking. Live a godly, holy life so that condemnation will not dog your steps. Live above sin and keep your mind clean. This will ensure that when you lie down at night, you will be at peace with your Maker. There is no greater assurance than knowing that your life is pleasing to your God.

Memorize the following verses of Scripture and apply them to your life: "Be careful for nothing; but in every thing by prayer and supplication with thanksgiving let your requests be made known unto God. And the peace of God, which passeth all understanding, shall keep your hearts and minds through Christ Jesus. Finally, brethren, whatsoever things are true, whatsoever things are honest, whatsoever things are just, whatsoever things are pure, whatsoever things are lovely, whatsoever things are of good report; if there be any virtue, and if there be any praise, think on these things" (Philippians 4:6-8).

People who do not rest well at night because of worry are not resting in God during the day. Jesus said, "Come unto me, all ye that labour and are heavy laden, and I will give you rest. Take my yoke upon you, and learn of me; for I am meek and lowly in heart: and ye shall find rest unto your souls. For my yoke is easy, and my burden is light" (Matthew 11:28-30). The Lord refers to His people as children. Yoke up with Jesus for spiritual rest, which will have you waking up in the morning happy, optimistic, and refreshed.

When babies and children are ready to go to sleep, they don't worry about getting along with the pesky neighbors and paying the electric bill. They don't fret about politics, the weather, and the possibility of a nuclear attack. Do your best to work to pay the bills and create harmony with others during the daytime. If you are doing all you can do and your life is still stressful, ask Jesus to take up the slack and work miracles on your behalf. Your faith and trust will grow as you watch Him do the impossible. Let Jesus take care of all the stuff that is out of your control and you will find yourself sleeping like a baby too.

DON'T DO DRUGS

Do not use prescription sleeping pills. Instead, try the tips mentioned above, especially the one about prayer and reading the Word of God. Sleeping pills sometimes cause a rebound effect because they lose their effectiveness and only worsen insomnia. They have also been known to cause addiction.

Choose natural, homeopathic sleeping disorder remedies over prescription drugs. Some natural sleeping aids to consider are California poppy, passionflower, chamomile, nux vomica, coffea, melatonin, and valerian. Natural methods will have you waking up alert and ready to dive into your day instead of shuffling through the grogginess commonly produced by conventional drugs.

Some over-the-counter drugs such as allergy and cold medications, painkillers, and appetite suppressants contain stimulating compounds that promote insomnia.

SLEEP WELL

Try to go to bed about the same time every night and get up about the same time every morning. Going to bed early, well before midnight, promotes better sleep than going to bed after midnight. Keep your bedroom clean and tidy. Most people sleep better when the room is quiet and dark. Lose excess weight. Even a few extra pounds make breathing more difficult. Almost every person I have met with sleep apnea has been at least somewhat overweight.

We spend one-third of our lives sleeping. It is worthwhile to make it as restful as possible so that the other two-thirds can be productive and fulfilling. If we eat well, we will be less sluggish throughout the day and may even need less sleep. God designed us to sleep so that our energy could be replenished. Unless we get more than we actually need, it is *not* a waste of time.

TWENTY-NINE

PARTING THOUGHTS

MAKE SMALL CHANGES

As you have been reading this book, you may have at times felt overwhelmed when you realized all of the changes you need to make. But Rome wasn't built in a day and changing our eating habits takes time too.

Making dietary changes can be uncomfortable because you are breaking out of your comfortable paradigm. Eating oatmeal instead of a toaster pastry, steamed broccoli instead of French fries, and substituting water for soft drinks might seem like massive changes to you.

Gradually replace the refined and processed foods in your cupboard. If you will make small changes, a little at a time, changing your diet won't seem like such a big ship to turn. Don't become overwhelmed. Just do the best that you can do.

The small steps we take to better our own health will not just affect us. They will affect our family, friends, and our work for God. The benefits of change start with one step, whether that step is on the treadmill, at the health food store, or in the kitchen preparing delicious, healthful food.

Again, make one small change at a time. Cement that small change into your lifestyle and then make another small change.

SET GOALS – SMALL GOALS

It may be helpful to make a list of goals. For example, if you drink four sodas a day, list a goal to drink only two a day. If you never exercise, list a goal of walking 10 minutes, five days a week. These written goals are small steps that can provide you with something to aim for. Make them achievable. Don't decide that you are going to climb Mt. Everest tomorrow if you do absolutely no exercise now. Make your goals attainable. As you reach your goals, you can add new ones. These goals are small steps to health.

Also, for one week, list everything you eat. Cross off one or two unhealthy foods and don't eat those the following week. Do the same thing for the second week. Do this until you have eliminated the really bad aspects of your diet and replaced them with healthy foods.

BE CONSISTENT – DON'T GIVE UP

Change is not usually easy and it requires consistency. Serious and long-term health issues will not change overnight, after the first day of healthy eating. Anticipate progressive, not immediate results. Though you will experience positive effects right away, consistency is required for long-term results.

It takes a long time to become unhealthy. In an instant-minded generation, we should not throw in the towel if we aren't in shape and minus all of our health problems in a week. Quick weight loss pills and plans and "miracle" cures are in the same category as get-rich-quick schemes. In our computerized society, we have been programmed to expect instantaneous results.

Keep your goals in view at all times. If you mess up, don't stay down. Begin again. Don't get upset at yourself and give up just because you mess up.

You must want to be healthy, feel good physically, and have greater energy *more* than you want to continue the sluggish, unhealthy lifestyle you're comfortable with. Weigh the benefits and you will realize that change, no matter how challenging it may be, is worth the effort.

DON'T PROCRASTINATE

Procrastination is the enemy of progress and the friend of failure. "I'll start exercising next week." "I'll start eating right after I finish this chocolate cake." Procrastination ensures that the illusionary "tomorrow" never arrives. Exercise your ability to choose to change – today.

SAVVY SUPPLEMENTATION

You may want to buy a good multivitamin/mineral supplement and any other supplements that you may personally need. Many people find whole food and "green food" supplements particularly beneficial.

Homeopathic remedies can be effective at treating a variety of ailments. Homeopathy treats the source of the problem, not just symptoms. Keep in mind that homeopathic remedies are usually slower acting than their over-the-counter and prescription counterparts.

All supplements are not created equal. There is a vast difference in the quality and potency of supplements.

Many health food stores have an employee that specializes in dispensing advice about supplements for particular health and nutritional needs. Also, a visit to a naturopathic physician can help you determine exactly what supplements will benefit you the most. It is vital that you take the correct amounts to keep your body in balance.

Especially when using herbs it is crucial that you seek the advice of a trained, qualified herbal specialist. Herbs work synergistically. Conversely, they can counteract one another and they can clash with prescription drugs. There is no single herb that is a panacea for perfect health and when it comes to herbs, you can get too much of a good thing. Use extreme caution and follow the advice of a skilled professional.

Remember that a quality multi will never be a good replacement for a healthy diet. These products are called "supplements" because they are intended to supplement an overall healthy diet. Don't expect supplements to make you healthy if your diet is lousy.

I met a man who once had rheumatoid arthritis.

He attributed his healing to three things: a miracle from God, fasting, and a change of diet. He continued to trust in God, fast regularly, and eat properly. Not only did he never have any more problems with rheumatoid arthritis, he did not use supplements because his diet was exceptionally pure and healthy. Certainly this is the ideal situation and his story reminds us that our commitment to making proper food choices should never be preempted by the availability of food supplements.

FOR THE SAKE OF THE GOSPEL

Paul wrote to the Philippian church about Epaphroditus, a man who was his assistant and companion. Paul said that "for the work of Christ [Epaphroditus] was nigh unto death, not regarding his life" (Philippians 2:30). Epaphroditus was deathly sick because of his labor in the kingdom of God. The Lord mercifully restored his health to him.

This is a scenario that is sometimes seen in those who are in full time service for the Lord. Pastors, evangelists, missionaries, and their spouses juggle church, family, and personal responsibilities. Some are bivocational, working secular jobs to make a living.

It is not a sin to take a break. It is not unspiritual to get away from routine and responsibilities to rekindle your relationship with your spouse and have fun with your children. You are not being lazy if you occasionally take time to regroup and renew. As a matter of fact, relaxing your mind and body will give you greater energy to work for the Lord and help prevent burnout. I was gratified to recently hear Rev. Art Hodges advocate setting aside time to rest. His three-part plan recommends that we 1) divert daily, 2) withdraw weekly and 3) abandon annually.

Our bodies are not yet celestial in nature and they can only operate on overload capacity for so long. Even Jesus realized that His disciples needed a break now and then. Mark 6:31 records Jesus saying, "Come ye yourselves apart into a desert place, and rest a

while." With all of the hustle and bustle and the demands placed upon them, they didn't even have time to
sit down and enjoy a decent meal. Sound familiar?
Sometimes life gets so hectic that we forget how to relax
our minds and bodies. But mental and physical rest is a
necessity if we want to maintain our vigor, stay positive,
and keep our focus.

I know of people who have been mightily used of
God. In time, their intense prayer, fasting, and dedication to the work of God took its toll on their health. It is
indisputable that spiritual battles are won because of
spiritual, physical, and mental exertion. I am grateful for
people that lay their lives on the line for the sake of the
gospel. Just as was the case with Epaphroditus, many
times God spares these precious people so they can continue to labor in kingdom work, but they sometimes
have to take time to heal and repair before they launch
into the next level of ministry.

Spiritual warfare is a necessity if we are to be
good soldiers for our King's cause. However, even
earthly military commanders understand that their soldiers will get mentally and physically exhausted if they
are on the front lines too long. Soldiers are provided
with reprieves so that their minds and bodies can stay
keen, alert, and perform optimally. Weary troops are
prone to make mistakes. Such mistakes endanger the
weary soldier and his comrades and compromise the ac-
complishment of the King's mission.

We must be willing to give our all yet we must
remember that our human minds and bodies sometimes
need rest. When Epaphroditus became sick from over-
exertion, his productivity in the Kingdom came to a
grinding halt.

We will be more of a blessing to the Kingdom of
God if we get proper rest and take care of our bodies
and our own spiritual lives before attempting to meet
the needs of others. Each time a commercial airplane
prepares to embark on a journey, passengers are told
what to do if the cabin should become depressurized. If
they have a child next to them, they are not supposed to

put the child's mask on first, but their own. The reason for this is simple: if the adult becomes incapacitated, they will be unable to help the dependant child in any way.

While our human desires tell us to set aside our own needs to help others, in reality this is neither sensible nor biblical. How can we rescue others from destruction if we are not whole, healthy, and strong spiritually, physically, and mentally? If we are tired, burned out, depressed, anxious, sick, or fearful, just how encouraging and helpful will we be to those who are struggling with some of those same issues?

God created man with a need to rest. The Old Testament law commanded the people to work for six days and rest on the seventh. During Creation Week God set the example for Sabbath rest "for in six days the Lord made heaven and earth, and on the seventh day he rested, and was refreshed" (Exodus 31:12-17). Even during harvest time (i.e., really busy and hectic times, when life was filled with pressure and time restraints) they were to keep the Sabbath and not neglect it (Exodus 34:21).

In addition to this weekly break from labor, the Lord implemented other extended rest periods. The purpose of these times was to celebrate the end of a period of strenuous work and to remember the goodness of God to His people. For example, the end of barley harvest was marked by the Feast of Unleavened Bread (Passover), the end of the wheat harvest was celebrated by the Feast of Weeks (Pentecost), and the grape harvest concluded with the Feast of Tabernacles, which commemorated the 40 years when the people of God lived in tents in the wilderness.

It is vital to keep in mind that these God-instituted "vacations" were centered around Him. They were celebrations of His love, provisional power, and goodness. These joyous, festive times were intended to give people not just physical and mental rest, but spiritual rest as well. These were opportunities for the children of Israel to grow closer to God, to grow in their relationship with Him, to refocus on what was really important in life.

Once my husband and I took several days off from traveling because I insisted that the reason I was irritable and impatient was because I was exhausted and tired due to the fast pace of our lives. This mini-vacation, however, did little for me. I was still irritable and unhappy. A couple of days into the vacation, my husband suggested that the problem just might possibly be that I needed to spend some time with the Lord. Once I humbled myself and prayed, releasing to the Lord my frustrations and acknowledging to Him that I had been neglecting Him, I felt His reassurance, love, acceptance, and peace.

You see, I had been praying, but most of my prayers were for the sake of others. I had been neglecting my own spiritual needs. I had been depriving myself of communication with my Maker. Once I got things back into proper perspective, I was able to properly enjoy our little vacation. The peace that was lost as a result of my disconnected relationship with God was restored.

Now when we go on vacation, I don't expect "getting away from it all" to be the cure-all for my problems. I don't take a vacation from God. What I need most is spiritual refreshing and renewal, even more than physical rest. I need God's peace to consume my mind and heart.

Sometimes we can be so focused on the harvest and the needs of others that we neglect our own needs. It is not wrong, but rather it is needful and important that we take time for ourselves and our families. When we keep our "time off" in proper perspective, it can renew us spiritually, recharge us mentally and emotionally, and help preserve the health of our temples.

BETTER WITH AGE
Ponce de Leon searched for it – that elusive Fountain of Youth from which he could drink and defy the

natural processes of aging. He searched in vain, yet his story is repeated over and over in the lives of many people today. No longer do people dream of a mystical fountain, however. Their dreams are not quite so obviously starry-eyed and magical.

Instead, people who are desperate to avoid the inevitable effects of growing older cling to the philosophical ideologies of seemingly intelligent and knowledgeable people who propagate their "secrets" of youthful longevity. Each year, books of this nature become bestsellers because people are eager to believe that there is a way to be exempt from old age. A sampling of such titles is *The Anti-Aging Plan* (Roy Walford), *Ageless Body, Timeless Mind – The Quantum Alternative to Growing Old* (Deepak Chopra), and *Shed 10 Years in 10 Weeks* (Julian Whitaker). It doesn't take long, though, before these types of books find their way to the dusty shelves of cluttered secondhand bookstores. The reason for the short lifespan of books on longevity is because humanistic approaches are simply pie-in-the-sky pipedreams. No matter how much people long to forever look and feel like a 16-year-old, they instinctively know that it just won't happen.

In and of itself, the expression "anti-aging" is a very misleading phrase. Walk down the aisles of the health and beauty department of your local store and you will see products with labels telling you that you can "Look ten years younger in seven days." Nearly every mainstream women's magazine routinely features miracle makeovers. Before and after pictures continue to enthrall people hopeful for an age-defying change. It seems like people want to look young forever.

However, Jesus wants us to live in reality. We're not going to live forever and we're not going to look young forever.

As fatalistic as it may seem, death begins with life. No one can escape the process of physical degeneration. For the born again believer, this is not a defeatist topic, but a topic that produces joy. II Corinthians 4:16

says that "though our outward man perish, yet the inward man is renewed day by day" because "we look not at the things which are seen, but at the things which are not seen: for the things which are seen are temporal; but the things which are not seen are eternal. For we know that if our earthly house of this tabernacle were dissolved, we have a building of God, an house not made with hands, eternal in the heavens" (II Corinthians 4:18-5:1). What is more gratifying than to be spiritually renewed day by day and anticipate a glorious reunion with our precious Lord and Savior?

Desiring to live a long life simply for the sake of longevity places an unbalanced emphasis on the body. This desire does not reflect a God-centered view of life and life after death. When we die, then will "the dust return to the earth as it was: and the spirit shall return unto God who gave it" (Ecclesiastes 12:7).

I recently heard a minister say that our bodies are nothing but shells. They are simply vehicles that will take us to our destination. Understanding the importance of the body compared to the importance of determining the everlasting destination of our spiritual man puts our view of long life into perspective.

Death is only a brief corridor into eternal life. Our purpose on this earth is to please God and to get ready for the next life. Ecclesiastes 12:13-14 sums it all up: "Let us hear the conclusion of the whole matter: Fear God, and keep his commandments: for this is the whole duty of man. For God shall bring every work into judgment, with every secret thing, whether it be good, or whether it be evil."

The Bible teaches that, while we progress closer and closer to death, serving God has tremendous benefits. Our elder years can be our most fruitful years. Contrary to our convoluted society's philosophy, old age is highly esteemed in the Bible.

In America, we have been conditioned to accept that old age will be filled with sickness. According to Psalm 90:10 and Ecclesiastes 12:1-7, we may experience changes in our physical strength and ability.

These changes serve as reminders that our days are drawing to a close.

Yet it is encouraging to know that there were men in the Old Testament who, aside from experiencing ordinary physical decline, apparently did not endure debilitating diseases during their latter years. Abraham "died in a good old age, an old man, and full of years" (Genesis 25:8). Isaac "died, and was gathered unto his people, being old and full of days" (Genesis 35:29). "Job died, being old and full of days" (Job 42:17). Chronicles of prolonged illness did not mark the end of these men's lives.

In the New Testament, excluding when He encountered overwhelming skepticism and doubt, Jesus "healed all that were sick" (Matthew 8:16; 12:15; Luke 6:19). The Bible does not say that He asked people how old they were before He healed them. If that were the case, the Scripture might have read, "He healed all that were sick – except the elderly." If you are elderly, Jesus still wants to heal you.

When we live for the Lord, we can anticipate having joy and being useful in Kingdom work to our very last day of life. I love what Nona Freeman wrote in her book *Keeper of the House*: "I have a word for you folks out there who think you went over the hill when you turned forty. BOSH! My most productive years began in my sixties. And you folks pining for retirement day to come need a change of heart and a change of mind – and a change of diet."[1]

David encourages us to bless the Lord because He is the one who satisfies our mouths with good things, so that our youth is renewed like an eagle's (Psalm 103:5). Living for God is the ultimate anti-aging plan. It's a win-win situation. Some things really do get better with age.

CHERISH YOUR CROWN

America's obsession with youth has Americans, especially American women, living in a state of denial.

It's strange to hear a 50-year old woman say, "I don't like my gray hair. It makes me look old." Well, what does she think she is? 16-years old?

We need to wake up and smell the roses. And closely examine our birth certificates. We ARE getting older. Instead of wishing that we were younger and looked like Hollywood stars, we should be enjoying every second of our lives. Why waste our time bemoaning the unchangeable fact that we are getting older just like everyone else in the world? Why not enjoy every stage of life? This approach will ensure that we age gracefully and happily, instead of fighting it every step of the way.

God's idea about gray hair: "The hoary [gray] head is a crown of glory, if it be found in the way of righteousness (Proverbs 16:31). Why do so many women try to cover up their crowns? What we consider so reproachable because of society's concepts is glorious to God.

Jesus said, "Thou canst not make one hair white or black" (Matthew 5:36). He was not telling them that they were *incapable* of dying their hair; plant derived dyes were in use at that time. Although they had the ability to cover up their natural hair color, they could not actually change it. In other words, underneath all of those chemical dyes, gray hair is still gray hair.

Dyed hair creates an artificial look because as our hair color and texture changes, so does our skin. It changes in color and elasticity and (horror of horrors!) wrinkles form. So many times, the resultant appearance of dyed hair is a harsh look. The hair does not match the face.

Anne Kreamer, a professional in the entertainment industry, was 49 years old when she examined a picture of herself and was shocked by what she saw. Over a 25-year period, she had spent $65,000.00 keeping her gray hair hidden, trying to be something she was not. She believed that by dyeing her hair she could feel and look younger than she was and hoped others were drawing the same conclusions.

In her book *Going Gray*, she reveals that she did not realize that her dyed hair "might have had a subtle but even more profound aging effect. I chose not to register the fact that hair dye, inevitably, faintly stains the skin around the hairline, tipping off anyone who looks closely that what you are presenting is a simulation of youth."[2]

Due to special lighting, makeup, and video and photography techniques available to entertainment stars, "it's literally impossible for us to measure up to the preternaturally youthful faces we see on TV or in magazines." "It's a given that every visible pore, wrinkle, splotch, sag, and bag will be airbrushed from the photographs of celebrities in magazines."[3]

Yet that is what Kreamer had been doing for years. She states that "the desire to look as young as possible is permanently entrenched in our culture."[4] While contemplating the plunge into honesty, she remembers asking herself, "Would I continue holding on to some dream of youthfulness or could I end the game of denial and move more honestly into middle age?"[5] She decided to live in reality. She quit dying her hair and experienced liberation.

True beauty is not found in a bottle or jar. True beauty is having the Lord's favor rest upon your life. "Favour is deceitful, and beauty is vain: but a woman that feareth the LORD, she shall be praised" (Proverbs 31:30). So ladies, instead of despising your crown, cherish it, for it is a crown of righteousness.

TRUE BEAUTY

In his book *The Maker's* Diet, Jordan Rubin writes "Current fashion fads aside, we don't need to look as muscular as the people we see on television or on magazine covers, but *anyone* can certainly be a lot healthier with a nutritious diet and moderate exercise."[6]

In a mixed up society that places so much emphasis on outward appearance, from time to time we must remind ourselves that God's idea of beauty differs greatly from our ideas of beauty. We should become more concerned about the One who knows the condition of our minds and hearts rather than worrying about those who can only see the shell of who we really are.

While looking our very best speaks of the value we place upon the temple that God dwells in, our ultimate goal should be to please the Lord, not the world around us.

It has been said that beauty is in the eye of the beholder. Proverbs 15:3 lets us know that "the eyes of the LORD are in every place, beholding the evil and the good."

Never do I feel so beautiful as when I am broken in the presence of the Lord. This is true beauty: beholding the One who is so beautiful and being so entangled with His love and acceptance that I shine forth with His beauty.

DO THE RIGHT THING

I am aware that some people will dismiss the information in this book as inconsequential. Some will see the facts but make light of them. Others will know what they need to do but simply be unwilling to change – and try to discourage others from changing too.

However, the attitude and actions of the masses has never been the standard by which my life is guided. The need for widespread approval has never been an accurate, automatic gauge of truth. Truth is truth, whether the masses accept it or not.

Yes, the majority of America is entangled in a perilous love affair with food. But I *choose* to swim upstream. It's difficult to grow when you go with the flow. Go upstream, do what is right, and you will build muscles you don't even know you have!

Nona Freeman wrote the following in her book *Keeper of the House*: "Our tastes and our eating choices become firmly fixed habits and courage is required to break the mold. It is not easy to go against the grain and against the crowd, but I've decided living to be eighty and feeling like thirty-six is worth it. Of course, I know the calendar will catch up with me one day, but I refuse to sit around and wait for it."[7]

"Isn't it remarkable, folks take better care of their cars and lawn mowers than they do of their bodies? The same people who would not consider using inadequate fuel for their vehicles, poke constant fun at the few "health nuts" who realize that trying to maintain a healthy body on junk is a sad story."[8]

At the time of this writing, Nona Freeman is 92. She travels hither and yon, ministering the Word and encouraging believers. She writes a column in a ladies' magazine. Taking care of our temples is simply the right thing to do. The following short poem, author unknown, contains a powerful message and encourages us to do what Nona Freeman adopted as a lifelong attitude.

Dare to be a Daniel.
Dare to stand alone.
Dare to have a purpose firm.
Dare to make it known.

THIRTY

JESUS LAST

I am Alpha and Omega, the beginning and the end,
the first and the <u>last</u>.
Revelation 22:13

As we began our discussion about health and nutrition, we based our study on Jesus, within the framework of desiring to cultivate a healthy habitat for His Spirit. We have discovered that the answers to our questions about physical wellness are found within the pages of the Word of God. Since we began this book by crediting Jesus as the Source of life and health, is it appropriate that we conclude it by giving Him thanks for the understanding He has imparted and once again emphasize the importance of keeping our pursuit of health God-centered.

SPIRITUAL HUNGER

Have you ever walked to the refrigerator just after you have eaten a big meal, opened it up and gazed inside? From time to time, we have all tried to find something to eat when we were not really hungry at all. At such times, our natural man probably doesn't need more natural food but our desire to eat something is an indicator that our spiritual man is craving to be fed some good, wholesome *spiritual* food.

Spiritual sustenance is obtained through spiritual means, not natural means. We absorb spiritual nutrients and become strong when we partake of the Word of God and spend time in prayer, which is simply communication with God. Job said, "I have esteemed the words of his mouth more than my necessary food" (Job

23:12). Job understood that hearing from his Maker – ingesting spiritual things – was more important than eating natural food.

Food has been a source of temptation throughout the history of mankind. The first sin in the history of man involved food. Satan used the fruit of the tree to tempt Eve. He's still using food to distract man from God. He would love for us to overeat, rarely fast, and become disconnected from God because we are more connected to earthly food than we are to heavenly food.

Prior to beginning His ministry, Jesus fasted forty days and nights. Afterward, the devil, the "tempter," came to Jesus and challenged Him by saying, "If thou be the Son of God, command that these stones be made bread." Jesus responded, "It is written, Man shall not live by bread alone, but by every word that proceedeth out of the mouth of God" (Matthew 4:1-4).

In the Garden of Eden, Eve was faced with a choice. In the wilderness, Jesus was faced with a choice. The proper use of the Word made the difference between Eve's failure and Jesus' triumph. Eve gave in to her carnal desires and partook of forbidden fruit; we are still suffering the consequences of her choice. Jesus trusted in the Word of God; as a result, we have the opportunity to enjoy spiritual life and salvation.

Inside each human being is a place that only Jesus can fill. Once His Spirit takes up residence in our bodies, we discover that He was what we were missing all of our lives. He is the missing link, the last piece of the puzzle. Without Him, life never makes sense and we are incomplete. With Him, we are satisfied and whole. He "satisfieth the longing soul, and filleth the hungry soul with goodness" (Psalm 107:9). Jesus gives meaning and purpose to our existence and makes life really worth living.

Time and time again, Jesus referred to food, something everyone can relate to, in order to reveal Himself to us. He desires a close relationship with us. He used various foods as object lessons to portray the different aspects of the relationship He is building with us. We will examine the two primary examples He used: bread and water.

THE BREAD OF LIFE

In the Bible the word "bread" is used hundreds of times. From Genesis to Revelation it refers to the prominent means by which life is sustained, both physically and spiritually speaking. Bread was such a dietary staple of Bible times that the word "bread" was also sometimes used in a generic sense to simply refer to "food." Biblical people equated "bread" with "life." It was a basic necessity.

In John chapter 6 Jesus used five barley loaves and two small fish to feed five thousand people. The next day men that had been the recipients of that miraculous meal sought Jesus. They discussed with Him the historical miracle of manna, or bread, that came down from heaven, providing food for the children of Israel while they wandered in the wilderness. Jesus told them, "I am the bread of life: he that cometh to me shall never hunger" (verse 35).

Later in the discussion he elaborated on that statement by saying, "I am the living bread which came down from heaven: if any man eat of this bread, he shall live for ever: and the bread that I will give is my flesh, which I will give for the life of the world" (verse 51). The Jews believed in the bread that their forefathers received in the wilderness but they could not comprehend what Jesus was saying about the necessity of them eating His "flesh." They were thinking in natural terms but He was talking about supernatural matters. This "hard saying" caused many to stop following Him (verses 60, 66).

When these people turned away from Him, Jesus asked His twelve disciples, "Will ye also go away?" (verse 67). Peter responded, "Lord, to whom shall we go? thou hast the words of eternal life. And we believe and are sure that thou art the Christ, the Son of the living God" (verses 68-69). Out of thousands, only a few comprehended who Jesus really was. They understood that Jesus was no ordinary man; He was the child that Isaiah prophesied about many years earlier. He was "the mighty God" temporarily dwelling within the confines of human flesh (Isaiah 9:6). His mission was to give His life, His flesh, for the sins of the world. Jesus said that the people that ate the manna in the wilderness were dead but those that would partake of Him, the Bread from Heaven, would live forever (verse 58).

How do we eat this Bread, so that we might live forever, in a spiritual sense?

The Passover was the feast of unleavened bread (Luke 22:1). This was a time set aside to celebrate the Israelites' deliverance from 400 years of Egyptian bondage. It was during this time that Jesus ate a final meal with His disciples, then went to the Garden of Gethsemane where He passionately prayed to submit His human will to the will of the Father. Jesus was fully God and fully man (Colossians 2:9). As the sinless man who would soon bear the sins of the entire world, He had to crucify His will before His flesh could be crucified.

Galatians 5:24 says that "they that are Christ's have crucified the flesh with the affections and lusts."

We partake of Christ's life when our fleshly, carnal nature dies. We do His will instead of our own. Until we are in complete submission to the will of God, we will never be completely satisfied. It is when our will is dead that we are the happiest. When we are not full of our self-will is when we can most enjoy and appreciate the wholesomeness and purity of the Bread of Life. When we are empty of ourselves, God can then fill us with Himself. He is the Bread of Life.

LIVING WATER

Our bodies are comprised of approximately 65% water. Water plays a vital role in all bodily processes, including circulation, digestion, and excretion. Water is the means by which our bodies receive and absorb nutrients. Water also helps our bodies stay at a normal temperature.

Thirst is our body's method of communicating to us that it needs more water to function properly. Many people drink only enough water to appease their thirst when they actually need much more. In fact, some people are dehydrated but don't realize it. Water is so important that without it we will die within just a few days.

In the desert lands of the Bible, springs, streams, and wells were very important. People and tribes protected their water supplies. A dispute over a well's ownership was considered a matter worth fighting about (Genesis 26:19-22).

So when Jesus came on the scene and began telling people about water that they could drink and never again be thirsty, He got their attention. He had to differentiate, however, between the natural water with which they were familiar and the never-ending "well of water springing up into everlasting life" (John 4:9-15).

In John 7:37-39 Jesus explained exactly what this living water is: "If any man thirst, let him come unto me, and drink. He that believeth on me, as the scripture hath said, out of his belly shall flow rivers of living water." Jesus was talking about the Holy Ghost that would be given to believers after His death and resurrection.

A group of 120 of Jesus' disciples were the first people to experience this Living Water. Just prior to His ascension, Jesus told them to go to Jerusalem and wait for the promise of the Holy Ghost (Acts 1:4-5). On the day of Pentecost, "they were all filled with the Holy Ghost, and began to speak with other tongues, as the Spirit gave them utterance" (Acts 2:4).

The Living Water is still available today. Those who are thirsty can receive the gift of the Holy Ghost, which is the Spirit of God that takes up residence within our mortal bodies. Jesus is still inviting anyone who is thirsty to take a drink of this Living Water. He said, "I will give unto him that is athirst of the fountain of the water of life freely" (Revelation 21:6)

David of the Old Testament cried out to God from the depths of his being: "As the hart [deer] panteth after the water brooks, so panteth my soul after thee, O God. My soul thirsteth for God, for the living God" (Psalm 42:1-2). A modern day song writer, Richard Blanchard, echoed David's craving for a deep relationship with God: "Fill my cup, Lord. I lift it up Lord. Come and quench this thirsting of my soul. Here's my cup, fill it up, and make me whole."

Jesus and only Jesus can quench our thirst. Drinking from earthly sources will never satisfy the longing of our souls to be connected and in tune with our Creator.

WHAT ARE YOU HUNGRY FOR?

When my husband assumed the interim pastorate of a home missions church our prayer was not "Lord, lead us to hungry people" but rather "Lord, lead us to people that are hungry for You, for truth, and for righteousness." A lot of people *say* that they want God but their words are just a mask hiding their true intentions. It's kind of like the guy that stands on the street corner with a sign that says, "Will Work for Food." From our experience, most of those guys are no more interested in working than they are in paying taxes. They want something (usually cold, hard cash) for nothing.

There are many people who want God, *if* He fits into their plans and their agendas. If He requires anything of them, they'll walk away from Him in a heartbeat. It is a scenario strangely reminiscent of what happened 2,000 years ago when Jesus said some hard things. As long as he was distributing free lunches, the people were ready to crown Him king (John 6:14-15). But as soon as He told them that there would be a price to pay to follow Him, they rejected Him (John 6:66).

All that some people want is attention. They have no compunction about draining others of all of their energy and resources. They feel like the world owes them a living and they don't feel compelled to do anything in return, even say "thank you." They are takers, not givers.

While this mentality is pathetic, socially speaking, it is even worse spiritually speaking. We must be certain of our motives. When we are born again and are newly adopted into the family of God, it is expected that we will be needy and dependent upon others, just as it is natural for infants and toddlers to be dependent upon their mothers for survival. However, normal growth dictates that in time we mature, become less selfish, and learn to give.

It's not that, as we grow in our relationship with God, that we no longer have needs or that it is wrong to want Jesus to meet those needs. He is both able and willing to meet our needs. But maturity brings with it patience and an understanding that God will do what is best for us. We understand that if we will just keep our lives focused on serving and loving Him and meeting the needs of others, we will be free from the bondage of self-centeredness.

Ecclesiastes 11:1 says, "Cast thy bread upon the waters: for thou shalt find it after many days." This is a reference to the practice of liberally casting seed into a marshy or flooded area. Eventually a crop would spring up where that seed was cast. When we liberally give to God and others, our needs will be met. God will make sure that our selflessness and hard work are rewarded with a bountiful harvest just when we need it.

So when Jesus requires sacrifice of us, we should not throw a temper tantrum and demand our own way. Our hunger for Him should be sincere. We should desire a relationship with Him, not solely for what we can get from Him, but because we view a close relationship with Him as the means by which we can love Him, setting aside our will for His, doing the things He asks us to do.

When He requires something of us that opposes our plans and our agendas, our response will be a true gauge of our intentions. In spite of what we say, our actions will prove if we are hungry for Him and His will or more interested in gratifying ourselves and fulfilling our own will.

When we try to appease our carnal hunger, we will never be satisfied. But if we hunger for God, He will satisfy us. We will leave His table nourished and strengthened. God will never feed us anything that will harm us spiritually, whereas eating the spiritually unhealthy convenience and quick-energy foods of the sinful world around us will have devastating effects on us and our families.

Are you hungry for God? Or are you satiated with the things of this world? Our love of pride-producing popularity, intoxicating intellectualism, and euphoric education must all be purged from our souls if we want to make room for Jesus. We must be hungrier for God and His righteousness than we are for manmade imitation carnal food that bloats us up but adds nothing substantial to our lives.

If there is a possibility that you may be serving God for the wrong reasons or your hunger for Him is not sincere, pray and ask Him to change your desires. He can help you to love and crave the things that are good for you. Before you know it, you will be addicted to righteousness and holiness. You will crave His presence and will fight against sin and anything that tries to keep you away from Him. Your hunger will drive you to sacrifice anything He asks, to go anywhere He wants you to go – all because you know that He will never lead you astray.

TASTE TEST

God created us with taste buds. These little sensors can detect about a dozen different groups of flavors. We have taste buds to help us discern if a food is good or bad for us. Unfortunately, we can develop a taste for things that are harmful to our bodies. We can program ourselves to like the taste of packaged, additive filled foods and dislike fresh fruits and vegetables. Most kids will choose a candy bar over an apple because they have developed an attachment to the candy bar and associate it with good taste.

Likewise, our spiritual taste buds are capable of adjusting to new flavors. We instinctively know that some foods are good for us and some foods are bad for us. To our detriment, we sometimes resist changing and doing what is good for us because we like to remain in our comfort zones.

There is a single principle in the Word of God which, when applied, can change our lives. It is: Love God and Hate Sin. When we love God with all our heart, soul, mind, and strength, and passionately hate sin, we have succeeded in altering our spiritual taste buds to like what is good for us.

Sometimes all it takes to change our taste buds is to shun the bad and ingest the good. The more fruits and vegetables you eat, the less you will crave Oreos and donuts. Someone will offer you a big slice of pie or cake and you will eat it, secretly wishing that it was a fresh grapefruit or a bowlful of organic strawberries. Sound farfetched? It isn't. You can get addicted to how whole foods make you feel. You will like the energy, stamina, and clean feeling you get.

We instinctively know that sin will pollute our temples and destroy us yet we sometimes give in to it. Ask God to help you change what your spiritual taste buds identify as enjoyable. Ask Him to help you start doing what is good for your temple, rather than giving in to what your taste buds have been conditioned to think tastes good through years of exposure. God can help you to hate what you once liked. You will find those things repulsive. As soon as you taste them, you will spit them back out before you can ingest them and they pollute your soul.

Sin will never satisfy us. But when the Holy Ghost, which is the Spirit of God, takes up residence in our bodies, nagging discontentment is replaced by complete satisfaction. Baptism in Jesus' name remits our sins and lifts the burden of guilt and sin from our lives.

Jesus replaces sadness, depression, and loneliness with joy, peace, and fulfillment. He takes you from feeling like you don't have a friend in the world to waking up every morning delighted to be alive because Jesus lives inside.

Once we have received this New Birth experience, we can compromise our access to peace, joy, and contentment if we begin to ingest the things that made us miserable to begin with. What are you feeding yourself?

Whatever we allow to enter our soul through our eyes and ears will affect our health. Just as it is unrealistic to expect to be physically healthy if we subsist on junk food void of nutritive value, so we should not expect to be spiritual if we are feeding ourselves spiritual junk food most of the time.

God pleaded with His people to quit wasting their time and energy. In Isaiah 55:2 He said, "Wherefore do ye spend money for that which is not bread? and your labour for that which satisfieth not? hearken diligently unto me, and eat ye that which is good, and let your soul delight itself in fatness."

If we want to enjoy Kingdom benefits, we must deny our carnal desires and separate ourselves from the uncleanness of the world. The best life is one that is pure, clean, and uncontaminated, free of poisons and additives.

Ask the Lord to give you a desire for purity. Ask Him to help your taste buds to crave that which is beneficial to your spirituality.

Then go ahead...take the taste test. You'll find that the Lord is good (Psalm 34:8)!

PICKY EATERS

When people are desperately hungry, they'll eat anything. It is crucial that, when we are hungry for the things of God, we correctly identify what we are hungry for and go to Him to satisfy our hunger. Otherwise, we will eat anything that is set before us and that could be deadly to our soul.

People who get hungry enough will turn into beggars. Beggars take the leftovers, the handouts, the scraps that others throw away. The apostle Paul told the

Galatians who wanted to return to their former lifestyle that they were desiring the "weak and beggarly elements" that would put them back into bondage (Galatians 4:9).

We should be picky about the type of spiritual food we eat. Not everything that is labeled "healthy" is good for us. Sometimes slick advertising conceals the truth with glamorous half-truths but we can't identify the lies because the packaging is so deceptive. Just because something is labeled "Christian" does not mean that it really is Christ-like and pleasing to God. False doctrine comes in many forms and can easily lead us astray.

We must read every word of the fine print before we invest in something. We must compare all new products and ideas to the Bible, which is the final authority for spiritual matters. We must stay connected to the body of Christ, like minded believers who eat the same foods that we eat and desire purity of doctrine and lifestyle. We must have a balanced diet of prayer, fasting, and the Word of God.

Be cautious and selective about what you eat. Prevent hunger and you won't be tempted to eat beggar's rations. You can keep yourself full of the Holy Ghost by making daily prayer and time in the Word the top priority in your life. The secret of successful Christians is their daily renewal in the presence of God. They are refreshed by the presence of God in intimate fellowship with Him.

During your lunch break at work, enjoy a five minute "Word" snack to energize you. Meditate on a certain Scripture throughout the day and keep your mind on God. Instead of spending all of your reading time engrossed in a news magazine or a novel, feast on the Word. Tune out the talk show babble and tune in the voice of God. Fast from physical food. When you withhold food from your fleshly nature, your spirit is fed and nourished as you pray and read the Word.

We get irritable when we get hungry, both naturally and spiritually. Sometimes our agitation can very easily be remedied by stepping into God's kitchen, pulling up to the table and enjoying the meal He has prepared for us. It's okay to be picky as long as we make choices that will truly strengthen our walk with God.

A HOLY GOD – A HOLY TEMPLE

God was impressed by Solomon's humility and sincerity that prompted him to meticulously build the temple. After the temple was dedicated to God, the Lord responded by saying "Now mine eyes shall be open, and mine ears attent unto the prayer that is made in this place. For now have I chosen and sanctified this house, that my name may be there for ever: and mine eyes and mine heart shall be there perpetually" (II Chronicles 7:15-16).

God said that He chose and sanctified the temple. It would be a place where His name would live. As such, it was no ordinary structure. It was magnificent and beautiful but what really set it apart from all other buildings was that, because it had been dedicated to God, it was a place where He directed His focus.

Today, if we are filled with the Holy Ghost and baptized in Jesus' name, our bodies are chosen and sanctified as a place to house His name. Our entire being should emanate our awe at being chosen to bear His name and be a habitat for His glory. Our attitude, life focus, and physical health should all show to Him our appreciation. Our lives should be an unspoken witness to the world of our love for Him.

We are not ordinary people. Our temples – bodies – are special because of Who lives in them. Our love and gratitude should prompt us to show forth the praises of Him who has called us out of darkness into His marvelous light (I Peter 2:9). "Ye also, as lively stones, are built up a spiritual house, an holy priesthood, to offer up spiritual sacrifices, acceptable to God by Jesus Christ" (I Peter 2:5).

THE GOOD LIFE

When God created Adam, the first man, He designed him to live forever. Physical and spiritual death were the consequences of sin. At first, though man eventually died a physical death, his lifespan was long. The longest recorded lifespan was 969 years, enjoyed by a man named Methuselah (Genesis 5:27). Probably due to mankind's insistence on doing evil, God shortened man's lifespan to 120 years just prior to the worldwide flood of Noah's time, and after that the lifespan gradually decreased (Genesis 6:3). Sometime later, God again shortened man's life to 70 years (Psalm 90:10). The Lord blesses some people with even longer lives. When such elders are godly and righteous, their examples and wisdom are invaluable to succeeding generations (Deuteronomy 11:21; Proverbs 16:31). Their longevity is a testimony to God's goodness and they are a blessing to the kingdom of God.

Whether we live to be fifty or one hundred, however, life is short. Before we know it, the time will come for us to leave this life behind and enter the corridor that leads to eternal life. Many people spend their entire lives building on sinking sand. While there is nothing wrong with developing a successful career, starting a business, and accumulating an estate and assets, these endeavors have no lasting value unless our lives are firmly rooted in Jesus Christ. The brevity of life demands that we make wise choices every single day, choices that will bring joy and not regret when we are nearing the end of our journey.

The purpose of this book is not to manufacture a magical formula for longevity. It is to improve our health so that we can be better equipped to develop our relationship with God and fulfill His will for our lives. Living a long, healthy life is a blessing from God but we should not desire to live a long time for the sake of simply existing.

A BRAND NEW LIFE

If you do not know God in the fullness of His saving power – the greatest miracle known to man – I encourage you to seek Him with all your heart. If you will seek Him from your heart, *with* all your heart, He will do awesome things for you that you cannot yet even imagine.

A man by the name of Peter, who walked with Jesus for over three years, had this to say, "Repent, and be baptized every one of you in the name of Jesus Christ for the remission of sins, and ye shall receive the gift of the Holy Ghost" (Acts 2:38). This simple formula, when applied, will change your life.

Repentance means to acknowledge, not just by your words, but your actions, that you are willing to make a change in your life. If you do this, then you understand that you *need* God. This is a step of humility which always gets God's attention. Repentance is also understanding that, as Deuteronomy 6:4 states, "The Lord our God is one Lord" and Jesus Christ is the name of this one God. Someone stated, "My life changed when I realized that there was only one God and I quit applying for the position!"

When you understand that Jesus is truly God made visible in human flesh, you will naturally follow Peter's second step and be baptized in the name of Jesus Christ for the remission (removal) of your sins (I Timothy 3:16). This is an awesome event that is better experienced than told. The load you may not even realize you are carrying will be suddenly lifted from your life. Baptism in the name of Jesus identifies us with Jesus, and we can access all of the benefits of being a part of His family – and they are many!

Receiving the Holy Ghost, which is *always* evidenced by speaking in a language unknown to us as *God* enables, is then a promise to us. The Holy Ghost is the Spirit of God living inside us, inhabiting our temples. Receiving the Holy Ghost restores us to communion with God.

If you have never had this wonderful experience called the New Birth, life has probably never really made sense to you. You struggle with understanding what your purpose on this earth is. Peace evades you and contentment eludes you. You wonder why deep down you feel so empty. Please seek God and allow Him to fill the void in your life. Let Him do for you all the good things that He wants to do. Don't let self-will hinder you from letting God give you things that you will never be able to give yourself. He loves you with a pure love – truly loves you as *nobody* else can.

Why do I discuss these things in a book about nutrition? Because you can be the healthiest person alive and still be miserable. You can live to be over 100, but if you have fear on your deathbed, what has been the point of your longevity? I discuss these things because a deep sense of satisfaction, contentment, and peace is absent from the hearts of the majority of the people in the world. Pockets of people throughout the world who have amazing health and longevity because of their regional diet are not exempt from the spiritual barrenness that comes from being estranged from God. Walking with God gives us purpose.

THE TREE OF LIFE

When God designed the Garden of Eden, He placed the tree of life in the middle of it (Genesis 2:9). When Adam sinned by partaking of the fruit of the tree of the knowledge of good and evil, he was no longer innocent. Sin severed Adam's direct communion with God. Spiritual and physical death was the penalty for disobedience. So that Adam would not eat of the tree of life and live forever in his sinful state, God expelled him from the Garden (Genesis 3:22-24).

Thousands of years passed and the second Adam, righteous and sinless, came on the scene (Romans 5:14-19). Jesus Christ was the spotless Lamb that paid the price once and for all so that all humanity might be restored into communion with God.

There is a promise for those that choose to be restored to relationship with God and keep His commandments. Referring to the place that is being prepared for those that love God, Revelation 22:14 says "Blessed are they that do his commandments, that they may have right to the tree of life, and may enter in through the gates into the city." Jesus said that "to him that overcometh will I give to eat of the tree of life, which is in the midst of the paradise of God" (Revelation 2:7).

In every decision that we make regarding the care of our spirits, souls, and bodies, we must keep the life beyond our short sojourn on this earth in view. The fruit of the tree of life will be sweetness beyond compare. Maintaining the health of our temples, minds, and hearts will be worth every sacrifice – when we see Jesus face to face.

So in your pursuit of spiritual and physical health, keep your goal in mind: A holy God deserves a healthy and holy house. Do your best to please Him with your temporary temple; one day He will usher you into a perfect eternal paradise, specially prepared for you.

ENDNOTES

Three
NEW LAWS IN THE NEW TESTAMENT
1. Gwyn Oakes, *The Front Row* (Dover, DE: Classic Publishing, 2002), 134-136.

Four
OUR BODIES – GOD'S TEMPLES
1. Patsy G. Harrison, *The Great Balancing Act* (Tulsa, OK: Harrison House Publishers, © 2002), 30-31.
2. Patrick Quinn, Ph.D., R.D., C.N.S., *Healing Secrets from the Bible* (North Canton, OH: The Leader Company, Inc., 1995), 3.
3. Nona Freeman, *Keeper of the House* (Fort Worth, TX, 1995).

Six
OVERFED AND UNDERNOURISHED
1. John Buell, "Obesity and the new prohibition," *Bangor Daily News*, 5 April 2005.
2. Eric Schlosser and Charles Wilson, *Chew on This* (Boston, MA: Houghton Mifflin Company, 2006), 209.
3. "Obesity Affects X-Rays," *Nature's Place* (December 2006): 6.
4. William Clower, Ph.D., *The Fat Fallacy* (New York, NY: Random House, Inc., 2003), 109.
5. Clay Jackson, M.D., "Obesity," *The Pentecostal Herald* (September 2004): 38.
6. Erik Steele, D.O., "Tackling obesity – if not in our schools, where?" *Bangor Daily News*, 12 April 2005.

Seven
THE "ACCEPTABLE" SIN
1. *Easton's Bible Dictionary*, Power Bible CD v4.0a, (Bronson, MI: Online Publishing Inc., 2003).
2. Daniel L. Segraves, *Proverbs: Ancient Wisdom for Today's World* (Hazelwood, MO: Word Aflame Press, 1990), 247.

Eight
PORTION CONTROL
1. Nanci Hellmich, "Low-fat foods pack caloric punch,"
USA Today, 25 October 2006.

Ten
AN INTERVIEW WITH MOSHE MYEROWITZ
1. Author Telephone Interviews with Moshe Myerowitz,
5 December 2006 and 24 October 2007. Dr Myerowitz
may be contacted at (207) 947-3333 - Myerowitz Chiropractic Natural Care Bangor, 1570 Broadway, Bangor,
ME, 04401.

Eleven
WHY DO WE EAT?
1. Travis Reed, "Chief ousted for urging weight loss,"
Bangor Daily News, 2 November 2006.

Thirteen
THE MIND-BODY CONNECTION
1. Stephen Gullo, Ph.D., *The Thin Commandments Diet*
(Emmaus, PA: Rodale, 2005), 117.

Fourteen
THE MEDICAL WORLD AND YOUR HEALTH
1. Rob Stein, "Americans' Health Care More Costly,
Treatment Substandard, Survey Finds," *Bangor Daily
News*, 4 November 2005.
2. *Better Nutrition* (July 2002): 21.
3. "Drug Cautions," *Taste for Life* (May 2005): 14.
4. Alexander Macalister, *International Standard Bible
Encyclopedia* (Biblesoft, PC Study Bible, 1996.)
5. Daniel L. Steinke, D.D.S., "Is it Your Turn Yet? Aren't
Drugs Wonderful?," *The Eastern Gazette*, 31 March to 6
April 2007, 2.
6. Erik Steele, D.O., "Protect Yourself: Be Your Own
FDA," *Bangor Daily News*, 29 March 2005.
7. Roon Frost, Editor, "Going to Extremes," *Taste for
Life* (June 2005): 4.

8. *Energy Times* (September 2002): 14 and (March 2003): 16. Reprinted by permission of *Energy Times*.
9. "New Risks in Kids' Meds," *Taste for Life* (August 2005): 10.
10. Tedd Mitchell, M.D., "The Truth about ADHD in Children," *USA Weekend*, 11-13 August 2006, 8.
11. Jordan S. Rubin, N.M.D., Ph.D., *The Maker's Diet* (Lake Mary, FL: Siloam, A Strang Company, 2004), 94.
12. www.thekansascitychannel.com, KMBC-TV (Kansas City, MO): 21 March 2007.
13. *Webster's New Universal Unabridged Dictionary*, 2nd ed. (New York, NY: Simon and Schuster, 1983), 1413.
14. Quinn, 14.

Fifteen
WHAT ARE WE EATING?
1. James B. LaValle, R.Ph., C.C.N., N.D., *Cracking the Metabolic Code* (North Bergen, NJ: Basic Health Publications, Inc., 2004) 290.
2. Ruth Winter, M.S., *A Consumer's Dictionary of Food Additives*, 5th ed. (New York, NY: Three Rivers Press, 1999), 397.
3. Schlosser, 104.
4. www.westonprice.org
5. Don Colbert, M.D., *What Would Jesus Eat?* (Nashville, TN: Thomas Nelson Publishers, 2002), 6.
6. Geri Harrington, *Real Food Fake Food* (New York, NY: Macmillan Publishing Company, 1987), 107.
7. "Irradiation and your Food," Whole Foods Market Informational Brochure.
8. Gabriel Cousens, *Conscious Eating* (Berkeley, CA: North Atlantic Books, 2000), 302.
9. Cousens, 300.
10. Cousens, 301.
11. Cousens, 302.
12. LaValle, 292.
13. "Everybody's Talking," *Coffee News*, Maine Highlands Edition, Volume 4, Issue 35, 19 March 2007.
14. Segraves, 318.

Sixteen
DON'T DIET – DO IT RIGHT FOR LIFE
1. Barb Jarmoska, "Freshnews," *Freshlife* (Williamsport, PA: Newsletter) April 2004, 1, 9. Barb may be contacted at www.road-2-health.com.
2. Clower, 22.
3. Clower, 224.
4. Clower, 24-25.
5. www.hacres.com/faq.html.
6. Peter D'Adamo, *Eat Right & Cook Right 4 Your Type* (Paramus, NJ: Prentice Hall, 2001), 4.
7. D'Adamo, 5, 421-424.
8. Sally Fallon, *Nourishing Traditions* (Washington, DC: New Trends Publishing, Inc., 2001), 61. www.newtrendspublishing.com - (877) 707-1776.
9. Fallon, 61.
10. Randall Neustaedter, O.M.D., *Let's Live*, (August 2007): 5.
11. Oakes, 134-136.

Seventeen
GREAT GRAINS
1. Bernard Ward, *Healing Foods from the Bible* (Boca Raton, FL: Globe Communications Corp., 1996), 85.
2. Christopher S. Kilman, *The Bread and Circus Whole Food Bible: How to Select and Prepare Safe, Healthful Foods without Pesticides or Chemical Additives* (Reading, MA: Addison-Wesley Publishing Company, Inc., 1991), 36.

Eighteen
SIMPLY SWEET
1. William Dufty, *Sugar Blues* (New York, NY: Warner Books Inc., 1975), 40.
2. *The World Book Encyclopedia*, Volume 18, 1991: 1960.
3. www.sugar.org.
4. Joseph D. Beasley, M.D. and Jerry J. Swift, M.A., *The Kellogg Report, The Impact of Nutrition, Environment*

and Lifestyle on the Health of Americans (Annandale-on-Hudson, NY: The Institute of Health Policy and Practice, the Bard College Center, 1989), 131.

5. Dufty, 18.
6. Clower, 201.
7. www.fda.gov/bbs/topics/ANSWERS/ANS00772. html.
8. Phyllis A. Balch, C.N.C., *Prescription for Nutritional Healing* (New York, NY: Avery, 2000), 552.
9. Liz Biro, "Increase Your Bottom Line When you Embrace the Latest Beverage Trends," *Sam's Club Source* (August-September 2006): 74.
10. Marina Kushner, *Life Without Caffeine* (Brooklyn, NY: SCR Publications, 2004), 31. scrbooks@yahoo.com - (877) 872-4718.
11. Kushner, 34.
12. Kushner, 125.
13. Clower, 118.

Nineteen
THE DELIGHTS OF DAIRY

1. www.raw-milk-facts.com.
2. www.answers.com/topic/dairy-industry.html.
3. www.agebb.missouri.edu/commag/dairy/audit/3hist.html.
4. Marcea Weber, *Whole Meals* (Paulton, Bristol, Australia: Prism Press, 1983), 20-21.
5. www.biology.clc.uc.edu/courses/bio106/earlymod.html.
6. Ron Schmid, N.D., *The Untold Story of Milk* (Washington, DC: New Trends Publishing, Inc., 2007), 231. www.newtrendspublishing.com - (877) 707-1776.
7. Schmid, *The Untold Story of Milk*, 234.
8. Nina Planck, *Real Food, What to Eat and Why* (New York, NY: Bloomsbury USA, 2007), 85.
9. Paul Kindstedt with the Vermont Cheese Council, *American Farmstead Cheese* (White River Junction, VT: Chelsea Green Publishing Company, 2005), 178.
10. Christopher Vasey, N.D., *The Whey Prescription* (Rochester, VT: Healing Arts Press, 1998), 4.

11. www.raw-milk-facts.com/raw_milk_health_benefits.html.
12. Steven Novil, Ph.D., "Kefir," (Morton Grove, IL: Lifeway Foods, Inc., 1997), paper.
13. Schmid, *The Untold Story of Milk*, 78-80.
14. Ron Schmid, *Traditional Foods are your Best Medicine* (Rochester, VT: Healing Arts Press, 1997), 109.

Twenty-One
THE SKINNY ON FATS
1. A. P. Simopoulos, *American Journal of Clinical Nutrition* (1992): 55, 411-414.
2. Carol Ferguson, "Getting the Right Fats?," *Nature's Place*, June 2005, 19.
3. Fallon, 13-14.
4. Annie Graves, "Weighing in on Trans Fat," *Taste for Life* (August 2005): 39-40.

Twenty-Two
FRESH PRODUCE
1. Madeleine S. Miller, *Encyclopedia of Bible Life* (New York and London: Harper and Brothers Publishers, 1944), 12-13.
2. Gene Spiller, *Nutrition Secrets of the Ancients* (Rocklin, CA: Prima Publishing, 1996), 129.
3. Dianne Onstad, *Whole Foods Companion* (White River Junction, VT: Chelsea Green Publishing Company, 2004), 434.
4. Colbert, 90.
5. Ralph Gower, *The New Manners and Customs of Bible Times* (Chicago, IL: Moody Press, 1987), 113.
6. James A. Duke, Ph.D., *Herbs of the Bible* (Loveland CO: Interweave Press, 1999), 67.
7. Kristy Erickson, "In a Nutshell," *Taste for Life* (November 2002): 58.
8. Ward, 68.
9. "Study Confirms Variety Key to Healthful Diet," *Environmental Nutrition* Volume 29, Issue 10 (October 2006): 3 (From *Journal of Nutrition*, August 2006).

10. www.usda.gov/factbook.html.

Twenty-Three
HERBS AND SPICES
1. Duke, 35.
2. *Jamieson, Fausset, and Brown Commentary* (Bible-soft, PC Study Bible, 1997).
3. J. O. Swahn, *The Lore of Spices* (London: Senate Publishing Ltd, 1991), 38.

Twenty-Five
PLAN OF ACTION
1. *Coffee News*, Maine Highlands Edition, Volume 4, Issue 1, 21 July 2006.
2. Eric Neuhaus, *Taste for Life* (October 2005): 50-51.
3. Balch, 707-708.

Twenty-Six
CLEANING THE TEMPLE
1. LaValle, 137-138.

Twenty-Seven
RESIDENT THIEF
1. Michelle Dangiuro, *Powerful Effects, Powerful Choices* (Carlisle, PA: Rosh Pinnah Publications, 1999), 24.
2. Dangiuro, 24.
3. Dangiuro, 23.
4. Dangiuro, 23.
5. Dangiuro, 22.
6. "Couch Potatoes: tube-ers," *Better Nutrition* (June 2002): 26.
7. "Watch TV Time," *Wild Harvest* (October 2003): 8.
8. Dangiuro, 81.
9. Dangiuro, 80.
10. Dangiuro, 80.
11. Clower, 114-115.
12. Clower, 115.
13. Clower, 114.
14. Clower, 113.
15. Dangiuro, 42.

16. Dangiuro, 80.

17. Schlosser, 57.

18. www.hollyscoop.com, 22 February 2007.

19. Elysa Gardner, "Madonna at a Crossroads," *People.* Online. Internet. 27 October 2005, www.usatoday.com.

20. Ed McMahon, *When Television was Young* (Nashville, TN: Thomas Nelson, 2007), 15-16.

Twenty-Nine
PARTING THOUGHTS

1. Nona Freeman, 21.

2. Anne Kreamer, *Going Gray* (New York, NY: Little, Brown and Company, 2007), 12.

3. Kreamer, 41.

4. Kreamer, 40.

5. Kreamer, 5.

6. Rubin, 173.

7. Freeman, 20.

8. Freeman, 19.

RECOMMENDED READING

Chew on This, Eric Schlosser, Houghton Mifflin, Boston, MA

Cracking the Metabolic Code, James B. LaValle, Basic Health Publications, North Bergen, NJ

How to Have Radiant Health, Joy Haney, Radiant Life Publications, Stockton, CA

Juicing for Life, Cherie Calbom, Avery, New York, NY

Keeper of the House, Nona Freeman, Fort Worth, TX

Prescription for Nutritional Healing, Phyllis A. Balch, Avery, New York, NY

The Fat Fallacy, William Clower, Random House, Inc., New York, NY

The Maker's Diet, Jordan S. Rubin, Siloam, Lake Mary, FL

The New Birth, David K. Bernard, Word Aflame Press, Hazelwood, MO

The Sons of Oil, David A. Huston, Rosh Pinnah Publications, Carlisle, PA

The Untold Story of Milk, Ron Schmid, New Trends Publishing, Washington, DC

Whole Foods Companion, Dianne Onstad, Chelsea Green Publishing Company, White River Junction, VT